Drugs,
Diseases,
and Anesthesia

Ronald J. Stern, M.D.
Anesthesiologist
Department of Anesthesia
Holmes Regional Medical Center
Melbourne, Florida

Drugs, Diseases, and Anesthesia

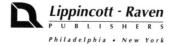

Lippincott - Raven
PUBLISHERS
Philadelphia • New York

Acquisitions Editor: R. Craig Percy
Developmental Editor: Melissa James
Manufacturing Manager: Dennis Teston
Production Manager: Larry Bernstein
Production Editor: Dee Josephson
Cover Designer: Ede Dreikers
Indexer: Leon Kremzner
Compositor: Lippincott-Raven Electronic Production
Printer: RR Donnelly

Printed in the United States of America

9 8 7 6 5 4 3 2 1

Library of Congress Cataloging-in-Publication Data

Stern, Ronald J.
    Drugs, diseases, and anesthesia / Ronald J. Stern.
        p.   cm.
    Includes index.
    ISBN 0-397-58736-8 (paper)
    1. Anesthesia–Side effects–Handbooks, manuals, etc.
2. Anesthesia–Complications–Handbook, manuals, etc.   3. Drug
interactions–Handbooks.   4. Drug Therapy–handbooks. QV 39
S8392d 1996]
RD82.7.S53S74   1996
617.9'6041—dc20
DNLM/DLC
for Library of Congress

CONTENTS

PREFACE

If you are responsible for health care of the anesthetized patient, whether your involvement is as the anesthesiologist, nurse anesthetist, medical or nursing student, or recovery room nurse, you are faced daily with potentially complex interactions between your patients' prescription drugs or diseases and the anesthetic agents that have been or are about to be administered.

For example, what are the possible significant interactions between anesthetic agents and your patient who has epilepsy and takes dilantin? What effects will different muscle relaxants have on your patient with multiple sclerosis? Does the fact that your patient has hypertension and takes a calcium channel blocker have any significance to the intraoperative or postoperative management of this patient?

This book and the computer program that preceded it were written to provide the answers to the preceding questions and many more. More precisely, this book developed out of the need to have these answers quickly, easily, and accurately at the bedside of our patients in the preoperative, intraoperative, and postoperative settings. The information in this book was extracted from the leading reference books in the fields of anesthesiology, pharmacology, internal medicine, and pediatrics. With the availability of *Drugs, Diseases, and Anesthesia,* it is hoped that a search through multiple sources will no longer be necessary for drug–anesthetic, disease–anesthetic, and anesthetic–anesthetic interactions.

For ease of use, this book is divided, as is the computer program, into three sections: Patient Drugs, Diseases, and Anesthetic Agents. In each section, the drug, disease, or anesthetic agent is followed by a description and then the anesthetic agents with which it may have potentially significant interactions. Because this book and computer program are written from the point of view of someone administering anesthesia, the significant interactions involve only anesthetic agents. Therefore, there are no interactions described between patient drugs and other patient drugs or between diseases and patient drugs.

The exhaustive literature search conducted during the writing of this book revealed significant contradictions as well as unsubstantiated anecdotal information in the reporting of interactions. This sort of information has either been identified or eliminated. Undoubtedly, there are significant interactions that have been missed, but the intent has been to present all drug–anesthetic, disease–anesthetic, and anesthetic–anesthetic interactions that are clinically relevant to the profession of anesthesiology. Therefore, if a prescription drug, a patient disease, or anesthetic agent is not listed in any of the sections, it was not found to have clinically significant interactions.

Drugs,
Diseases,
and Anesthesia

1

PATIENT DRUGS

ALPHA ADRENERGIC BLOCKERS

Classification and indications
—Alpha adrenergic blockers are a group of medications that block alpha receptors. This group includes phentolamine, phenoxybenzamine, prazosin, doxazosin, and terazosin.
—They are used to treat hypertension. Some of these agents (terazosin) are also used to treat benign prostatic hypertrophy.

Pharmacology
—Stimulation of alpha adrenergic receptors results in a number of responses including contraction of smooth muscle (vascular, bronchial, ureteral, ciliary), contraction of sphincters in the gastrointestinal and genitourinary systems, as well as control of pancreatic insulin release.
—The alpha receptors are classified into alpha 1 (and subtypes a, b, c) and alpha 2 (and subtypes a, b, c, d).
—Alpha 1 receptors are located primarily on smooth muscle where their stimulation results in vasoconstriction.
—Alpha 2 receptors are mainly in the cerebral cortex and medulla, and stimulation of these receptors results in inhibition of sympathetic outflow. There are, however, some alpha 2 receptors located in the peripheral nervous system, but their exact function is not clear.
—Alpha 1 blockers (such as phenoxybenzamine) produce hypotension whereas alpha 2 blockers (such as yohimbine) produce hypertension.
—Significant interactions with anesthetics can occur with patients who are receiving alpha blocking agents. Blockade of alpha 1 receptors can result in unresponsiveness to vasopressors, depending on the vasopressor being used.
—In patients receiving alpha 1 blockers, the response to vasopressors that are primarily alpha agonists (phenylephrine and methoxamine) can be suppressed.
—Vasopressors that stimulate both alpha and beta receptors can interact with alpha 1 blockers in different ways, depending on the amount of alpha and beta agonist activity.
—Epinephrine, at lower doses, stimulates beta receptors more than alpha receptors. When epinephrine is used to treat patients receiving alpha blockers, hypotension may occur due to the vasodilating effect from qepinephrine's prominent beta 2 stimulation.
—Norepinephrine differs from epinephrine by stimulating mainly beta 1 and alpha receptors, rather than beta 2 receptors. When norepinephrine is given to patients on alpha

blockers, the beta 1 stimulation may produce some increase in blood pressure. Hypotension is unlikely because of minimal beta 2 agonism. Metaraminol may have similar effects.

—Ephedrine and mephentermine are likely to have interactions similar to epinephrine with patients receiving alpha blockers. These agents have significant beta 2 stimulation along with beta 1 and alpha adrenergic activity.

Doxazosin (Cardura)
Classification and indications
—Doxazosin is an alpha 1 adrenergic blocking agent.

—It is indicated for treatment of hypertension.

Pharmacology
—Doxazosin is a competitive alpha 1 receptor blocking agent. It results in arterial and venous dilation and produces a decrease in both cardiac preload and afterload.

Prazosin (Minipress)
Classification and indications
—Prazosin is an alpha 1 adrenergic blocking agent.

—It is indicated for treatment of hypertension.

Pharmacology
—Prazosin is a very selective alpha 1 adrenergic antagonist. Alpha 1 blockade from prazosin results in both arterial and venous vasodilation and a decrease in both cardiac preload and afterload.

Phenoxybenzamine (Dibenzyline)
Classification and indications
—Phenoxybenzamine is an alpha adrenergic blocking agent.

—It is used orally for the management of hypertension and sweating in patients with pheochromocytoma.

Pharmacology
—Phenoxybenzamine is an irreversible inhibitor of alpha adrenergic receptor blockers.

Terazosin (Hytrin)
Classification and indications
—Terazosin is an alpha 1 adrenergic blocking agent.

—It is indicated for treatment of hypertension and for benign prostatic hypertrophy.

Pharmacology
—Terazosin is a selective alpha 1 adrenergic antagonist. Alpha 1 blockade from terazosin results in arterial and venous vasodilation and a decrease in both cardiac preload and afterload.

—Symptoms of bladder obstruction are relieved by terazosin because alpha 1 blockade causes smooth muscle relaxation (affecting mainly the bladder neck).

Alpha Adrenergic Blockers Interactions with Anesthetic Drugs

Alpha adrenergic blockers with vasopressors (ephedrine, epinephrine, metaraminol, methoxamine, norepinephrine, phenylephrine)

—Blockade of alpha 1 receptors can result in unresponsiveness to vasopressors, depending on the vasopressor being used.

—Ephedrine and mephentermine have significant beta 2 stimulation along with beta 1 and alpha adrenergic activity. As a result, it is possible that hypotension could worsen in patients on alpha blockers given ephedrine due to the unopposed vasodilation resulting from beta 2 stimulation.

—Although good documentation of this interaction is scarce, this is similar to the response that can be seen with epinephrine.

—Because norepinephrine has beta 1 activity, it is more likely to be effective in treating hypotension in patients on alpha blockers.

Ambenonium Chloride (Mytelase)

Classification and indications

—Ambenonium chloride is a synthetic medication similar to neostigmine and pyridostigmine.

—It is used in the treatment of myasthenia gravis to improve muscle strength.

Pharmacology

—Ambenonium is a reversible inhibitor of cholinesterase. As a result, acetylcholine accumulates at cholinergic nerve endings and at the neuromuscular junction.

—This results in improved muscle strength in myasthenics, but has some side effects, including gastrointestinal stimulation, hypersalivation, and miosis.

—Other side effects from excess acetylcholine may include bradycardia.

—Significant interactions can occur with procainamide that can worsen the status of patients with myasthenia gravis. This can occur because procainamide has neuromuscular blocking properties. Also, like quinidine, procainamide antagonizes the cholinergic effect of anticholinesterases.

Ambenonium Chloride Interactions with Anesthetic Drugs
Ambenonium chloride with procainamide
—Patients receiving cholinergic medications for myasthenia gravis may experience worsening muscle weakness with administration of procainamide.
—Procainamide, in addition to acting as an antagonist to the neuromuscular effects of cholinergic medications, has neuromuscular blocking properties.

AMINOGLYCOSIDE ANTIBIOTICS

Classification and indications
—Aminoglycosides are antibiotics derived from *Streptomyces* or *Micromonospora.* This group includes amikacin, gentamicin, kanamycin, netilmicin, and tobramycin.
—Aminoglycoside antibiotics are indicated for treatment of serious or potentially serious infections caused by gram-negative bacteria. They are sometimes indicated for treatment of susceptible gram-positive bacteria.

Pharmacology
—Aminoglycosides are usually bactericidal (as opposed to bacteriostatic). The mechanism of action is probably due to inhibition of protein synthesis.
—Since they are poorly absorbed from the gastrointestinal (GI) tract, aminoglycosides must be given IV or IM. However, they are almost completely absorbed through the peritoneum and irrigation of the abdomen with these agents results in significant plasma aminoglycoside levels.
—Aminoglycosides can cause ototoxicity and nephrotoxicity and can have significant interactions with neuromuscular blocking agents.
—Documented interactions with muscle relaxants have followed parenteral use of aminoglycosides as well as after irrigation of the of the peritoneum, pleura, and skin flaps. The severity of the interaction appears to be dose-related and self-limiting.

Amikacin (Amikin)
Classification and indications
—Amikacin is a semisynthetic aminoglycoside antibiotic. It is derived from kanamycin.
—Aminoglycoside antibiotics are indicated for treatment of serious or potentially serious infections caused by gram-neg-

ative bacteria. They are sometimes indicated for treatment of susceptible gram-positive bacteria.

Gentamicin (Garamycin, Jenamicin, Storz-G)
Classification and indications
—Gentamicin is an aminoglycoside antibiotic.
—It is used for treatment of infections caused by some gram-negative (*Acinetobacter, Enterobacter, E. coli, Klebsiella, Proteus,* and others) and gram-positive bacteria (*Staphylococcus aureus, S. epidermidis*).

Kanamycin (Kantrex)
Classification and indications
—Kanamycin is an aminoglycoside antibiotic.
—Aminoglycoside antibiotics are indicated for treatment of serious or potentially serious infections caused by gram-negative bacteria. They are sometimes indicated for treatment of susceptible gram-positive bacteria.

Netilmicin (Netromycin)
Classification and indications
—Netilmicin is an aminoglycoside antibiotic.
—Aminoglycoside antibiotics are indicated for treatment of serious or potentially serious infections caused by gram-negative bacteria. They are sometimes indicated for treatment of susceptible gram-positive bacteria.

Streptomycin
Classification and indications
—Streptomycin is an aminoglycoside antibiotic.
—It is used in the treatment of tuberculosis and other mycobacterial diseases, as well as tularemia and plague. It can also be used to treat some infections with susceptible gram-negative bacteria.

Tobramycin (Nebcin)
Classification and indications
—Tobramycin is an aminoglycoside antibiotic.
—Aminoglycoside antibiotics are indicated for treatment of serious or potentially serious infections caused by gram-negative bacteria. They are sometimes indicated for treatment of susceptible gram-positive bacteria.

Aminoglycoside Interactions with Anesthetic Drugs
Aminoglycoside antibiotics with furosemide
—Some sources suggest that furosemide may increase the potential for ototoxicity or nephrotoxicity of aminoglycoside

antibiotics. In fact, there is little persuasive evidence of this interaction.

Aminoglycoside antibiotics with muscle relaxants (atracurium, doxacurium, gallamine, metocurine, mivacurium, pancuronium, pipercuronium, rocuronium, succinylcholine, tubocurarine, vecuronium)

—A number of antibiotics have significant interactions with neuromuscular blocking agents. These include the aminoglycosides (amikacin, gentamicin, kanamycin, neomycin, paromomycin, netilmicin, neomycin, streptomycin, tobramycin), as well as polymyxin B, colistin, amphotericin B, clindamycin, bacitracin, and lincomycin.

—All of the above antibiotics may potentiate non-depolarizing agents, but some (aminoglycosides, amphotericin B, clindamycin, colistin) can also potentiate succinylcholine blockade.

—These antibiotics potentiate neuromuscular blockade by different mechanisms, making management of these problems difficult. Although treatment with anticholinesterases or calcium has been recommended, results are inconsistent.

AMINOPHYLLINE (Aerolate, Aquaphyllin, Asmalix, Bronkody, Dilor, Dyflex, Elixophyllin, Lanophyllin, Lufyllin, Neothylline, Quibron, Slo-Phyllin, Slo-Bid, Theo-Dur, Theobid, Theoclear, Theolair, Theovent, Truphylline)

Classification and indications

—Aminophylline is a xanthine derivative.

—It is used as a bronchodilator and to treat apnea in infants and patients with Cheyne–Stokes respiration.

Pharmacology

—Aminophylline is a compound of theophylline with ethylenediamene, which makes theophylline more water-soluble.

—Theophylline competitively inhibits phosphodiesterase and increases intracellular cyclic AMP, resulting in bronchodilation and pulmonary arteriolar dilation.

—Theophylline is a CNS and cardiovascular stimulant. Partially offsetting the stimulating effect on the cardiovascular system is systemic arteriolar and venous dilation (as well as coronary artery dilation).

—Optimal bronchodilation usually requires serum theophylline levels between 10 and 20 μg/mL. Above 20 μg/mL, adverse effects of theophylline are likely to manifest (tachycardia, nausea, delirium, seizures, etc.).

—Elimination of theophylline is impaired in patients with congestive heart failure, chronic obstructive pulmonary disease, liver disease, or in geriatric patients.

Aminophylline Interactions with Anesthetic Drugs
Aminophylline with adenosine

—Adenosine is a nucleoside that slows conduction through the atrioventricular node. Xanthines such as theophylline, aminophylline, and caffeine can reverse or block the physiologic effects of adenosine.

AMIODARONE (Cordarone)

Classification and indications

—Amiodarone is an antiarrhythmic agent. It is a benzofuran derivative.

—It is indicated for the management of life-threatening ventricular arrhythmias that cannot be treated with other agents.

Pharmacology

—It is considered a class III antiarrhythmic, but has some properties of class I agents.

—Although the precise mechanism is not known, amiodarone appears to delay repolarization, slow depolarization (both actions characteristic of class III agents), and inhibit alpha and beta activity.

—Long-term oral therapy can suppress sinus node function with a resultant decrease in heart rate.

—Significant interactions have been associated with calcium channel blockers, beta blockers, and other agents used by anesthesiologists.

—At this time, amiodarone is only available commercially for oral administration.

Amiodarone Interactions with Anesthetic Drugs
Amiodarone with beta blockers (esmolol, labetalol, propranolol)

—Metoprolol and propranolol have both been associated with life-threatening arrhythmias (severe bradycardia, cardiac arrest, or ventricular fibrillation) in patients taking amiodarone. In all cases, these arrhythmias developed within 1 to several hours after initiation of these beta blockers and after only one or two doses.

—Although these cases involved oral beta blockers, intravenous propranolol could have similar results.

—Other beta blockers have not been associated with this interaction.

Amiodarone with inhalational anesthetics (desflurane, enflurane, halothane, isoflurane, sevoflurane)

—Amiodarone, an antiarrhythmic which increases refractoriness and slows conduction in most cardiac tissue, has been associated with severe cardiac complications including arrhythmias, low cardiac output, and decreased systemic vascular resistance in patients having general anesthesia with inhalational agents.

—The mechanism of these interactions is not known.

Amiodarone with calcium channel blockers (diltiazem, verapamil), lidocaine, procainamide)

—Amiodarone increases refractoriness and slows conduction in most cardiac tissue. A number of medications, including class I antiarrhythmics like lidocaine, calcium channel blockers, and beta blockers, which have similar effects, can precipitate severe bradycardia when given to a patient taking amiodarone.

—A case was reported of a patient with sick sinus syndrome on amiodarone who developed profound sinus bradycardia after local anesthesia with lidocaine.

AMPHOTERICIN B (Fungizone)

Classification and indications

—Amphotericin B is considered an antifungal antibiotic. It is produced by *Streptomyces nodosus.* It is administered intravenously.

—It is used in the treatment of severe systemic or meningeal fungal infections (such as blastomycosis, aspergillosis, candidiasis, etc.).

Pharmacology

—Amphotericin B is not effective against bacterial, rickettsial, or viral infections.

—Treatment with amphotericin B is frequently associated with nephrotoxicity and hypokalemia. The hypokalemia is felt to be responsible for the muscle weakness experienced by some patients.

—Prolonged neuromuscular blockade has been reported in patients receiving amphotericin and is believed to be related to hypokalemia.

Amphotericin B Interactions with Anesthetic Drugs
Amphotericin B with muscle relaxants (atracurium,
doxacurium, gallamine, metocurine, mivacurium,
pancuronium, pipercuronium, rocuronium, succinylcholine,
tubocurarine, vecuronium)

—A number of antibiotics have significant interactions with neuromuscular blocking agents. These include the aminoglycosides (amikacin, gentamicin, kanamycin, neomycin, paromomycin, netilmicin, neomycin, streptomycin, tobramycin), as well as polymyxin B, colistin, amphotericin B, clindamycin, bacitracin, and lincomycin.

—All of the above antibiotics may potentiate non-depolarizing agents, but some (aminoglycosides, amphotericin B, clindamycin, colistin) can also potentiate succinylcholine blockade.

—These antibiotics potentiate neuromuscular blockade by different mechanisms, making management of these problems difficult. Although treatment with anticholinesterases or calcium has been recommended, results are inconsistent.

ANTIBIOTICS

—A number of antibiotics have significant interactions with neuromuscular blocking agents. These include the aminoglycosides (amikacin, gentamicin, kanamycin, neomycin, paromomycin, netilmicin, neomycin, streptomycin, tobramycin), as well as polymyxin B, colistin, amphotericin B, clindamycin, bacitracin, and lincomycin.

—These antibiotics potentiate neuromuscular blockade by different mechanisms, making management of these problems difficult.

—All of the above antibiotics may potentiate non-depolarizing agents, but some (aminoglycosides, amphotericin B, clindamycin, colistin) can also potentiate succinylcholine blockade.

—Some other antibiotics (such as tetracyclines) have also been implicated in interactions with muscle relaxants, but good documentation is not available.

—Reversal of antibiotic neuromuscular blockade is unreliable. Though anticholinesterases may be useful, they may worsen some cases of antibiotic-induced neuromuscular block. Calcium has been suggested in some cases, but it is unreliable.

Antibiotics Interactions with Anesthetic Drugs
Antibiotics with muscle relaxants (atracurium, doxacurium, gallamine, metocurine, mivacurium, pancuronium, pipercuronium, rocuronium, succinylcholine, tubocurarine, vecuronium)

—A number of antibiotics have significant interactions with neuromuscular blocking agents. These include the aminoglycosides (amikacin, gentamicin, kanamycin, neomycin, paromomycin, netilmicin, neomycin, streptomycin, tobramycin), as well as polymyxin B, colistin, amphotericin B, clindamycin, bacitracin, and lincomycin.

—All of the above antibiotics may potentiate non-depolarizing agents, but some (aminoglycosides, amphotericin B, clindamycin, colistin) can also potentiate succinylcholine blockade.

—These antibiotics potentiate neuromuscular blockade by different mechanisms, making management of these problems difficult. Although treatment with anticholinesterases or calcium has been recommended, results are inconsistent.

BACITRACIN (Baci-IM)

Classification and indications
—Bacitracin is an antibiotic produced by *Bacillus subtilis.*
—It is used to treat infection with gram-positive bacteria (*Staphylococcus, Streptococcus, Corynebacterium, Clostridium*).

Pharmacology
—Bacitracin appears to function by interfering with cell wall synthesis.
—It may be either bactericidal or bacteriostatic, depending on the concentration of antibiotic or the susceptibility of the bacteria.
—It may be administered IM, intrathecally, or in the peritoneum, pleura, or synovium. Because it is not absorbed from the gastrointestinal tract, it can be used to treat intestinal infections that do not require systemic blood levels.
—Like some other antibiotics, bacitracin may potentiate neuromuscular blockade. This interaction appears to mainly involve non-depolarizing agents.

Bacitracin Interactions with Anesthetic Drugs

Bacitracin with muscle relaxants (atracurium, doxacurium, gallamine, metocurine, mivacurium, pancuronium, pipercuronium, rocuronium, succinylcholine, tubocurarine, vecuronium)

—A number of antibiotics have significant interactions with neuromuscular blocking agents. These include the aminoglycosides (amikacin, gentamicin, kanamycin, neomycin, paromomycin, netilmicin, neomycin, streptomycin, tobramycin), as well as polymyxin B, colistin, amphotericin B, clindamycin, bacitracin, and lincomycin.

—All of the above antibiotics may potentiate non-depolarizing agents, but some (aminoglycosides, amphotericin B, clindamycin, colistin) can also potentiate succinylcholine blockade.

—These antibiotics potentiate neuromuscular blockade by different mechanisms, making management of these problems difficult. Although treatment with anticholinesterases or calcium has been recommended, results are inconsistent.

BETA BLOCKERS

Classification and indications

—Beta blockers are a group of drugs that competitively inhibit beta receptors. Some agents are selective (esmolol) whereas others are nonselective (propranolol).

—These agents are used in the treatment of hypertension, angina, and cardiac arrhythmias.

Pharmacology

—Effects of beta 1 blockade include decreased heart rate and contractility, slowed conduction through the atrioventricular and sinus node, decreased automaticity, and decreased myocardial oxygen consumption.

—Beta 2 blockade results in some increase in peripheral vascular resistance (due to unopposed alpha stimulation). The overall effect of beta blockade and other less understood mechanisms causes a decrease in blood pressure.

—Some beta-blocking agents have mild beta adrenergic stimulating effects which can partly offset resting bradycardia in some patients without interfering in control of hypertension.

—This partial agonist activity is called intrinsic sympathomimetic activity (ISA) or partial agonist activity (PAA).

—Bronchial constriction from beta 2 blockade may result in increased airway resistance, especially in patients with reactive airway disease (asthma, coronary obstructive pulmonary disease, bronchitis).

—Significant interactions can occur with calcium channel blockers, cocaine, vasopressors, and other agents used during anesthesia.

Acebutolol (Sectral)
Classification and indications
—Acebutolol is a beta 1 selective blocker.

—It is used for treatment of hypertension, cardiac arrhythmias, and angina.

Atenolol (Tenormin)
Classification and indications
—Atenolol is a beta antagonist that is mainly selective for beta 1 receptors.

—It is used in the treatment of hypertension, angina, and myocardial infarction.

Pharmacology
—Atenolol is a selective inhibitor of beta 1 receptors and has little effect on beta 2 receptors unless administered in high doses (>100 mg/day).

Betaxolol (Betoptic, Kerlone)
Classification and indications
—Betaxolol is a beta antagonist that is mainly selective for beta 1 receptors.

—It is used in the treatment of hypertension and as an ophthalmic preparation for the treatment of elevated intraocular pressure.

Pharmacology
—Betaxolol is a selective inhibitor of beta 1 receptors and has little effect on beta 2 receptors.

—It is about 9 times more potent than atenolol.

Carteolol (Cartrol)
Classification and indications
—Carteolol is a nonselective beta adrenergic blocker with intrinsic sympathomimetic activity.

—It is indicated for treatment of hypertension.

Labetalol (Normodyne, Normozide, Trandate)
Classification and indications
—Labetalol is an alpha and beta adrenergic blocking agent.

—It is indicated for the treatment of hypertension.

Pharmacology

—Labetalol is a nonselective beta blocker (both beta 1 and beta 2) and a selective alpha 1 blocker. After intravenous administration, the ratio of alpha to beta blockade is about 1:7.

Levobunolol (Betagen)
Classification and indications

—Levobunolol is a nonselective beta adrenergic blocker that is used topically in the eye.

—It is used to treat elevated intraocular pressure of different causes.

Pharmacology

—Timolol and levobunolol are nonselective (beta 1 and beta 2) blockers. They are potent agents (compared to oral propranolol, oral levobunolol is 20–50 times more potent).

—These agents probably reduce intraocular pressure by reducing formation of aqueous humor, but the exact mechanism is not known.

—Because they can be absorbed systemically from the ocular conjunctiva, symptoms of beta blockade can occur.

Metoprolol (Tenoretic, Tenormin)
Classification and indications

—Metoprolol is a beta antagonist that is mainly selective for beta 1 receptors.

—It is used in the treatment of hypertension, angina, and myocardial infarction.

Pharmacology

—Metoprolol is a selective inhibitor of beta 1 receptors and has little effect on beta 2 receptors unless administered in high doses (>100 mg/day).

Nadolol (Corgard, Corzide)
Classification and indications

—Nadolol is a nonselective beta blocker, similar to propranolol.

—It is used to treat hypertension and angina. Other uses have included arrhythmias and migraine headache.

Penbutolol (Levatol)
Classification and indications

—Penbutolol is a nonselective beta blocker.

—It is used to treat hypertension

Pharmacology

—The pharmacology of penbutolol is similar to that of other nonselective beta blockers (like propranolol).

Pindolol (Visken)
Classification and indications
—Pindolol is a nonselective beta adrenergic blocker with intrinsic sympathomimetic activity.

—It is indicated for treatment of hypertension.

Pharmacology
—Some beta blocking agents have mild beta adrenergic stimulating effects that can partially offset resting bradycardia in some patients without interfering in control of hypertension.

—This partial agonist activity is called intrinsic sympathomimetic activity (ISA) or partial agonist activity (PAA).

Propranolol (Betachron, Inderal, Inderide)
Classification and indications
—Propranolol is a nonselective beta blocker, similar to nadolol.

—It is used to treat hypertension and angina. Other uses have included arrhythmias and migraine headache.

Timolol (Timoptic)
Classification and indications
—Timolol is a nonselective beta adrenergic blocker that is used topically in the eye.

—It is used to treat elevated intraocular pressure of different causes.

Pharmacology
—Timolol and levobunolol are nonselective (beta 1 and beta 2) blockers.

—These agents probably reduce intraocular pressure by reducing formation of aqueous humor, but the exact mechanism is not known.

—Because they can be absorbed systemically from the ocular conjunctiva, symptoms of beta blockade can occur.

Beta Blockers Interactions with Anesthetic Drugs
Beta blockers with calcium channel blockers (diltiazem, verapamil)
—Verapamil and diltiazem, particularly when used intravenously, can significantly potentiate the effects of beta blockers on cardiac conduction and contractility.

—Severe bradycardia and hypotension can occur when these medications are used concomitantly, especially in patients with abnormalities of cardiac conduction (sick sinus syndrome) or ventricular function (congestive heart failure).

Beta blockers with cocaine

—Coronary vasoconstriction has been demonstrated in patients receiving infusions of a beta blocker (propranolol) after intranasal cocaine. The significance of this to clinical practice and particularly for patients on chronic beta blocker therapy is not clear.

—Patients who develop hypertension, tachycardia, and angina from cocaine may be best treated by an agent such as labetalol, which has alpha blocking properties.

Beta blockers with diazoxide

—The hypotensive response to diazoxide may be accentuated in patients taking beta blockers. This may be due to the blunting of the normal sympathetic response that would otherwise occur.

Beta blockers with epinephrine

—Patients who are receiving beta blockers may be more resistant to the bronchodilator effects of isoproterenol. The nonselective beta blockers, such as propranolol, are more likely to have an interaction of greater magnitude than selective blockers, such as metoprolol.

Beta blockers with isoproterenol

—Patients who are receiving beta blockers may be more resistant to the bronchodilator effects of isoproterenol. The nonselective beta blockers, such as propranolol, are more likely to have an interaction of greater magnitude than selective blockers, such as metoprolol.

Beta blockers with ketamine

—Ketamine may produce myocardial depression if there is interference with the normal sympathetic response, as seen in patients on beta blockers.

Beta blockers with lidocaine

—Lidocaine clearance is reduced in patients taking beta blockers, which may result in higher serum levels of lidocaine than anticipated. This is attributed to a decreased cardiac output and decreased hepatic blood flow seen in patients taking beta blockers.

—Lidocaine with epinephrine used as a local anesthetic in large amounts can cause extreme hypertension in patients on chronic beta blocker therapy. This occurs because of unrestricted alpha stimulation in patients on beta blockers.

—Cardioselective beta blockers like acebutolol, atenolol, and metoprolol are less likely to be associated with a severe hypertensive with epinephrine.

Beta blockers with muscle relaxants (atracurium, doxacurium, gallamine, metocurine, mivacurium, pancuronium, pipercuronium, rocuronium, tubocurarine, vecuronium)

—Beta blockers may potentiate non-depolarizing neuromuscular blocking agents. This interaction has been reported between propranolol and tubocurarine.

—Other beta blockers are also capable of causing weakness in patients with myasthenia gravis, but the mechanism or significance of these interactions is unclear.

Beta blockers with phenylephrine

—Phenylephrine produces mostly alpha stimulation, and in patients who are receiving beta blockers it has been associated with exaggerated hypertensive responses. This is due to the unopposed vasoconstriction from beta blockade. A similar response is seen with epinephrine.

—This interaction is more likely to occur with nonselective beta blockers such as propranolol, nadolol, timolol, or pindolol.

BUMETANIDE (Bumex)

Classification and indications

—Bumetanide is a diuretic that is structurally related to furosemide.

—It is indicated for the treatment of edema resulting from different causes including congestive heart failure, hepatic disease, and renal dysfunction. It is also used to treat hypertension.

Pharmacology

—Bumetanide, like other loop diuretics, functions by blocking reabsorption of sodium and chloride ions in the ascending limb of the loop of Henle. This results in an osmotic diuresis from the increased solute load (unabsorbed ions). Also, by decreasing ion reabsorption, the concentration of medullary interstitial fluid decreases and therefore promotes diuresis.

—The result of interference with ion reabsorption is loss of sodium, potassium, chloride, and hydrogen ions (as well as others). Patients on chronic therapy or who are receiving very large doses usually require some replacement of these ions.

—Bumetanide decreases both renal and peripheral vascular resistance as well as increasing venous capacitance. This results in increased renal blood flow, decreased venous return to the heart and decreased blood pressure.

—In patients with chronic renal insufficiency, large doses may increase the glomerular filtration rate temporarily.

—Tinnitus and permanent or reversible hearing loss has been associated with rapid IV or IM administration of furosemide, usually with doses much >20–40 mg. Also, coadministration of bumetanide and aminoglycoside antibiotics may increase ototoxicity.

Bumetanide Interactions with Anesthetic Drugs
Bumetanide with enalapril (enalaprilat)

—Angiotensin-converting enzyme (ACE) inhibitors used to treat hypertension in a patient who is being diuresed with the loop diuretics may produce a profound drop in blood pressure. This response has been seen as early as 2–3 hours after initiation of ACE inhibitors.

—The mechanisms of this interaction may include hypovolemia from diuretic therapy or, in some patients, high levels of renin and angiotensin.

—The setting in which this interaction may be significant for anesthesiologists might be a hypertensive patient who presents for urgent surgery while receiving intensive diuretic treatment for cardiac decompensation. Use of ACE inhibitor therapy in the perioperative setting may precipitate the interaction described.

CALCIUM CHANNEL BLOCKERS

Classification and indications

—Calcium channel blockers are a group of medications that interfere with calcium movement in cardiac and vascular smooth muscle cells.

—They are indicated for treatment of hypertension and arrhythmias, depending on the agent (some have more pronounced cardiac conduction effects whereas others are more potent antihypertensives).

Pharmacology

—Depolarization of cardiac and smooth muscle cells is associated with ion movement (sodium, calcium, potassium, chloride) through ion channels. These channels are voltage-gated, meaning that they are opened and closed according to changes in transmembrane potentials.

—With depolarization, there is rapid movement of sodium through "fast" channels, whereas calcium moves much more slowly through "slow" channels. It is by interfering with calcium movement through these slow calcium channels that calcium channel blockers mainly exert their effects.

—Some of the calcium channel blockers have more pronounced effects on cardiac conduction (verapamil, diltiazem), whereas others have greater effects on vascular smooth muscle, resulting in lower blood pressure and coronary vasodilation (nifedipine, nicardipine).

—Calcium channel blockers slow conduction through the AV node (verapamil, diltiazem) and increase nodal refractoriness. As a result, these agents can slow ventricular rate in patients with atrial fibrillation or flutter and in patients with paroxysmal supraventricular tachycardia.

—A negative inotropic effect (decreased myocardial contractility) is associated mainly with verapamil but can also be seen with diltiazem and nicardipine.

Amlodipine (Norvasc)
Classification and indications
—Amlodipine is a calcium channel blocker.
—It is used in the treatment of hypertension as an oral medication.

Bepridil (Vasocor)
Classification and indications
—Bepridil is a calcium channel blocker available in oral form. It is not chemically related to the other calcium channel blockers such as verapamil, diltiazem, or nifedipine.
—It is indicated in the management of angina. Its antiarrhythmic and antihypertensive properties are less pronounced than those of some other calcium channel blockers.

Diltiazem (Cardizem)
Classification and indications
—Diltiazem is a calcium channel blocker.
—When used orally, it is indicated for the management of hypertension and angina.

Felodipine (Plendil)
Classification and indications
—Felodipine is a calcium channel blocker.
—It is used to treat hypertension.

Isradipine (DynaCirc)
Classification and indications
—Isradipine is a calcium channel blocker.

—It is used in the treatment of hypertension as an oral medication.

Nicardipine (Cardene)
Classification and indications
—Nicardipine is a calcium channel blocker.

—It is indicated for the management of hypertension.

Nifedipine (Adalat, Procardia)
Classification and indications
—Nifedipine is a calcium channel blocker.

—It is indicated for the management of hypertension.

Nimodipine (Nimotop)
Classification and indications
—Nimodipine is a calcium channel blocker that is structurally similar to nifedipine.

—It is used for treatment of subarachnoid hemorrhage. In this situation, nimodipine may reduce neurologic damage resulting from ischemia.

Pharmacology
—Nimodipine appears to function like some other calcium channel blockers (nifedipine), but it affects the cerebral vasculature preferentially. This may occur because of the high lipid solubility of this drug.

Verapamil (Calan, Isoptin, Verelan)
Classification and indications
—Verapamil is a calcium channel blocker.

—When used orally, it is indicated for the management of hypertension, angina, and to control the ventricular rate in patients with atrial fibrillation or flutter.

Calcium Channel Blockers Interactions with Anesthetic Drugs
Calcium channel blockers with calcium chloride, calcium gluconate
—Calcium may antagonize some effects of calcium channel blockers.

—In some patients, intravenous calcium has reduced the hypotensive effects of nifedipine but not its ability to prevent angina. In other cases, calcium has caused a return of an arrhythmia that had been controlled with a calcium channel blocker.

—Because the response to calcium may not be completely pre-dictable in patients treated with calcium channel blockers, caution should be used when using intravenous calcium in such patients.

Calcium channel blockers with muscle relaxants (atracurium, doxacurium, gallamine, metocurine, mivacurium, pancuronium, pipercuronium, rocuronium, tubocurarine, vecuronium)

—Calcium channel blockers have been associated with prolon-gation of neuromuscular blockade from non-depolarizing agents.

—This interaction is probably related to the depletion of intra-cellular calcium associated with chronic therapy. This can result in a decrease in acetylcholine release at the neuromus-cular junction.

CARBAMAZEPINE (Epitol, Tegretol)

Classification and indications

—Carbamazepine is an anticonvulsant that is an iminiostilbene derivative.

—It is used in the treatment of generalized (grand mal), partial (psychomotor), and mixed seizure disorders. It is also used to treat trigeminal neuralgia and some other disorders.

Pharmacology

—Carbamazepine is chemically unrelated to other anticonvul-sants but is structurally related to the tricyclic antidepres-sants.

—Functionally, it seems to inhibit seizure activity by suppress-ing propagation of seizures (similar to phenytoin).

—Significant cardiovascular effects include the ability to aug-ment atrioventricular block with adenosine.

—It is administered only in oral form.

Carbamazepine Interactions with Anesthetic Drugs

Carbamazepine with adenosine

—Adenosine when used in patients taking carbamazepine may produce a greater blockade than anticipated. A decrease in adenosine dosage may be appropriate in such patients.

Carbidopa (Lodosyn, Sinemet)

Classification and indications

—Carbidopa is a decarboxylase inhibitor that prevents destruc-tion of levodopa.

—It is used to treat Parkinson's disease.

Pharmacology

—Levodopa and the decarboxylase inhibitor, carbidopa, are believed to function by increasing dopamine concentrations in the basal ganglia of the brain. It is thought that depletion of dopamine is the etiology of Parkinsonism.

—Levodopa, unlike dopamine, is able to cross the blood-brain barrier where it may be converted to dopamine by the enzyme, dopa decarboxylase.

—Carbidopa inhibits peripheral decarboxylation of levodopa (which otherwise occurs rapidly and reduces the amount available to enter the CNS).

—Butyrophenones (droperidol) block the dopaminergic effects of dopamine and can antagonize levodopa and carbidopa.

Carbidopa Interactions with Anesthetic Drugs
Carbidopa with droperidol

—Carbidopa is used to increase dopamine concentrations in the brain. Butyrophenones (such as droperidol) block the dopaminergic effects of dopamine and can antagonize levodopa and carbidopa.

CHLORAMBUCIL (Leukeran)

Classification and indications

—Chlorambucil is an alkylating agent. It is one of the nitrogen mustards.

—It is used to treat leukemias, lymphomas, and other malignancies.

Pharmacology

—Alkylating agents form bonds with nucleic acids (DNA and RNA). As a result, growth of rapidly proliferating cells is disrupted.

—Adverse reactions to chlorambucil include nausea and vomiting, alopecia, and leukopenia.

—Interstitial pulmonary fibrosis has occurred in patients receiving alkylating agents.

—Plasma pseudocholinesterase levels may be depressed in some patients receiving this medication. As a result, prolonged blockade from succinylcholine may occur.

Chlorambucil Interactions with Anesthetic Drugs
Chlorambucil with succinylcholine

—Some patients receiving chlorambucil may have depressed levels of plasma pseudocholinesterase. In some cases, the result may be delayed metabolism of succinylcholine and a prolonged neuromuscular blockade.

CIMETIDINE (Tagamet)

Classification and indications
—Cimetidine is a histamine H2 receptor antagonist.
—It is used as treatment for a variety of conditions including gastric, duodenal, and stress ulcers, as well as gastroesophageal reflux. It is also used preoperatively to reduce gastric volume and acidity.

Pharmacology
—Cimetidine is a competitive inhibitor of histamine at the H2 receptor of parietal cells found in the gastric mucosa.
—Histamine, by stimulating the H2 receptors, stimulates production of gastric acid by the parietal cells.
—Maximal effect on acid production occurs in 60–90 minutes after oral, intravenous, or intramuscular administration.
—Following a dose of 300 mg PO, blood levels sufficient to reduce gastric acidity by 80% persist for 4–5 hours.
—The half-life of the drug is approximately 2 hours in patients with normal renal function. Depending on the level of renal dysfunction, the half-life may increase to as much as 5 hours.
—Cimetidine has been associated with many drug interactions due to several complex metabolic alterations. These include interference with hepatic metabolism and renal clearance.

Cimetidine Interactions with Anesthetic Drugs
Cimetidine with narcotics (alfentanil, buprenorphine, butorphanol, fentanyl, meperidine, morphine, nalbuphine, sufentanil)
—Cimetidine may potentiate narcotics, causing greater respiratory depression and sedation than expected. This may be related to the alteration of hepatic metabolism of narcotics produced by cimetidine.
—This effect is seen less with morphine than other narcotics and is probably related to the fact that morphine undergoes a different metabolic process than some other narcotics such as fentanyl or meperidine.
—Ranitidine is not associated with this interaction.

Cimetidine with lidocaine
—In patients receiving oral but not intravenous cimetidine, acute intravenous infusion of lidocaine may result in early

signs of toxicity. This is due to the decrease in hepatic clearance of lidocaine caused by cimetidine.

—This interaction has been documented after single oral doses of cimetidine and may decrease lidocaine clearance by up to 30%.

—This interaction is not seen with other H2 receptor antagonists.

CLINDAMYCIN (Cleocin)

Classification and indications

—Clindamycin is an antibiotic derived from lincomycin.

—It is indicated for treatment of infection with most aerobic gram-positive organisms including staphylococci, streptococci, and some other gram-negative and gram-positive organisms.

Pharmacology

—Clindamycin is thought to be active by interfering with protein synthesis of the susceptible organisms. It may be either bacteriostatic or bactericidal.

—It may be administered orally, intramuscularly, or intravenously.

—Like some other antibiotics, clindamycin can potentiate neuromuscular blockade. The mechanism of action is not clear. Potentiation appears to mainly involve non-depolarizing agents.

Clindamycin Interactions with Anesthetic Drugs
Clindamycin with muscle relaxants (atracurium, doxacurium, gallamine, metocurine, mivacurium, pancuronium, pipercuronium, rocuronium, succinylcholine, tubocurarine, vecuronium)

—A number of antibiotics have significant interactions with neuromuscular blocking agents. These include the aminoglycosides (amikacin, gentamicin, kanamycin, neomycin, paromomycin, netilmicin, neomycin, streptomycin, tobramycin), as well as polymyxin B, colistin, amphotericin B, clindamycin, bacitracin, and lincomycin.

—All of the above antibiotics may potentiate non-depolarizing agents, but some (aminoglycosides, amphotericin B, clindamycin, colistin) can also potentiate succinylcholine blockade.

—These antibiotics potentiate neuromuscular blockade by different mechanisms, making management of these problems difficult. Although treatment with anticholinesterases or calcium has been recommended, results are inconsistent.

CLONIDINE (Catapress, Combipress)

Classification and indications
—Clonidine is an antihypertensive agent.
—It is used to treat hypertension.

Pharmacology
—Clonidine is an alpha 2 adrenergic receptor stimulant. Alpha 2 receptors are located mainly in the medulla oblongata where they modify sympathetic vasomotor centers; stimulation of these receptors causes inhibition of the central sympathetic centers, resulting in lower blood pressure and heart rate. Cardiovascular effects include a decline in cardiac output.

—Sedation may be seen with administration of clonidine and is thought to be related to the central alpha 2 receptor agonism.

—Clonidine has been shown to decrease minimal alveaolar concentration (MAC) of inhaled and opioid anesthetics, also attributed to its effect on alpha 2 receptors. Use of naloxone (Narcan) may result in reversal of the antihypertensive effects of clonidine and may precipitate the exaggerated hypertension associated with sudden clonidine withdrawal.

—Clonidine is well absorbed via the GI tract and is also administered transdermally. After an oral dose, declines in blood pressure occur usually within 30–60 minutes. Transdermal blood levels require longer to achieve therapeutic levels and are used for outpatient management of hypertension.

—Elimination depends on hepatic metabolism and renal excretion. Patients with renal dysfunction may have prolonged elimination times, since the majority of the drug is excreted via the kidneys.

Clonidine Interactions with Anesthetic Drugs
Clonidine with inhalational anesthetics, narcotics*
—Clonidine has been shown to potentiate narcotics and reduce the MAC of inhaled anesthetics.

---

* Inhalational anesthetics (desflurane, enflurane, halothane, isoflurane, nitrous oxide, sevoflurane)
Narcotics (alfentanil, buprenorphine, butorphanol, fentanyl, meperidine, morphine, nalbuphine, sufentanil)

—This effect may be related to clonidine's inhibition of the sympathetic outflow from the vasomotor center in the medulla (clonidine is a central alpha 2 receptor agonist, which results in inhibition of CNS sympathetic centers).

CYCLOPHOSPHAMIDE (Cytoxan, Neosar)

Classification and indications
—Cyclophosphamide is a chemotherapeutic alkylating agent derived from nitrogen mustard.
—It is used in the treatment of different malignancies including Hodgkin's disease, multiple myeloma, leukemias, and breast cancer. It also has been used for minimal change nephrotic syndrome in children who have not responded to other therapy.

Pharmacology
—Cyclophosphamide is an alkylating agent, meaning it forms bonds with nucleic acids (DNA and RNA). As a result, growth of rapidly proliferating cells is disrupted.
—Adverse reactions to cyclophosphamide include nausea and vomiting, alopecia, and leukopenia.
—At high doses, cyclophosphamide can be cardiotoxic.
—Interstitial pulmonary fibrosis has occurred in patients receiving high doses of cyclophosphamide for prolonged periods.
—Plasma pseudocholinesterase levels may be depressed in some patients receiving this medication. As a result, prolonged blockade from succinylcholine may occur.

Cyclophosphamide Interactions with Anesthetic Drugs
Cyclophosphamide with succinylcholine
—Antipseudocholinesterases (echothiophate, phenelzine, nitrogen mustard, cyclophosphamide) prevent the metabolic destruction of succinylcholine and thus prolong its neuromuscular blocking properties.

DEMECARIUM BROMIDE (Humorsol)

Classification and indications
—Demecarium bromide is a long-acting anticholinesterase.
—It is used to treat glaucoma (both angle closure and open angle forms). It may also be used to diagnose and treat some forms of strabismus.

Pharmacology

—Demecarium is an anticholinesterase that is structurally related to neostigmine.

—The miotic (pupillary constriction) drugs are parasympathomimetic agents with different mechanisms of action.

—Direct-acting agents are drugs like acetylcholine. Indirect-acting drugs inhibit acetylcholinesterase either reversibly (physostigmine, demecarium) or irreversibly (the organophosphates echothiophate, isoflurophate).

—The anticholinesterases used to reverse neuromuscular blockers are shorter acting, competitive inhibitors of acetylcholinesterase.

—It is thought that these drugs, by producing miosis (pupillary constriction), allow greater flow of aqueous humor from the anterior chamber of the eye. This seems to occur in both open angle and angle closure forms.

—Because these drugs are nonspecific anticholinesterases, they inhibit not only acetylcholinesterase but plasma pseudocholinesterase as well. This may result in prolonged blockade from succinylcholine.

—Even though demecarium is considered a reversible anticholinesterase, it behaves much like the organophosphates. Therefore, as long as 2 weeks may be required to achieve adequate pseudocholinesterase levels after treatment has been stopped.

Demacarium Bromide Interactions with Anesthetic Drugs
Demecarium bromide with succinylcholine

—The nonspecific anticholinesterase miotics (echothiophate, demecarium bromide, isoflurophate) used in treatment of glaucoma can result in significant depression of plasma pseudocholinesterase levels.

—Prolonged neuromuscular blockade can occur with succinylcholine in these patients. A period of 2–4 weeks may be necessary to restore plasma cholinesterase levels after discontinuing the anticholinesterase miotics.

DIGITALIS (Crystodigin, Lanoxicaps, Lanoxin)

Classification and indications

—Digitalis can be a term used to refer to the entire class of cardiac glycosides, which includes digoxin, digitoxin, deslanoside, and digitalis.

—All of the cardiac glycosides have a positive inotropic action and slow conduction through the atrioventricular node. They are used for treatment of heart failure and to control ventricular rate in patients with atrial fibrillation or flutter or paroxysmal supraventricular tachycardia.

Pharmacology

—The increased contractility of the myocardium appears to be related to inhibition of the sodium-potassium pump by digitalis. The net result of this action is an accumulation of intracellular calcium, which improves contractility.

—Slowed conduction through the atrioventricular (AV) node is a result of a direct action as well as an increase in vagal tone and a decrease in sympathetic stimulation.

—Digitalis also lengthens the effective refractory period of the AV node. However, in patients with Wolf–Parkinson–White syndrome, digitalis reduces the refractory period of the bypass tracts and may result in worsening tachycardia.

—Digitalis toxicity affects several organ systems, but most seriously the cardiovascular system. Excessive vagal tone from digitalis may cause severe sinus bradycardia. Tachyarrhythmias and premature atrial or ventricular contractions can be seen and may be explained partly by increased automaticity from excess digitalis.

—Hypokalemia is a frequent causative factor in digitalis toxicity. Potassium reduces the binding of digitalis to the Na-K-ATPase enzyme in the myocardium and reduces toxicity. In any patient with bradycardia receiving digitalis and especially in patients with normo- or hyperkalemia and sinus bradycardia, potassium infusions may worsen bradycardia and conduction block.

—Potassium infusions are most effective for the digitalis-toxic patient with tachyarrhythmias and hypokalemia.

—Other treatments for digitalis-related arrhythmias include phenytoin, lidocaine, procainamide, and propranolol.

—Digitalis toxicity may also cause hyperkalemia, probably a result of inhibition of the Na-K pump by digitalis. Hyperkalemia may be severe enough to cause AV block or asystole.

—Elimination of digitalis is mainly through urinary excretion. Patients with impaired renal function will have prolonged digitalis elimination times.

Digitalis Interactions with Anesthetic Drugs

Digitalis with albuterol

—Acute administration of albuterol either intravenously or orally resulted in a 16% reduction of digoxin concentration within 30 minutes in a number of patients with stable digoxin levels. Additionally, serum potassium concentrations also declined approximately 15% within 10 minutes of the albuterol dose.

Digitalis with bretylium

—Digitalis-induced arrhythmias generally should not be treated with bretylium. This is because bretylium initially releases catecholamines that may potentiate the arrhythmias seen with digitalis toxicity.

Digitalis with calcium gluconate

—Intravenous calcium has been reported to precipitate severe arrhythmias in patients taking digitalis glycosides. If such arrhythmias should occur, lowering of calcium levels may be effective.

Digitalis with calcium chloride

—Intravenous calcium has been reported to precipitate severe arrhythmias in patients taking digitalis glycosides. If such arrhythmias should occur, lowering of calcium levels may be effective.

Digitalis with succinylcholine

—Succinylcholine may precipitate cardiac arrhythmias in digitalized patients.

—Possible explanations of this interaction include the potential of succinylcholine to cause a shift of potassium from the intracellular to extracellular compartments in muscle tissue.

Digitalis with ketamine

—Ketamine may have a protective effect against digitalis-induced arrhythmias by decreasing phase 4 automaticity.

Digitalis with verapamil

—When verapamil is given to patients taking digoxin, toxic digoxin levels may occur. This may be due to several different mechanisms including displacement of digoxin from tissue binding sites.

DIPHENYLHYDANTOIN (Dilantin)

Classification and indications

—Diphenylhydantoin (phenytoin) is an anticonvulsant that also has antiarrhythmic properties.

—It is indicated for the management of seizures and atrial and ventricular tachycardias. It is considered a class IB antiarrhythmic (affecting only phase 4 depolarization).

Pharmacology

—The anticonvulsant property of diphenylhydantoin results mainly from its ability to limit propagation of seizure activity (other agents may work by elevating seizure threshold).

—The antiarrhythmic properties involve a decrease in automaticity as well as a decrease in excitability of Purkinje fibers. Because of this effect, phenytoin is contraindicated in patients with sinus bradycardia, sinoatrial block, as well as patients with second- and third-degree heart block, or with Stokes–Adams syndrome.

—Diphenylhydantoin is particularly effective for the treatment of ventricular arrhythmias caused by digitalis intoxication but is not very useful for atrial arrhythmias.

—Toxicity associated with phenytoin administration includes hypotension, CNS depression, and cardiovascular collapse.

—Therapeutic concentrations for phenytoin are between 7.5 and 20 μg/mL. Intramuscular administration is not recommended due to erratic absorption.

—Following IV administration of 1–1.5 g, therapeutic concentrations are achieved in 1–2 hours.

—The average half-life is about 10–15 hours after intravenous administration and elimination is a result of hepatic metabolism.

Diphenylhydantoin Interactions with Anesthetic Drugs
Diphenylhydantoin with benzodiazepines
(chlordiazepoxide, diazepam, lorazepam, midazolam)

—Benzodiazepines, when given to a patient on chronic diphenylhydantoin therapy, may cause an increased serum level of diphenylhydantoin. This may be due to a decrease in the metabolism of diphenylhydantoin caused by benzodiazepines.

—The half-life of benzodiazepines can be decreased in patients on chronic diphenylhydantoin therapy.

Diphenylhydantoin with muscle relaxants (atracurium, doxacurium, gallamine, metocurine, mivacurium, pancuronium, pipercuronium, rocuronium, tubocurarine, vecuronium)

—Patients on chronic phenytoin therapy may be resistant to non-depolarizing muscle blockade. The studies involved metocurine and vecuronium, but may involve other non-depolarizing agents.

—The mechanism of this interaction is not known.

—Acute infusions of phenytoin may prolong non-depolarizing blockade. This was studied prospectively in a small number of patients who received a 10 mg/kg loading dose of phenytoin during steady-state muscle blockade with vecuronium. They had significant potentiation of their neuromuscular block compared to control patients.

DIPYRIDAMOLE (Persantine)

Classification and indications
—Dipyridamole is a platelet inhibitor.
—It is used mainly as an adjunct to coumarin anticoagulation for patients who have had cardiac valve replacement. Other uses are not proven to be effective, but include:
    —Prevention of thromboembolism for patients with TIA, hip replacement surgery, MI, etc.
    —Chronic angina (dipyridamole has some coronary artery vasodilating properties).

Pharmacology
—Dipyridamole decreases platelet adhesiveness on prosthetic valves, but probably not on biological surfaces.
—The mechanism of this action probably involves increasing serum adenosine levels. This occurs because dipyridamole interferes with adenosine metabolism by inhibiting phosphodiesterase (the enzyme that metabolizes adenosine monophosphate) and by blocking uptake and destruction of adenosine by erythrocytes and other cells.
—Adenosine is a platelet function inhibitor and also causes vasodilation.
—Significant interactions can occur between adenosine (used to control tachyarrhythmias) and dipyridamole.

Dipyridamole Interactions with Anesthetic Drugs
Dipyridamole with adenosine
—Dipyridamole blocks the uptake and metabolism of adenosine by erythrocytes and some other cells. As a result, the dose necessary to produce hemodynamic changes from adenosine may be significantly decreased.
—In one study, pretreatment of patients with dipyridamole decreased the required dose of adenosine by 75–90%.

DISULFIRAM (Antabuse)

Classification and indications
—Disulfiram is a thiuram derivative.
—It is used to treat alcohol dependence by functioning as an alcohol deterrent.

Pharmacology
—Disulfiram treatment results in hypersensitivity to alcohol. Unpleasant and sometimes severe reactions to alcohol occur in patients receiving disulfiram.
—These symptoms include headache, nausea and vomiting, palpitation, anxiety, vertigo, and confusion. Reactions can occur at alcohol levels as low as 5–10 mg/dL.
—The mechanism of action is inhibition of the enzyme aldehyde dehydrogenase, which is responsible for degradation of acetaldehyde to acetic acid (acetaldehyde is a normal product of alcohol metabolism). Accumulation of acetaldehyde is thought to result in the above symptoms.
—Normal elimination of alcohol is otherwise unaffected.
—In some patients, the severity of symptoms form alcohol–disulfiram interactions may be life threatening.

Disulfiram Interactions with Anesthetic Drugs
Disulfiram with inhalational anesthetics (enflurane, desflurane, halothane, isoflurane, sevoflurane)
—Profound hypotension may occur when patients taking disulfiram are exposed to halogenated anesthetics.

DOPAMINE (Intropin)

Classification and indications
—Dopamine is an endogenous catecholamine. It is the immediate precursor of norepinephrine.
—It is indicated for the management of low cardiac output resulting from myocardial infarction or cardiac surgery, for example.

Pharmacology
—Dopamine stimulates beta 1, alpha, and dopaminergic receptors. Also, unlike dobutamine, it causes release of endogenous norepinephrine from storage sites.
—Stimulation of the receptors is partly related to dose. At a dose of 0.5–2 μg/kg/min, there is primarily stimulation of

dopaminergic receptors, producing vasodilation of coronary, renal, mesenteric, and cerebral vasculature.

—At doses of 2–10 μg/kg/min, there is also stimulation of beta 1 receptors resulting in increased myocardial contractility and some vasodilation. At doses above 10 μg/kg/min, alpha adrenergic receptor stimulation causes peripheral vasoconstriction.

—In summary, low or moderate doses cause increased urinary blood flow and variable levels of myocardial stimulation, whereas higher doses increase peripheral resistance by vasoconstriction. The vasoconstriction may affect the renal and mesenteric vasculature, depending on the dose.

—Dopamine may cause tachycardia, ectopy, and hypertension in some patients. Also, patients with depletion of catecholamines (such as chronic congestive heart failure) may not respond as well to dopamine because release of endogenous catecholamines is an important mechanism of its action. In such cases, dobutamine may be more effective.

Dopamine Interactions with Anesthetic Drugs
Dopamine with beta blockers (esmolol, labetalol, propranolol)

—Use of beta blockers for treatment of supraventricular tachycardia may have undesirable effects in some patients; specifically, in patients requiring cardiovascular support with agents that are both inotropic and vasoconstrictive (dopamine, epinephrine, norepinephrine), blockade of beta receptors may result in decreased cardiac contractility in the face of systemic vasoconstriction, resulting in cardiac failure.

Dopamine with diphenylhydantoin

—Several patients have developed profound hypotension after receiving intravenous diphenylhydantoin while on dopamine infusions.

—The mechanism of this interaction is not known, and not all patients will experience this interaction.

ECOTHIOPHATE (Phospholine Iodide)

Classification and indications

—Ecothiophate is a long-acting anticholinesterase.

—It is used to treat glaucoma (both angle closure and open angle forms). It may also be used to diagnose and treat some forms of strabismus.

Pharmacology

—Ecothiophate is an organophosphate anticholinesterase. As a result, it is a parasympathomimetic agent and causes miosis (pupillary constriction).

—It is thought that these drugs, by producing miosis (pupillary constriction), allow greater flow of aqueous humor from the anterior chamber of the eye. This seems to occur in both open angle and angle closure forms.

—Organophosphates are considered irreversible inhibitors of acetylcholinesterase (except by pralidoxime, an acetylcholinesterase reactivator). As long as 2 weeks may be required to achieve adequate pseudocholinesterase levels after treatment has been stopped.

—The anticholinesterases used to reverse neuromuscular blockers are shorter acting, competitive inhibitors of acetylcholinesterase.

—Since these drugs are nonspecific anticholinesterases, they inhibit not only acetylcholinesterase but plasma pseudocholinesterase as well. This may result in prolonged blockade from succinylcholine.

Ecothiophate Interactions with Anesthetic Drugs
Ecothiophate with procaine

—Ecothiophate, an antagonist of plasma pseudocholinesterase, may interact with procaine to cause procaine toxicity.

—Because procaine depends on pseudocholinesterase for its metabolism, reduced activity of this enzyme could lead to toxicity. Although patients with inherited deficiencies of plasma cholinesterase have been reported to experience severe toxicity with procaine, there is no documentation of this reaction with ecothiophate.

Ecothiophate with succinylcholine

—The nonspecific anticholinesterase miotics (ecothiophate, demacarium bromide, isoflurophate) used in treatment of glaucoma can result in significant depression of plasma pseudocholinesterase levels.

—Prolonged neuromuscular blockade can occur with succinylcholine in these patients. A period of 2–4 weeks may be necessary to restore plasma cholinesterase levels after discontinuing the anticholinesterase miotics.

ERGOT ALKALOIDS

Classification and indications

—Ergot alkaloids are a group of compounds derived from a fungus (*Claviceps purpurea*). The clinically useful alkaloids that have significant interactions with anesthetic agents are ergotamine, dihydroergotamine, ergonovine, and methylergonovine.

—These agents are used mainly either for obstetrics (ergonovine, methylergonovine) or for treatment of migraine (ergotamine, dihydroergotamine).

Pharmacology

—The pharmacology of the ergot alkaloids is complex, but the significant interactions with agents used during anesthesia are related to the cardiovascular effects of the ergot alkaloids.

—Peripheral vasoconstriction results from stimulation of alpha adrenergic receptors and blockade of the reuptake of norepinephrine.

—Vasoconstriction of the dilated carotid artery vascular bed (thought to be the cause of migraine headaches) occurs with therapeutic doses of ergotamine and dihydroergotamine.

—To be most effective in the treatment of migraines, these agents should be administered in the early, prodromal stages (when vascular dilation begins).

—Methysergide is also an ergot alkaloid used for migraine, but its mechanism of action is related to its antiserotonin activity. It has little vasoconstrictive action.

—Ergonovine and methylergonovine are both potent stimulators of uterine contractions. They also can produce vasoconstriction of both arteries and veins.

—Significant interactions can occur between the vasoactive ergot alkaloids (ergotamine, dihydroergotamine, ergonovine, methylergonovine) and vasoactive agents, the result of which may be severe hypertension.

Dihydroergotamine (DHE 45)

Classification and indications

—Dihydroergotamine is an ergot alkaloid.

—It is indicated for the treatment of migraine headaches. It is used parenterally.

Ergonovine (Ergotrate Maleate)

Classification and indications

—Ergonovine is an ergot alkaloid

—It is used in obstetrics to treat or prevent hemorrhage either postpartum or postabortion.

Pharmacology

—Both ergonovine and methylergonovine directly stimulate contractions of uterine muscle. For this reason, they are useful in controlling bleeding from a hypotonic uterus postpartum or postabortion.

Ergotamine Tartrate (Bellergal, Cafergot, Ercaf, Ergo-Caff, Ergostat, Lanatrate, Medihaler Ergotamine, Migergot, Phenerbel, Wigraine)

Classification and indications

—Ergotamine is an ergot alkaloid.

—It is indicated for the treatment of migraine headaches.

Methylergonovine (Methergine)

Classification and indications

—Methylergonovine is an ergot alkaloid.

—It is used in obstetrics to treat or prevent hemorrhage either postpartum or postabortion.

Pharmacology

—Both ergonovine and methylergonovine directly stimulate contractions of uterine muscle. For this reason, they are useful in controlling bleeding from a hypotonic uterus postpartum or postabortion.

Ergot Alkaloids Interactions with Anesthetic Drugs

Ergot alkaloids with dopamine

—A case report of gangrene of the extremities was reported in a patient who received infusions intravenously of both dopamine and ergonovine.

—The proposed mechanism of this interaction is that the vasoconstrictive properties of these medications can be additive.

—Although the other ergot alkaloids have not specifically been identified as interacting in such a way with dopamine, it is reasonable to use caution with this combination.

Ergot alkaloids with vasopressors (ephedrine, epinephrine, metaraminol, methoxamine, norepinephrine, phenylephrine)

—Ergot alkaloids may interact with vasopressors to produce hypertension that is more likely to be severe in patients with a predisposition to hypertension.

—Because of possibly additive vasoconstrictive effects, the administration of vasopressors to patients receiving ergot alkaloids may produce unexpected degrees of hypertension.

ERYTHROMYCIN (E-Mycin, EES, ERYC, Ery-Tab, EryPed, Eryzole, Ilosone, Ilotycin, PCE Dispertab, Pediazole, Sulfimycin, Wyamycin)

Classification and indications

—The erythromycins are macrolide antibiotics produced by *Streptomyces erythreus.*

—They are use to treat susceptible strains of gram-positive cocci (*Staphylococcus, Streptococcus*), gram-positive bacilli (*Corynebacterium, Clostridium, Listeria,* etc.), some gram-negative cocci (*Neisseria)*, and some gram-negative bacilli (*Haemophilus, Legionella, Pasteurella,* etc.).

Pharmacology

—Erythromycins include different forms of the antibiotic including e. estolate, e. ethylsuccinate, e. gluceptate, and e. lactobionate.

—They are usually bacteriostatic and function by interfering with protein synthesis.

—Significant interactions have been reported in patients receiving erythromycin who are given alfentanil or midazolam.

Erythromycin Interactions with Anesthetic Drugs
Erythromycin with alfentanil

—Patients who are receiving erythromycin may demonstrate prolonged, unexpected respiratory depression following alfentanil. Single doses of erythromycin do not appear to have this with alfentanil.

—The proposed mechanism of this interaction is that several doses of erythromycin are necessary to produce a metabolite that delays alfentanil metabolism.

Erythromycin with midazolam

—Erythromycin may potentiate and prolong the effects of midazolam. This effect has been documented in both a controlled study and a case report of orally administered midazolam. The interaction can apparently occur with both oral and intravenous erythromycin and, in the case report, the intravenous erythromycin altered midazolam pharmacokinetics even when given shortly following the midazolam.

—Erythromycin may alter midazolam metabolism by interfering with the cytochrome P450 isoenzyme that affects midazolam metabolism.

ETHACRYNIC ACID (Edecrin)

Classification and indications

—Ethacrynic acid is a loop diuretic (as is furosemide).

—It is indicated for the treatment of edema resulting from different causes including congestive heart failure, hepatic disease, and renal dysfunction. It is also used to treat hypertension.

Pharmacology

—Ethacrynic acid, like other loop diuretics, functions by blocking reabsorption of sodium and chloride ions in the ascending limb of the loop of Henle. This results in an osmotic diuresis from the increased solute load (unabsorbed ions). Also, by decreasing ion reabsorption, the concentration of medullary interstitial fluid decreases and therefore promotes diuresis.

—The result of interference with ion reabsorption is loss of sodium, potassium, chloride, and hydrogen ions (as well as others). Patients on chronic therapy or those who are receiving very large doses usually require some replacement of these ions.

—Tinnitus and permanent or reversible hearing loss have been associated with rapid IV administration of ethacrynic acid. Coadministration of aminoglycoside antibiotics may increase ototoxicity.

Ethacrynic Acid Interactions with Anesthetic Drugs
Ethacrynic acid with enalapril

—Angiotensin-converting enzyme (ACE) inhibitors used to treat hypertension in a patient who is being diuresed with the loop diuretics may produce a profound drop in blood pressure. This response has been seen as early as 2–3 hours after initiation of ACE inhibitors.

—The mechanisms of this interaction may include hypovolemia from diuretic therapy or, in some patients, high levels of renin and angiotensin.

—The setting in which this interaction may be significant for anesthesiologists might be a hypertensive patient who presents for urgent surgery while receiving intensive diuretic treatment for cardiac decompensation. Use of ACE inhibitor therapy in the perioperative setting may precipitate the interaction described.

FLECAINIDE (Tambocor)

Classification and indications

—Flecainide acetate is an antiarrhythmic agent structurally related to procainamide and encainide. It is considered a class IC antiarrhythmic along with encainide and propafenone.

—Because of its potential toxicity, it is indicated only for oral treatment or prevention of life-threatening ventricular arrhythmias that are not responsive to other medications.

Pharmacology

—Class 1C antiarrhythmic agents bind to the fast sodium channels and are the most potent agents for suppressing ventricular premature impulses and decreasing conduction, particularly in the His-Purkinje system.

—Flecainide has significant arrhythmogenic properties and can worsen existing arrhythmias or produce new ones. For this reason, it is reserved for prevention or treatment of only life-threatening ventricular arrhythmias.

—Because flecainide can significantly decrease myocardial contractility, agents with similar effects (beta blockers and some calcium channel blockers) may potentiate this effect.

—Although encainide and propafenone are also class IC antiarrhythmics, they have not been demonstrated to have significant interactions with beta blockers or calcium channel blockers.

Flecainide Interactions with Anesthetic Drugs
Flecainide with beta blockers and calcium channel blockers *

—Flecainide can cause decreased myocardial contractility, particularly at the onset of intravenous therapy. Patients most significantly affected are those with compromised left ventricular function (ejection fraction less than 30%).

—Beta blockers and some calcium channel blockers may have added negative inotropic effects with flecainide.

—Verapamil has more negative inotropic effect than diltiazem, nicardipine, or nifedipine.

FUROSEMIDE (Lasix)

Classification and indications

—Furosemide is a loop diuretic.

—It is indicated for the treatment of edema resulting from different causes including congestive heart failure, hepatic disease, and renal dysfunction. It is also used to treat hypertension.

Pharmacology

—Furosemide, like other loop diuretics, functions by blocking reabsorption of sodium and chloride ions in the ascending

---

* Beta blockers (esmolol, labetalol, propranolol)
Calcium channel blockers (diltiazem, nicardipine, nifedipine, verapamil)

limb of the loop of Henle. This results in an osmotic diuresis from the increased solute load (unabsorbed ions). Also, by decreasing ion reabsorption, the concentration of medullary interstitial fluid decreases and therefore promotes diuresis.

—The result of interference with ion reabsorption is loss of sodium, potassium, chloride, and hydrogen ions (as well as others). Patients on chronic therapy or who are receiving very large doses usually require some replacement of these ions.

—Furosemide decreases both renal and peripheral vascular resistance as well as increasing venous capacitance. This results in increased renal blood flow, decreased venous return to the heart, and decreased blood pressure.

—In patients with chronic renal insufficiency, large doses may increase glomerular filtration rate temporarily.

—Tinnitus and permanent or reversible hearing loss have been associated with rapid IV or IM administration of furosemide, usually with doses much greater than 20–40 mg. Also, coadministration of furosemide and aminoglycoside antibiotics may increase ototoxicity.

Furosemide Interactions with Anesthetic Drugs
Furosemide with enalapril

—Angiotensin-converting enzyme (ACE) inhibitors used to treat hypertension in a patient who is being diuresed with the loop diuretics may produce a profound drop in blood pressure. This response has been seen as early as 2–3 hours after initiation of ACE inhibitors.

—The mechanisms of this interaction may include hypovolemia from diuretic therapy or, in some patients, high levels of renin and angiotensin.

—The setting in which this interaction may be significant for anesthesiologists might be a hypertensive patient who presents for urgent surgery while receiving intensive diuretic treatment for cardiac decompensation. Use of ACE inhibitor therapy in the perioperative setting may precipitate the interaction described.

GUANADREL (Hylorel)

Classification and indications

—Guanadrel and guanethidine are postganglionic blocking agents.

—They are used to treat hypertension.

Pharmacology

—Guanadrel and guanethidine cause depletion of cate-cholamines from sympathetic nerve endings. As a result, sympathetic nervous stimulation that would normally cause vasoconstriction is blocked.

—Because of catecholamine depletion and reduced end-organ stimulation, there is greater sensitivity than normal to direct-acting amines (phenylephrine, epinephrine, dobutamine).

—Indirect-acting amines (metaraminol, mephentermine, ephed-rine) may have less response than expected. Dopamine has both direct and indirect actions and should be used cautiously.

Guanadrel Interactions with Anesthetic Drugs

Guanadrel with vasopressors (dobutamine, dopamine, ephedrine, epinephrine, metaraminol, methoxamine, norepinephrine, phenylephrine)

—Patients receiving guanethidine and guanadrel can have an exaggerated hypertensive response to norepinephrine and other direct-acting catecholamines such as phenylephrine, dobutamine, and epinephrine.

—Indirect-acting catecholamines, such as ephedrine, metaram-inol, mephentermine, and dopamine, may have fewer pressor effects than expected.

—Guanethidine and guanadrel deplete intraneuronal norepi-nephrine in postganglionic sympathetic neurons and in this way may diminish the response of indirect-acting cate-cholamines while sensitizing adrenergic receptors to direct-acting amines.

GUANETHIDINE (Esimil, Ismelin)

Classification and indications

—Guanadrel and guanethidine are postganglionic blocking agents.

—They are used to treat hypertension.

Pharmacology

—Guanadrel and guanethidine cause depletion of cate-cholamines from sympathetic nerve endings. As a result, sympathetic nervous stimulation that would normally cause vasoconstriction is blocked.

—Because of catecholamine depletion and reduced end-organ stimulation, there is greater sensitivity than normal to direct-acting amines (phenylephrine, epinephrine, dobutamine).

—Indirect-acting amines (metaraminol, mephentermine, ephedrine) may have less response than expected. Dopamine has both direct and indirect actions and should be used cautiously.

Guanethidine Interactions with Anesthetic Drugs
Guanethidine with chlorpromazine
—Chlorpromazine can reverse the antihypertensive effects of guanethidine if given in doses larger than 100 mg/day.
Guanethidine with vasopressors (dobutamine, dopamine, ephedrine, epinephrine, metaraminol, methoxamine, norepinephrine, phenylephrine)
—Patients receiving guanethidine and guanadrel can have an exaggerated hypertensive response to norepinephrine and other direct-acting catecholamines such as phenylephrine, dobutamine, and epinephrine.
—Indirect-acting catecholamines, such as ephedrine, metaraminol, mephentermine, and dopamine may have less pressor effects than expected.
—Guanethidine and guanadrel deplete intraneuronal norepinephrine in postganglionic sympathetic neurons and in this way may diminish the response of indirect acting catecholamines, while sensitizing adrenergic receptors to direct-acting amines.

IFOSFAMIDE (Ifex)

Classification and indications
—Ifosfamide is an alkylating agent. It is one of the nitrogen mustards.
—It is used to treat leukemias, lymphomas, and other malignancies.
Pharmacology
—Alkylating agents form bonds with nucleic acids (DNA and RNA). As a result, growth of rapidly proliferating cells is disrupted.
—Adverse reactions to chlorambucil include nausea and vomiting, alopecia, and leukopenia.
—Hemorrhagic cystitis can be a serious adverse reaction to ifosfamide.
—Interstitial pulmonary fibrosis has occurred in patients receiving alkylating agents.

—Plasma pseudocholinesterase levels may be depressed in some patients receiving this medication. As a result, prolonged blockade from succinylcholine may occur.

Ifosfamide Interactions with Anesthetic Drugs
Ifosfamide with succinylcholine
—Some patients receiving the drug, ifosfamide, may have depressed levels of plasma pseudocholinesterase. In some cases, the result may be delayed metabolism of succinylcholine and a prolonged neuromuscular blockade.

ISOFLUROPHATE (Floropryl)

Classification and indications
—Isoflurophate is a long-acting anticholinesterase.
—It is used to treat glaucoma (both angle closure and open angle forms). It may also be used to diagnose and treat some forms of strabismus.

Pharmacology
—The miotic (pupillary constriction) drugs are parasympathomimetic agents with different mechanisms of action.
—Direct-acting agents are drugs like acetylcholine. Indirect-acting drugs inhibit acetylcholinesterase either reversibly (physostigmine, demecarium) or irreversibly (the organophosphates echothiophate, isoflurophate).
—The anticholinesterases used to reverse neuromuscular blockers are shorter acting, competitive inhibitors of acetylcholinesterase.
—It is thought that these drugs, by producing miosis (pupillary constriction), allow greater flow of aqueous humor from the anterior chamber of the eye. This seems to occur in both open angle and angle closure forms.
—Because these drugs are nonspecific anticholinesterases, they inhibit not only acetylcholinesterase, but plasma pseudocholinesterase as well. This may result in prolonged blockade from succinylcholine.
—Because it is rapidly hydrolyzed in the serum, isoflurophate usually reduces serum cholinesterases only slightly. However, it is an irreversible inhibitor of acetylcholinesterase and up to 2 weeks are required for cholinesterase levels to return to normal.

Isoflurophate Interactions with Anesthetic Drugs
Isoflurophate with succinylcholine
—The nonspecific anticholinesterase miotics (ecothiophate, demacarium bromide, isoflurophate) used in treatment of glaucoma can result in significant depression of plasma pseudocholinesterase levels.
—Prolonged neuromuscular blockade can occur with succinylcholine in these patients. A period of 2–4 weeks may be necessary to restore plasma cholinesterase levels after discontinuing the anticholinesterase miotics.

ISONIAZID (Laniazid, Nydrazid, Rifamate, Rimactane, Tubizid)

Classification and indications
—Isoniazid is an antituberculosis agent.
—It is used to treat tuberculosis and some other mycobacterial diseases.

Pharmacology
—The exact mechanism of action of isoniazid is not known, but it appears to be bacteriostatic or bactericidal to mycobacteria by interfering with cell-wall synthesis and protein metabolism.
—When used to treat tuberculosis, it is used with at least one other agent. If used as prophylaxis, it can be used alone.
—Isoniazid can affect metabolism of enflurane, resulting in higher fluoride levels. In some cases, this may result in nephrotoxic levels of fluoride. The mechanism of this interaction is not known.

Isoniazid Interactions with Anesthetic Drugs
Isoniazid with enflurane
—Normally, fluoride levels with enflurane use remain well below nephrotoxic levels. In patients taking isoniazid, however, fluoride levels may reach nephrotoxic levels.

LEVODOPA (Dopar, Larodopa, Sinemet)

Classification and indications
—Levodopa is a metabolic precursor of dopamine.
—It is used to treat Parkinson's disease.

Pharmacology

—Levodopa and the decarboxylase inhibitor, carbidopa, are believed to function by increasing dopamine concentrations in the basal ganglia of the brain. It is thought that depletion of dopamine is the etiology of Parkinsonism.

—Levodopa, unlike dopamine, is able to cross the blood–brain barrier where it may be converted to dopamine by the enzyme dopa decarboxylase.

—Carbidopa inhibits peripheral decarboxylation of levodopa (which otherwise occurs rapidly and reduces the amount available to enter the CNS).

—Butyrophenones (droperidol) block the dopaminergic effects of dopamine and can antagonize levodopa and carbidopa.

Levodopa Interactions with Anesthetic Drugs

Levodopa with droperidol

—Levodopa is used to treat patients with Parkinson's disease. Droperidol and phenothiazines antagonize the effects of dopamine in the basal ganglia. Patients with Parkinson's disease who receive the dopamine precursor levodopa may be adversely affected by administration of these drugs.

LIDOCAINE (LidoPen, Xylocaine)

Classification and indications

—Lidocaine is a local anesthetic and a class IB antiarrhythmic agent.

—It is indicated for treatment of ventricular arrhythmias. It is also indicated for use as a local anesthetic for infiltration, nerve block, spinal, epidural, and caudal anesthesia.

Pharmacology

—Like all local anesthetics, lidocaine prevents the generation and conduction of nerve impulses by blocking the normal increase in sodium permeability that accompanies depolarization of nerve axons.

—The antiarrhythmic activity of lidocaine is a result of interference with phase 4 depolarization, like all class IB drugs (lidocaine, tocainide, phenytoin, mexilitene). Class IA drugs are local anesthetics that interfere with phase 0 and phase 4 depolarization (quinidine, procainamide, disopyramide).

—Onset of activity after intravenous administration of 50–100 mg is within 45–90 seconds and has a duration of 10–20 minutes. Loading doses are required to achieve therapeutic levels rapidly.

—Lidocaine can potentiate the action of non-depolarizing muscle relaxants.

Lidocaine Interactions with Anesthetic Drugs

Lidocaine with muscle relaxants (atracurium, doxacurium, gallamine, metocurine, mivacurium, pancuronium, pipercuronium, rocuronium, succinylcholine, tubocurarine, vecuronium)

—Most local anesthetics can block neuromuscular transmission from non-depolarizing agents as well as depolarizing muscle relaxants. Of clinical significance to the anesthesiologist, lidocaine, given as a 50- to 100-mg bolus or even by infusion, can significantly increase a nondepolarizer block or a phase II block from succinylcholine.

LINCOMYCIN (Lincocin)

Classification and indications

—Lincomycin is an antibiotic derived from *Streptomyces lincolnensis.*

—It is used to treat infections with gram-positive cocci (*Staphylococcus, Streptococcus*). It is not considered a first-line drug but is used as an alternative to less toxic medications.

Pharmacology

—Lincomycin functions like several other antibiotics (clindamycin, erythromycin, and others) by interfering with bacterial protein synthesis.

—It can be administered IV, IM, or PO and is bacteriostatic or bactericidal depending on the concentration achieved.

—A number of antibiotics have neuromuscular blocking properties, including lincomycin. As a result, these antibiotics can potentiate neuromuscular blockers. Although some agents potentiate both succinylcholine and non-depolarizing agents, lincomycin, like most antibiotics, affects non-depolarizing agents.

Lincomycin Interactions with Anesthetic Drugs
Lincomycin with muscle relaxants (atracurium, doxacurium, gallamine, metocurine, mivacurium, pancuronium, pipercuronium, rocuronium, succinylcholine, tubocurarine, vecuronium)

—A number of antibiotics have significant interactions with neuromuscular blocking agents. These include the aminoglycosides (amikacin, gentamicin, kanamycin, neomycin, paromomycin, netilmicin, neomycin, streptomycin, tobramycin), as well as polymyxin B, colistin, amphotericin B, clindamycin, bacitracin, and lincomycin.

—All of the above antibiotics may potentiate non-depolarizing agents, but some (aminoglycosides, amphotericin B, clindamycin, colistin) can also potentiate succinylcholine blockade.

—These antibiotics potentiate neuromuscular blockade by different mechanisms, making management of these problems difficult. Although treatment with anticholinesterases or calcium has been recommended, results are inconsistent.

LITHIUM (Cibalith-S, Eskalith, Lithane, Lithobid, Lithonate, Lithotabs)

Classification and indications
—Lithium is an antimanic agent.

—It is used to treat psychiatric disorders such as bipolar (a mixture of mania and depression) and unipolar (major depression) disorders, as well as schizophrenia, impulsivity, and alcohol dependence. It has also been used to treat myelosuppression from chemotherapy.

Pharmacology
—The mechanism of action of lithium is not completely understood. It appears to affect neurotransmitter (such as serotonin) function in the brain, which is felt to be important in the pathogenesis of mania and depression.

—Lithium may have significant interactions with some muscle relaxants. Though there is controversy about the clinical significance, it seems that lithium may prolong the neuromuscular blockade from succinylcholine and some non-depolarizing agents (pancuronium).

Lithium Interactions with Anesthetic Drugs

Lithium with muscle relaxants (atracurium, doxacurium, gallamine, metocurine, mivacurium, pancuronium, pipercuronium, rocuronium, succinylcholine, tubocurarine, vecuronium)

—Lithium has been reported to increase the duration of both non-depolarizing and depolarizing neuromuscular blocking drugs.

—The mechanism of this interaction is unknown and the clinical significance of this interaction is uncertain.

MAGNESIUM SULFATE

Classification and indications

—Magnesium sulfate, when administered parenterally, is an anticonvulsant.

—It is used mainly in the prevention or treatment of seizures during severe eclampsia.

Pharmacology

—Magnesium sulfate, at serum magnesium concentrations of >2.5 meq/L, is a CNS depressant. Although the precise mechanism of action is not clear, this CNS depression is thought to be the basis for its anticonvulsant properties.

—Interference with neuromuscular transmission by magnesium is due to:

  —Decreased acetylcholine released by motor nerve endings.

  —Decreased depolarization of the motor endplate.

  —Decreased excitability of the muscle membrane.

—As a result, patients receiving magnesium sulfate are more sensitive to muscle blockade from both non-depolarizing and depolarizing agents.

—At serum levels of >4 meq/L, deep tendon reflexes (DTRs) diminish. Respiratory paralysis and loss of DTRs may occur at serum magnesium levels of 10 meq/L.

—Symptomatic muscle weakness can be partially reversed with intravenous calcium.

Magnesium Sulfate Interactions with Anesthetic Drugs

Magnesium sulfate with muscle relaxants (atracurium, doxacurium, gallamine, metocurine, mivacurium, pancuronium, pipercuronium, rocuronium, succinylcholine, tubocurarine, vecuronium)

—Neuromuscular blockade produced by both depolarizing and non-depolarizing agents can be potentiated in patients receiving magnesium sulfate. The mechanisms involved include a decreased amount of acetylcholine released by the nerve impulse at the motor nerve terminal and a decrease in the depolarizing action of acetylcholine on the muscle.

Magnesium sulfate with calcium channel blockers (diltiazem, nicardipine, nifedipine, verapamil)

—Magnesium potentiates the effect of calcium channel blockers and the combination may result in profound hypotension.

Magnesium sulfate with calcium chloride, calcium gluconate

—Calcium opposes the neuromuscular depressant effects of magnesium sulfate at the neuromuscular junction.

MECHLORETHAMINE (Mustargen)

Classification and indications

—Mechlorethamine is an alkylating agent. It is one of the nitrogen mustards.

—It is used to treat leukemias, lymphomas, and other malignancies.

Pharmacology

—Alkylating agents form bonds with nucleic acids (DNA and RNA). As a result, growth of rapidly proliferating cells is disrupted.

—Adverse reactions to chlorambucil include nausea and vomiting, alopecia, and leukopenia.

—Interstitial pulmonary fibrosis has occurred in patients receiving alkylating agents.

—Plasma pseudocholinesterase levels may be depressed in some patients receiving this medication. As a result, prolonged blockade from succinylcholine may occur.

Mechlorethamine Interactions with Anesthetic Drugs

Mechlorethamine with succinylcholine

—Some patients receiving mechlorethamine may have depressed levels of plasma pseudocholinesterase. In some cases, the result may be delayed metabolism of succinylcholine and a prolonged neuromuscular blockade.

MELPHALAN (Alkeran)

Classification and indications

—Melphalan is an alkylating agent. It is one of the nitrogen mustards.

—It is used to treat malignancies of the breast and ovary as well as other cancers.

Pharmacology

—Alkylating agents form bonds with nucleic acids (DNA and RNA). As a result, growth of rapidly proliferating cells is disrupted.

—Adverse reactions to chlorambucil include nausea and vomiting, and leukopenia.

—Interstitial pulmonary fibrosis has occurred in patients receiving alkylating agents.

—Plasma pseudocholinesterase levels may be depressed in some patients receiving this medication. As a result, prolonged blockade from succinylcholine may occur.

Melphalan Interactions with Anesthetic Drugs
Melphalan with succinylcholine

—Some patients receiving melphalan may have depressed levels of plasma pseudocholinesterase. In some cases, the result may be delayed metabolism of succinylcholine and a prolonged neuromuscular blockade.

MEPERIDINE (Demerol)

Classification and indications

—Meperidine is a synthetic opiate (phenylpiperidine derivative).

—It is used in anesthesia for preoperative sedation, as part of a general anesthetic, and for postoperative analgesia or control of shivering.

Pharmacology

—Meperidine, like other narcotics, exerts its analgesic effects through opioid receptors in the CNS (brain and spinal cord).

—Although narcotics used in anesthesia are potent analgesics, there is controversy about the level of amnesia induced with even large doses of narcotics. To avoid awareness during anesthesia, use of other anesthetic agents (benzodiazepines, inhalation agents, etc.) are recommended.

—Somatosensory evoked potentials (SEPs) are not significantly affected by narcotics.

—Although there is some controversy about increases in intracranial pressure from opioids, in general, opioids cause slight decreases in cerebral blood flow, metabolic rate, and intracranial pressure.

—Cardiovascular effects of meperidine include hypotension with anesthetic doses (resulting from histamine release) and tachycardia (probably related to structural similarity to atropine).

—Like other narcotics, meperidine causes respiratory depression and reduced hypoxic ventilatory drive.

—Muscle rigidity, particularly of the chest wall, has been associated with rapid administration of narcotics. The mechanism of this action is not clear, but older patients seem more prone to this response. It has also been associated most frequently with alfentanil.

—Muscle rigidity can occur not only during induction but also on emergence from anesthesia or, rarely, hours after the last opioid dose.

—Peak analgesia following parenteral meperidine occurs within 1 hour and lasts for 2–4 hours.

—Elimination depends mainly on hepatic metabolism with some renal excretion. Patients with hepatic or renal dysfunction may have drug accumulation after repeated high doses of meperidine.

Meperidine Interactions with Anesthetic Drugs
Meperidine with naloxone

—Cases of pulmonary edema, hypertension, and ventricular arrhythmias have occurred in postoperative patients receiving naloxone for reversal of respiratory depression induced by narcotics. The precise etiology of these reactions is not known.

—A patient who receives multiple doses of meperidine over a prolonged period will accumulate a metabolite called normeperidine, which is a CNS stimulant with few analgesic qualities.

—When naloxone is used in such patients, the result of reversing the primarily CNS depressant effect of meperidine may be seizure activity.

METHADONE (Dolophine, Methadose)

Classification and indications

—Methadone is a synthetic opioid.

—Its main use is as a replacement for heroin or other narcotics in patients who are drug-dependent. It may also be used as an analgesic for treatment of severe or chronic pain.

Pharmacology
—Methadone has similar actions to those of morphine (analgesia, respiratory depression, sedation). However, it may cause less euphoria and withdrawal from methadone is associated with a slower onset, longer course, and milder withdrawal symptoms than other narcotics.

—The duration of action is increased with repeated administration and a single oral dose may have a duration of 24–48 hours in patients who are physically dependent on methadone.

—Detoxification of narcotic addiction is accomplished with oral methadone during withdrawal stages. This may require up to 180 days.

—Patients who require longer than 180 days for detoxification are considered to be on a maintenance regimen. Such patients may receive oral methadone daily for prolonged periods.

—For treatment of narcotic addiction, methadone is administered orally. For management of severe or chronic pain, it may also be administered intramuscularly or subcutaneously.

—Administration of naloxone or butorphanol to patients receiving methadone can precipitate withdrawal symptoms.

Methadone Interactions with Anesthetic Drugs
Methadone with buprenorphine, butorphanol, nalbuphine
—Patients who are physically dependent on methadone or other narcotics may experience withdrawal symptoms when given a narcotic with agonist/antagonist properties. This includes buprenorphine, butorphanol, and nalbuphine.

Methadone with naloxone
—Naloxone reverses the respiratory depression as well as the analgesic effects of narcotics, including methadone. In patients who are receiving methadone for treatment of narcotic addiction, naloxone can precipitate withdrawal symptoms.

METHYLDOPA (Aldomet)

Classification and indications
—Methyldopa is an antihypertensive agent.
—It is used to treat hypertension.

Pharmacology
—Methyldopa has a number of known effects on the central nervous and cardiovascular systems, but the precise mechanism of its antihypertensive effect is not clear.

—Methyldopa is metabolized to alpha-methylnorepinephrine in the CNS where this metabolite stimulates central alpha adrenergic receptors. Stimulation of these central alpha receptors (as opposed to peripheral alpha receptors) causes a decrease in blood pressure.

—Other mechanisms of action may include false neurotransmission and reduced plasma renin activity.

—A report of a patient receiving methyldopa described a hypertensive response to propranolol. The mechanism of this interaction is not clear.

Methyldopa Interactions with Anesthetic Drugs
Methyldopa with beta blockers (esmolol, labetalol, propranolol)

—Patients taking methyldopa for hypertension may experience a hypertensive response when given beta blockers. This has been reported in a patient on methyldopa who was given a slow intravenous injection of propranolol.

—The mechanism for this response is thought to be related to the accumulation of methylnorepinephrine, which is a result of methyldopa therapy. This substance has both vasoconstricting and vasodilating properties. The latter, when blocked by beta blockers, could leave unopposed vasoconstriction, resulting in hypertension.

MEXILITENE (Mexitil)

Classification and indications

—Mexilitene is a local anesthetic that, like lidocaine, is a class IB antiarrhythmic agent.

—It is used to treat ventricular arrhythmias.

Pharmacology

—Like lidocaine, mexilitene prevents the generation and conduction of nerve impulses by blocking the normal increase in sodium permeability that accompanies depolarization of nerve axons.

—The antiarrhythmic activity of mexilitene is a result of interference with phase 4 depolarization, like all class IB drugs (lidocaine, tocainide, phenytoin, encainide). Class IA drugs are local anesthetics that interfere with phase 0 and phase 4 depolarization (quinidine, procainamide, flecainide).

—Unlike lidocaine, mexilitene is available as an oral preparation.

Mexilitene Interactions with Anesthetic Drugs
Mexilitene with muscle relaxants (atracurium, doxacurium, gallamine, metocurine, mivacurium, pancuronium, pipercuronium, rocuronium, succinylcholine, tubocurarine, vecuronium)
—Mexilitene, like lidocaine and most local anesthetics, can potentiate neuromuscular blockade from depolarizing and non-depolarizing agents.

MONOAMINE OXIDASE INHIBITORS

Classification and indications
—This is a group of medications that are antidepressants.
—They are used to treat depression that is not responsive to tricyclic antidepressants.

Pharmacology
—Monoamine oxidase (MAO) is an enzyme that inactivates several amines (epinephrine, norepinephrine, dopamine, serotonin). It is widely distributed in the body (nerve endings, intestine, liver, stomach, brain).
—MAO inhibitors, by inactivating this enzyme, cause an accumulation of endogenous amines. This is believed to be the mechanism of antidepressant activity.
—In addition to the endogenous amines listed above, exogenous amines like tyrosine or those found in cold medications are normally inactivated by monoamine oxidases in the gastrointestinal tract.
—When these MAOs are inactivated by MAO inhibitors, the exogenous amines can be absorbed and are then taken up by nerve endings where they displace norepinephrine and cause a potentially severe hypertensive response (the tyramine or "cheese" reaction).
—There are two forms of monoamine oxidase (A and B) that apparently have different affinities for different amines and different tissue distributions. MAO A is found mainly in the GI tract and MAO B is found mainly in the brain.
—Isocarboxazid and phenelzine are irreversible inhibitors of monoamine oxidase and tranylcypromine binds reversibly to the enzyme.
—Significant interactions with MAO inhibitors occur with meperidine (severe hypertension, rigidity, excitation), amines such as ephedrine, dopamine, etc. (hypertension), and general anesthetics (potentiated sedation).

Isocarboxazid (Marplan)
Classification and indications
—Isocarboxazid is a monoamine oxidase (MAO) inhibitor.
—It is used to treat depression that is not responsive to tricyclic antidepressants.

Phenelzine (Nardil)
Classification and indications
—Phenelzine is a monoamine oxidase (MAO) inhibitor.
—It is used to treat depression that is not responsive to tricyclic antidepressants.

Selegilene (Eldepryl)
Classification and indications
—Selegiline is a monamine oxidase (MAO) inhibitor.
—Unlike the other MAO inhibitors, which are mainly used for treatment of depression, selegiline is indicated for treatment of Parkinson's disease (it is not used alone, but with other agents).

Tranylcypromine (Parnate)
Classification and indications
—Tranylcypromine is a monoamine oxidase (MAO) inhibitor.
—It is used to treat depression that is not responsive to tricyclic antidepressants.

Monoamine Oxidase Inhibitors Interactions with Anesthetic Drugs
Monoamine oxidase inhibitors with barbiturates (methohexital, sodium pentothal)
—Barbiturates given to a patient receiving monoamine oxidase inhibitors may have a prolonged effect resulting in delayed awakening.

Monoamine oxidase inhibitors with doxapram HCl
—Doxapram, a CNS stimulant, can also produce tachycardia and hypertension. When used in patients taking monoamine oxidase inhibitors, exaggerated hypertension and arrhythmias can occur.

Monoamine oxidase inhibitors with meperidine
—A syndrome of CNS excitation, hyperpyrexia, and seizures may occur when meperidine is administered to a patient taking monoamine oxidase (MAO) inhibitors. The mechanism of this interaction is not clearly understood. Meperidine should be avoided in any patient receiving MAO inhibitors and morphine or other narcotics should be used instead.

—Alternatively, potentiation of the narcotic effect can occur, resulting in respiratory depression or even coma.

Monoamine oxidase inhibitors with succinylcholine

—Phenelzine, but not other monoamine oxidase inhibitors, has been associated with prolonged neuromuscular blockade from succinylcholine.

—The mechanism for this interaction is reportedly from phenelzine's ability to decrease plasma pseudocholinesterase.

Monoamine oxidase inhibitors with vasopressors (dobutamine, dopamine, ephedrine, epinephrine, metaraminol, methoxamine, norepinephrine, phenylephrine)

—Indirect-acting vasopressors (ephedrine, mephentermine, and metaraminol) act by releasing intraneuronal monoamines such as dopamine and norepinephrine. This is the explanation of the hypertensive crises seen when patients receiving monamine oxidase (MAO) inhibitors are given these vasopressors.

—Direct-acting vasopressors such as phenylephrine, epinephrine, norepinephrine, and dobutamine may be potentiated by MAO inhibitors and should be used in smaller amounts than normally used.

—Dopamine has both direct and indirect actions and must be used with caution (perhaps one-tenth of the normal dose).

MORPHINE (Astramorph, Duramorph, Infumorph, MS Contin, MSIR, Oramorph, RMS, Roxanol)

Classification and indications

—Morphine is an opium alkaloid derived from the poppy plant (heroin is a derivative of morphine).

—It is used as an analgesic for both acute and chronic pain, as well as for preoperative sedation.

Pharmacology

—Morphine, like other narcotics, exerts its analgesic effects through opioid receptors in the CNS (brain and spinal cord).

—Cardiovascular effects of morphine include hypotension, which results from histamine release (causing arteriolar dilation) and venodilation. Bradycardia, especially after rapid administration, probably results from decreased central sympathetic outflow and/or central vagal stimulation.

—Onset of analgesia following intravenous morphine is within minutes, with an elimination half-life of 2–4 hours, but peak analgesia occurs after about 20 minutes.

—Following oral administration, peak analgesia occurs after about 60 minutes. Absorption from the GI tract is variable.

—Epidural injection of morphine results in prolonged (up to 20 hours) levels in the CSF. Peak CSF concentrations occur after about 60–90 minutes following epidural injection of morphine.

—Subarachnoid (intrathecal) injection of morphine requires much lower doses for analgesia than other routes because of the lack of meningeal barriers with intrathecal dosing.

—Correlation of elimination half-life with clinical duration is unpredictable. In the case of IV morphine, clinical duration is about 4 hours, whereas that of meperidine is approximately 2–4 hours.

—For comparison, the elimination half-lives of fentanyl, sufentanil, and alfentanil are 219, 164, and 90 minutes, respectively.

—Elimination of morphine is mainly a result of hepatic metabolism.

Morphine Interactions with Anesthetic Drugs
Morphine with esmolol

—Coadministration of esmolol and morphine has resulted in significant increases (up to almost 50%) in steady-state levels of esmolol, but not morphine.

Morphine with naloxone

—Use of naloxone in postoperative patients for reversal of respiratory depression has resulted in cases of pulmonary edema in some cases.

—The etiology of this interaction is not completely understood.

NEOSTIGMINE (Prostigmin)

Classification and indications

—Neostigmine is a synthetic medication similar to ambenomium and pyridostigmine.

—It is used in the treatment of myasthenia gravis to improve muscle strength.

Pharmacology

—Neostigmine is a reversible inhibitor of cholinesterase. As a result, acetylcholine accumulates at cholinergic nerve endings and at the neuromuscular junction.

—This results in improved muscle strength in myasthenics but has some side effects, including GI stimulation, hypersalivation, and miosis.
—Other side effects from excess acetylcholine may include bradycardia.
—Significant interactions can occur with procainamide that can worsen the status of patients with myasthenia gravis. This can occur because procainamide has neuromuscular blocking properties. Also, like quinidine, procainamide antagonizes the cholinergic effect of anticholinesterases.

Neostigmine Interactions with Anesthetic Drugs
Neostigmine with procainamide
—Patients receiving cholinergic medications for myasthenia gravis may experience worsening muscle weakness with administration of procainamide.
—Procainamide, in addition to acting as an antagonist to the neuromuscular effects of cholinergic medications, has neuromuscular blocking properties.

NITROGEN MUSTARD

Classification and indications
—Nitrogen mustards are a group of alkylating agents (chlorambucil, cyclophosphamide, ifosfamide, mechlorethamine, melphalan).
—These drugs are used to treat lymphomas and other malignancies.

Pharmacology
—Alkylating agents are highly reactive drugs that form linkages with organic compounds. They primarily target the nucleic acids of the cell nucleus.
—Adverse reactions from these agents can include bone marrow suppression, nausea and vomiting, alopecia, cardiotoxicity, and pulmonary fibrosis.
—Apparently, nitrogen mustards can cause a significant and persistent inhibition of plasma cholinesterase. This may result in prolonged blockade from succinylcholine for up to 10 days after treatment with these agents.

Nitrogen Mustard Interactions with Anesthetic Drugs
Nitrogen mustard with succinylcholine
—Antipseudocholinesterases (echothiophate, phenelzine, nitrogen mustard, cyclophosphamide) prevent the metabolic

destruction of succinylcholine and thus prolong its neuro-muscular blocking properties.

OXYTOCIN (Pitocin, Syntocinon)

Classification and indications

—Oxytocin is a hormone that is secreted by the hypothalamus and stored in the posterior pituitary gland (as well as vaso-pressin). In medical practice, the oxytocin used is a synthetic form.

—It is indicated for obstetric use as a stimulant for uterine con-tractions to induce or augment labor, or to help control post-partum bleeding and expulsion of the uterus.

Pharmacology

—Oxytocin causes increased contraction of the uterus. This effect is most pronounced in the patient in labor, as opposed to patients in early pregnancy when large amounts of oxy-tocin are required to increase uterine tone.

—Cardiovascular effects include vasodilation, including renal, coronary, and cerebral vessels. If oxytocin is used in very large amounts, there may be a drop in blood pressure with a reflex tachycardia and increased cardiac output.

—Following intravenous administration, onset of increased uterine tone is almost immediate and lasts for about 1 hour.

Oxytocin Interactions with Anesthetic Drugs

Oxytocin with vasopressors (ephedrine, epinephrine, metaraminol, methoxamine, norepinephrine, phenylephrine)

—Oxytocin administration has been associated with severe hypertension in patients who had received a prophylactic vasoconstrictor up to 4 hours previously for a caudal block.

—Severe hypertension is more likely to occur in patients with existing mild hypertension and in those patients who receive an ergot alkaloid (such as methylergonovine), rather than a dilute solution of oxytocin.

PHENOTHIAZINES

Classification and indications

—Phenothiazines are antipsychotic agents.

—They are used to treat psychotic disorders. Other uses include the treatment of nausea and vomiting, hiccups, and anxiety.

Pharmacology
—Phenothiazines are one of a group of antihistamines that includes ethylenediamines, ethanolamines, propylamines, and piperazines.
—They competitively inhibit histamine at the H1 receptor and can diminish symptoms of H1 stimulation (bronchial smooth muscle contraction, increased mucous production, increased capillary permeability, pruritus).
—Antihistamines in the above classes do not inhibit H2 receptors of the gastric mucosa.
—The phenothiazine-type antihistamines (methdilazine, promethazine, trimeprazine), in addition to antihistamine effects, share the properties and interactions of phenothiazines.
—Phenothiazines are antipsychotic medications that are considered neuroleptic agents.
—The neuroleptic syndrome consists of decreased psychotic symptoms, flattened affect, and decreases in aggressiveness, impulsivity, and spontaneous movement.
—CNS effects are complex and incompletely understood. They may involve antidopaminergic activities, which may explain extrapyramidal symptoms in some patients.
—Although they can be useful for treatment of postoperative nausea and vomiting, they are not useful in motion sickness.
—Cardiovascular effects include alpha blockade which may result in hypotension. Interactions with epinephrine, because of alpha blockade, can result in profound hypotension. Also, this group of drugs may cause decreased myocardial contractility.

Chlorpromazine (Thorazine)
Classification and indications
—Chlorpromazine is a phenothiazine antipsychotic agent.
—It is used to treat psychotic disorders. Other uses include the treatment of nausea and vomiting, hiccups, and anxiety.

Clozapine (Clozaril)
Classification and indications
—Clozapine is an antipsychotic medication that differs from the other classes of antipsychotic drugs (phenothiazines, butyrophenones).
—It is used mainly in the treatment of schizophrenia.

Pharmacology

—Clozapine is considered an atypical antipsychotic drug that shares some of the pharmacologic properties of other antipsychotic medications.

—The mechanism of action is not well understood. Unlike the phenothiazines and butyrophenones, clozapine has mild antidopaminergic activities.

—Cardiovascular effects include an anticholinergic effect (like tricyclic antidepressants) that may result in tachycardia.

—Of greater potential importance is alpha adrenergic blockade, which may result in significant interactions with epinephrine (severe hypotension can occur).

—Similar responses to epinephrine can be seen with chlorpromazine and thioridazine.

Thioridazine (Mellaril)
Classification and indications

—Thioridazine is a phenothiazine.

—It is used to treat psychotic disorders (such as schizophrenia), depression, anxiety, agitation, and some other behavioral disorders.

Phenothiazine Interactions with Anesthetic Drugs
Phenothiazines with epinephrine

—Phenothiazines, particularly chlorpromazine, thioridazine, and clozapine, may produce an unexpected hypotensive response with epinephrine.

—The mechanism for this interaction involves the alpha receptor blockade associated with neuroleptic drugs, leaving the vasodilating beta receptors unopposed.

—Hypotension is possibly better treated with more selective alpha adrenergic agents such as phenylephrine.

—This interaction is not likely to be seen with phenothiazines other than the three listed above, although vasopressors other than epinephrine are recommended in patients taking these medications.

POLYMYXIN B (Aerosporin)

Classification and indications

—Polymyxin B is an antibiotic derived from *Bacillus* polymyxin. In addition to polymyxin B, there is also polymyxin A and E (colistin).

—It can be used in different forms: intravenous, intrathecal, intramuscular, ophthalmic, otic, or as an irrigant for bowel or bladder. It is indicated for infections with *Pseudomonas aeruginosa* and for some infections caused by other susceptible bacteria (*H. influenza, E. coli,* and others).

Pharmacology

—Polymyxin is bactericidal to susceptible bacteria (gram-negative) by binding to the cell membrane and causing damaging changes to its permeability.

—These drugs can cause serious adverse effects such as ototoxicity and nephrotoxicity, which are unlikely when used in topical form (otic, ophthalmic, skin).

—Polymyxin B apparently can inhibit neuromuscular function causing muscle weakness. As a result, potentiation of muscle relaxants used during anesthesia can occur. This interaction can affect non-depolarizing agents as well as succinylcholine.

—Normally, systemic absorption is not significant when polymyxin is used to irrigate bladder or bowel unless there is significant inflammation of these tissues.

Polymyxin B Interactions with Anesthetic Drugs
Polymyxin B with muscle relaxants (atracurium, doxacurium, gallamine, metocurine, mivacurium, pancuronium, pipecuronium, rocuronium, succinylcholine, tubocurarine, vecuronium)

—A number of antibiotics have significant interactions with neuromuscular blocking agents. These include the aminoglycosides (amikacin, gentamicin, kanamycin, neomycin, paromomycin, netilmicin, neomycin, streptomycin, tobramycin), as well as polymyxin B, colistin, amphotericin B, clindamycin, bacitracin, and lincomycin.

—All of the above antibiotics may potentiate non-depolarizing agents, but some (aminoglycosides, amphotericin B, clindamycin, colistin) can also potentiate succinylcholine blockade.

—These antibiotics potentiate neuromuscular blockade by different mechanisms, making management of these problems difficult. Although treatment with anticholinesterases or calcium have been recommended, results are inconsistent.

PROBENECID (Benemid, Col-Probenecid, Colbenemid, Probalan, Probampacin, Proben-C)

Classification and indications
—Probenecid is a uricosuric agent derived from sulfonamide.

—It is used to treat hyperuricemia (the cause of gout) and to increase the serum concentrations of some antibiotics.

Pharmacology

—Probenecid interferes with absorption and secretion of some substances in the renal tubules.

—In the proximal tubules, it competitively inhibits reabsorption of uric acid (high levels of which cause gout).

—In the proximal and distal tubules, weak organic acids such as penicillins, cephalosporins, and others are normally secreted. This secretion by the renal tubules is competitively inhibited by probenecid.

—The mechanism of the above actions is not known.

—Patients receiving probenecid may experience prolonged sedation when given sodium thiopental.

Probenecid Interactions with Anesthetic Drugs
Probenecid with sodium pentothal

—Patients receiving probenecid may experience prolonged sedation after thiopental anesthesia.

—This interaction was studied prospectively in more than 80 patients.

PROCAINAMIDE (Procan SR, Pronestyl)

Classification and indications

—Procainamide is a class IA antiarrhythmic agent (as are quinidine and lidocaine).

—It is indicated for the management of atrial and ventricular arrhythmias.

Pharmacology

—Cardiac conduction effects from procainamide include an increased refractory period of the atria, ventricles, and the His-Purkinje fibers. Also, there is decreased automaticity and excitability of these tissues.

—Conduction can be more rapid through the atrioventricular node, so that ventricular response to atrial tachyarrhythmias may be increased unless AV conduction is blocked first by other means (digoxin).

—At toxic levels, procainamide may cause prolonged AV conduction times, even producing AV block. This can be manifested as a widened QRS, prolonged QT and PR, and increasing AV block.

—In patients with impaired ventricular function, procainamide may worsen contractility.

—Procainamide can worsen the clinical status of patients with myasthenia gravis. This can occur because procainamide has neuromuscular blocking properties and also can interfere with the cholinergic effects of the anticholinesterases. Quinidine has similar effects.

—Elimination of procainamide is highly dependent on adequate renal function and patients with renal disease may show toxicity earlier than do normal patients.

Procainamide Interactions with Anesthetic Drugs
Procainamide with muscle relaxants (atracurium, doxacurium, gallamine, metocurine, mivacurium, pancuronium, pipercuronium, rocuronium, succinylcholine, tubocurarine, vecuronium)

—Procainamide can potentiate muscle relaxation from nondepolarizing agents. This is probably a result of decreased acetylcholine release at the neuromuscular junction caused by procainamide.

PYRIDOSTIGMINE BROMIDE (Mestinon)

Classification and indications
—Pyridostigmine is a synthetic medication similar to ambenomium and neostigmine.

—It is used in the treatment of myasthenia gravis to improve muscle strength.

Pharmacology
—Pyridostigmine is a reversible inhibitor of cholinesterase. As a result, acetylcholine accumulates at cholinergic nerve endings and at the neuromuscular junction.

—This results in improved muscle strength in myasthenics, but has some side effects, including GI stimulation, hypersalivation, and miosis.

—Other side effects from excess acetylcholine may include bradycardia.

—Significant interactions can occur with procainamide, which can worsen the status of patients with myasthenia gravis. This can occur because procainamide has neuromuscular blocking properties. Also, like quinidine, procainamide antagonizes the cholinergic effect of anticholinesterases.

Pyridostigmine Bromide Interactions with Anesthetic Drugs
Pyridostigmine bromide with procainamide

—Patients receiving cholinergic medications for myasthenia gravis may experience worsening muscle weakness with administration of procainamide.

—Procainamide, in addition to acting as an antagonist to the neuromuscular effects of cholinergic medications, has neuromuscular blocking properties.

QUINIDINE (Cardioquin, Cin-Quin, Duraquin, Quinaglute, Quinalan, Quinatime, Quinidex, Quinora)

Classification and indications

—Quinidine is a class IA antiarrhythmic agent prepared from quinine or plant sources.

—It is used for maintenance of normal sinus rhythm in patients who have been treated for different arrhythmias including atrial fibrillation or flutter, paroxysmal supraventricular tachycardias, and atrial or ventricular premature contractions. It is also considered the drug of choice for treatment of severe falciparum malaria (formerly this was treated with quinine).

Pharmacology

—The antiarrhythmic properties of quinidine are similar to those of procainamide.

—Automaticity is decreased in the His-Purkinje system (like lidocaine and procainamide) and there is a decrease in speed of conduction in these tissues and the atria and ventricles.

—Conduction through the atrioventricular node is either unaffected or increased. This is due to an anticholinergic effect. As with procainamide, patients with rapid atrial arrhythmias (atrial fibrillation/flutter) should receive treatment to slow AV conduction prior to receiving quinidine. This is often accomplished with digitalization.

—At toxic levels, quinidine may cause prolonged AV conduction times, even producing AV block. This can be manifested as a widened QRS, prolonged QT and PR, and increasing AV block.

—In patients with impaired ventricular function, quinidine may worsen contractility.

—Both quinidine and procainamide can worsen the clinical status of patients with myasthenia gravis. This can occur because they have neuromuscular blocking properties and also can interfere with the cholinergic effects of the anticholinesterases.-Potentiation of both non-depolarizing and depolarizing agents can occur.

Quinidine Interactions with Anesthetic Drugs
Quinidine with muscle relaxants (atracurium, doxacurium, gallamine, metocurine, mivacurium, pancuronium, pipercuronium, rocuronium, succinylcholine, tubocurarine, vecuronium)

—Quinidine and quinine can potentiate muscle relaxation from both depolarizing and non-depolarizing agents.

—The mechanism of this interaction is a curare-like action at the myoneural junction. Also, plasma pseudocholinesterase is inhibited by quinidine (and quinine), resulting in possible prolongation of muscle relaxation from succinylcholine.

RIFAMPIN (Rifadin, Rifamate, Rimactane)

Classification and indications
—Rifampin is an antibiotic.

—It is used with other agents to treat tuberculosis and other mycobacteria. It is also used to treat asymptomatic carriers of *Neisseria meningitidis.*

Pharmacology
—Rifampin inhibits bacterial RNA polymerase.

—It is available for oral or intravenous therapy.

—Significant interactions can occur with calcium channel blockers. Patients receiving rifampin may require higher than normal doses of intravenous and oral calcium channel blockers due to an alteration of their metabolism or protein binding by rifampin.

Rifampin Interactions with Anesthetic Drugs
Rifampin with calcium channel blockers (diltiazem, nicardipine, nifedipine, verapamil)

—Patients taking rifampin require significantly higher doses of calcium channel blockers. This interaction has been documented with verapamil, diltiazem, and nifedipine.

—The studies done demonstrated the increased requirement for both oral and intravenous forms of the calcium channel blockers, but requirements were higher for patients taking oral medications.

—The mechanisms of this interaction include an increased metabolism and reduced protein binding of the calcium channel blockers by rifampin.

RITODRINE (Yutopar)

Classification and indications
—Ritodrine is a beta adrenergic agonist.
—It is used to arrest premature labor.

Pharmacology
—Ritodrine is primarily a beta 2 adrenergic agonist. Results of beta 2 stimulation are relaxation of uterine and bronchial smooth muscle as well as vasodilation of skeletal muscle vasculature.
—Ritodrine also stimulates beta 1 receptors and may produce some increase in heart rate, contractility, and blood pressure.
—Interactions with ritodrine include potentiation of pressor effects by vasopressors such as phenylephrine and ephedrine. Also, beta blockers can oppose the uterine relaxation produced by ritodrine.
—Coadministration of ritodrine and corticosteroids has been associated with maternal pulmonary edema. This interaction is rare and of unknown etiology.

Ritodrine Interactions with Anesthetic Drugs

Ritodrine with atropine
—Atropine, a sympatholytic drug, may produce unexpected hypertension in patients receiving ritodrine.

Ritodrine with beta blockers (esmolol, labetalol, propranolol)
—Beta blockers may inhibit the effects of ritodrine, which is a beta 2 selective blocker used for uterine relaxation.

Ritodrine with isoproterenol
—Ritodrine may potentiate the pressor effects of sympathomimetic amines.
—The mechanism of this interaction is probably related to the beta 1 adrenergic stimulation that can be seen with ritodrine administration.

Ritodrine with vasopressors (ephedrine, epinephrine, metaraminol, methoxamine, norepinephrine, phenylephrine)
—Ritodrine may potentiate the pressor effects of sympathomimetic amines.
—The mechanism of this interaction is probably related to the beta 1 adrenergic stimulation that can be seen with ritodrine administration.

TERBUTALINE (Brethaire, Brethine, Bricanyl)

Classification and indications
—Terbutaline is a synthetic beta sympathomimetic agent which primarily affects beta 2 receptors.
—It is used for treatment of bronchospasm and to inhibit uterine contractions in preterm labor.

Pharmacology
—Terbutaline is primarily a beta 2 adrenergic agonist. Results of beta 2 stimulation are relaxation of uterine and bronchial smooth muscle as well as vasodilation of skeletal muscle vasculature.
—Terbutaline also stimulates beta 1 receptors and may produce some increase in heart rate, contractility, and blood pressure, especially when terbutaline is used at high doses.
—Interactions with terbutaline include potentiation of pressor effects by vasopressors such as phenylephrine and ephedrine. Also, beta blockers can oppose the uterine and bronchial relaxation produced by terbutaline.

Terbutaline Interactions with Anesthetic Drugs
Terbutaline with beta blockers (esmolol, labetalol, propranolol)
—Beta blockers may reverse the relaxation of bronchial and uterine smooth muscle produced by terbutaline.

Terbutaline with isoproterenol
—Terbutaline, a beta adrenergic agonist, may potentiate the cardiovascular effects of sympathomimetic agents.

Terbutaline with vasopressors (ephedrine, epinephrine, metaraminol, methoxamine, norepinephrine, phenylephrine)
—Terbutaline, a beta adrenergic agonist, may potentiate the cardiovascular effects of sympathomimetic agents.

THEOPHYLLINE (Aerolate, Asmalix, Dilor, Dyflex, Elixophyllin, Lanophyllin, Lufyllin, Neothylline, Quibron, Slo-Phyllin, Slo-bid, Theoclear, Theodur, Theolair, Theovent, Truphylline)

Classification and indications
—Aminophylline is a xanthine derivative.
—It is used as a bronchodilator and to treat apnea in infants and patients with Cheyne–Stokes respiration.

Pharmacology
—Aminophylline is a compound of theophylline with ethylenediamine, which makes theophylline more water soluble.
—Theophylline competitively inhibits phosphodiesterase and
increases intracellular cyclic AMP, resulting in bronchodilation and pulmonary arteriolar dilation.
—Theophylline is a CNS and cardiovascular stimulant. Partially offsetting the stimulating effect on the cardiovascular
system is systemic arteriolar and venous dilation (as well as
coronary artery dilation).
—Optimal bronchodilation usually requires serum theophylline levels between 10 and 20 μg/mL. Above 20 μg/mL,
adverse effects of theophylline are likely to manifest (tachycardia, nausea, delirium, seizures, etc.).
—Elimination of theophylline is impaired in patients with congestive heart failure, chronic obstructive pulmonary disease,
liver disease, or in geriatric patients.

Theophylline Interactions with Anesthetic Drugs
Theophylline with adenosine
—Adenosine is a nucleoside that slows conduction through the
atrioventricular node. Xanthines such as theophylline, aminophylline, and caffeine can reverse or block the physiologic
effects of adenosine.

THYROXINE (Cytomel (T3), Euthroid, Levothroid, Levothyroxine, Levoxine, Synthroid, Thyrolar)

Classification and indications
—Thyroxine is a synthetic replacement of endogenous thyroxine.
—It is used as replacement for diminished or absent thyroid
function. It is also used to suppress thyrotropin hormone
secretion in cases of goiter or thyroiditis.

Pharmacology
—Thyroid hormones stimulate cellular metabolism, resulting
in increases in energy used and heat produced.
—The two forms of thyroid hormone that are most clinically
important are triiodothyronine (T3) and tetraiodothyronine
(T4 or thyroxine).
—Control of thyroid hormone secretion is normally the result
of a feedback mechanism. When circulating thyroid levels are

low, the hypothalamus secretes thyrotropic releasing hormone (TRH), which stimulates the pituitary to secrete thyroid-stimulating hormone (TSH). TSH causes the thyroid gland to increase output of T3 and T4.

—The causes of hypothyroidism include autoimmune thyroiditis (the most common cause), postpartum thyroiditis, medications, and other causes.

—Administration of excessive amounts of thyroid hormone can produce symptoms of hyperthyroidism with tachycardia, myopathy, nervousness, angina, etc.

—Marked hypertension and tachycardia has occurred in patients receiving thyroxine who were given ketamine for anesthesia.

Thyroxine Interactions with Anesthetic Drugs
Thyroxine with ketamine
—Ketamine may produce unexpected hypertension and tachycardia in patients taking thyroid medication. This is based on a case report of two patients and the significance and mechanism of this interaction are unclear.

TOCAINIDE (Tonocard)

Classification and indications
—Tocainide is a local anesthetic and a class IB antiarrhythmic agent. It is a derivative of lidocaine, but it can be administered orally and intravenously.

—It is indicated for treatment of ventricular arrhythmias.

Pharmacology
—Like all local anesthetics, tocainide prevents the generation and conduction of nerve impulses by blocking the normal increase in sodium permeability that accompanies depolarization of nerve axons.

—The antiarrhythmic activity of tocainide is a result of interference with phase 4 depolarization, like all class IB drugs (lidocaine, tocainide, phenytoin, mexilitine). Class IA drugs are local anesthetics that interfere with phase 0 and phase 4 depolarization (quinidine, procainamide, disopyramide).

—Tocainide, like lidocaine, can potentiate non-depolarizing muscle relaxants.

Tocainide Interactions with Anesthetic Drugs
Tocainide with muscle relaxants (atracurium, doxacurium, gallamine, metocurine, mivacurium, pancuronium, pipercuronium, rocuronium, succinylcholine, tubocurarine, vecuronium)
—Tocainide, an orally active form of lidocaine, can potentiate both depolarizing and non-depolarizing neuromuscular blockade. This is a property of most local anesthetics as well as a number of other medications.

TRICYCLIC ANTIDEPRESSANTS
Classification and indications
—Tricyclics are a group of antidepressant medications.
—Tricyclic medications as a group are used to treat depressive disorders, including depressive stages of schizophrenia, some anxiety disorders, and phobias. Some of the TCAs are used to treat attention deficit disorder, enuresis in children, and eating disorders.
Pharmacology
—Tricyclic antidepressants interfere with the reuptake of catecholamines. This may explain the exaggerated response sometimes seen with exogenous pressors.
—Also, this group of drugs has an anticholinergic (vagolytic) effect which contributes to tachycardia associated with their use.
—Combination of tricyclic antidepressants and monoamine oxidase inhibitors can result in hyperpyrexia, convulsions, and death.
—Because of some documented interactions with anesthetic agents, some recommend discontinuing TCA medications for 2 weeks prior to elective surgery. However, this practice has been questioned and is no longer universally accepted.
Amitriptyline (Elavil, Endep, Enovil, Etraphon, Limbitrol, Triavil)
Classification and indications
—Amitriptyline is a tricyclic antidepressant medication.
—It is indicated for the treatment of depression.
Amoxapine (Asendin)
Classification and indications
—Amoxapine is a tricyclic antidepressant medication.
—It is indicated for treatment of depression.

Clomipramine (Anafranil)
Classification and indications
—Clomipramine is a tricyclic antidepressant.
—It is used in the treatment of obsessive-compulsive disorders.

Desipramine (Norpramin, Pertofrane)
Classification and indications
—Desipramine is a tricyclic antidepressant medication.
—It is used to treat depression.

Doxepin (Sinequan)
Classification and indications
—Doxepin is a tricyclic antidepressant medication.
—It is indicated for the treatment of depression and/or anxiety.

Imipramine (Janimine, Tofranil)
Classification and indications
—Imipramine is a tricyclic antidepressant medication.
—It is used as an antidepressant and also as a treatment of childhood enuresis.

Maprotilene (Ludiomil)
Classification and indications
—Maprotiline is a tricyclic antidepressant medication.
—It is used to treat manic-depression and depression with or without anxiety.

Nortriptyline (Aventyl, Pamelor)
Classification and indications
—Nortriptyline is a tricyclic antidepressant medication.
—It is used to treat depression.

Protriptyline (Vivactil)
Classification and indications
—Protriptyline is a tricyclic antidepressant medication.
—It is used for treatment of depressive disorders.

Trimipramine (Surmontil)
Classification and indications
—Trimipramine is a tricyclic antidepressant medication.
—It is indicated for treatment of depression.

Tricyclic antidepressants Interactions with Anesthetic Drugs
Tricyclic antidepressants with epinephrine
—Patients taking tricyclic antidepressant drugs develop an exaggerated pressor response, consisting of hypertension and cardiac arrhythmias, when given epinephrine intravenously. The mechanism of this interaction is unclear, but is probably related to blockade of norepinephrine reuptake that is caused by TCA medications.

—Although patient studies have documented the above interaction for intravenous epinephrine, it is possible that intramuscular, infiltration (for local anesthesia), or inhalational (for respiratory therapy) epinephrine could have the same results.

2

DISEASES

ACIDOSIS

—Acidosis exists if the pH of arterial blood is below 7.37 or if the pH is within a normal range (7.37–7.43) but there is respiratory or metabolic compensation. To determine if there is compensation for an acid–base disturbance, one must examine arterial pCO_2 and serum bicarbonate levels (base excess).

—Respiratory acidosis occurs as a result of inadequate elimination of CO_2 as a result of hypoventilation (such as severe asthma or chronic obstructive pulmonary disease). The accumulation of CO_2 causes an increase in the amount of carbonic acid.

—Metabolic acidosis is a result of accumulation of excess acids (such as lactic acid) or a loss of base, such as occurs in diarrhea or renal disease.

Acidosis Interactions with Anesthesia Drugs
Acidosis and edrophonium, neostigmine, pyridostigmine

—Alterations of the normal acid–base status may result in difficulty reversing non-depolarizing neuromuscular blockade.

—Respiratory acidosis ($pCO_2 > 50$) and metabolic alkalosis have been shown to prevent adequate reversal of pancuronium neuromuscular block. This interaction appears to be complex and is incompletely understood, but is probably related to changes in electrolytes and intracellular pH rather than simple changes in acid–base measurements.

ADVANCED AGE

—The term "advanced age" is used to describe patients who are 65 or older. In spite of the fact that there may be significant differences in the physiologic state of similarly aged patients, chronological age is nevertheless the most reliable predictor of age-related changes in organ system function.

—Relating physiologic changes from aging to changes in response to anesthetics can be difficult. However, certain effects on anesthetic requirements as a result of aging are less controversial.

—The minimal alveolar concentration (MAC) for inhaled anesthetics decreases progressively in adulthood by approximately 6% each decade. Very elderly patients may have a 30% decreased MAC compared to young adults.

—Induction doses of thiopental, propofol, and etomidate for elderly patients may need to be 20–40% lower than for young adult patients.

—Sensitivity of elderly patients to narcotics and benzodiazepines is probably greater and reduced doses are recommended for older patients.

—The above responses to anesthetics have been attributed to different mechanisms including decreased volumes of distribution, delayed hepatic and renal clearance, and increased brain sensitivity.

Advanced Age Interactions with Anesthesia Drugs
Advanced age and alfentanil
—Alfentanil is primarily metabolized in the liver (>99%).

—In elderly patients, clearance of alfentanil may be significantly reduced, increasing the half-life and causing prolongation of effects.

—Also, elderly patients demonstrate an increased central nervous system (CNS) sensitivity to alfentanil, reducing dosing requirements for this age group.

Advanced age and atracurium
—Age, obesity, liver, and renal dysfunction have no significant effect on metabolism of atracurium.

—Atracurium is metabolized by Hoffman elimination as well as by ester hydrolysis.

—Hoffman elimination is a nonenzymatic process that occurs at physiologic temperatures and pH. Ester hydrolysis occurs most rapidly in an acid pH and does not require plasma pseudocholinesterase.

Advanced age and doxacurium, mivacurium, rocuronium
—Prolonged duration of neuromuscular blockade can be seen in older patients with several different non-depolarizing agents, including doxacurium, mivacurium, and rocuronium.

—In some cases, delayed onset of muscle relaxation also occurs. This has been attributed to decreased perfusion of the neuromuscular junction as a result of advanced age.

Advanced age and etomidate, propofol, sodium pentothal
—A reduced induction dose is recommended for thiopental, etomidate, and propofol in most elderly patients.

—Reduction in the dose requirements for these drugs may be a result of a decreased volume of distribution, decreased elimination, or a combination of effects brought about by aging.

Advanced age and narcotics (buprenorphine, butorphanol, fentanyl, meperidine, nalbuphine, morphine, sufentanil)
—Elderly patients may require lower doses of narcotics than younger adults.

—This may be a result of reduced metabolism of this class of drugs or represent an increased brain sensitivity to narcotics as a result of aging.

Advanced age and benzodiazepines (chlordiazepoxide, diazepam, midazolam)

—Elderly patients may have decreased requirements for benzodiazepines.

—The exact mechanism for this response is controversial but may be related to decreased metabolism of this class of drugs. Alternatively, some elderly patients may be more sensitive to the central nervous system effects of these medications.

Advanced age and heparin

—Older patients may demonstrate resistance to anticoagulation from heparin compared to younger patients.

—This interaction is believed to result from lower antithrombin III levels seen in some older patients.

Advanced age and ketorolac

—Older patients (>65 years) should receive lower doses of ketorolac because age-related reductions in renal function place these patients at higher risk for renal damage from ketorolac.

—In these patients, whose renal function may be very dependent on renal vascular dilation from prostaglandins, inhibition of these prostaglandins by ketorolac may worsen kidney function.

Advanced age and lidocaine

—Patients with congestive heart failure or compromised cardiac function can experience delayed elimination of lidocaine. This is a result of decreased hepatic blood flow.

—This interaction is significant mainly for patients receiving prolonged infusions (>24 hours). Normal loading doses and short-term infusion doses are appropriate.

AIR EMBOLISM

—Venous air embolism can occur during surgery when an opened vein has pressure lower than atmospheric pressure. This most frequently occurs during neurosurgery of the brain with the patient in the sitting position. Because the opened vein can be from 20 to 65 cm above the heart, the intravenous pressure can be below atmospheric pressure, allowing entrainment of air. However, even patients having surgery in the supine or prone positions can experience venous air embolism if intravenous pressures are low.

—The clinical significance of the air embolism depends on several factors: the amount and rate of air entrainment, the presence of nitrous oxide, the right heart pressures, the presence of a patent foramen ovale, and the ability of the patient's cardiovascular system to compensate for the air embolism.

—While small amounts of air entrained via an open vein can be handled with slight physiologic derangement, large amounts of entrained air can result in cardiovascular collapse. This occurs because foaming in the heart can cause mechanical obstruction to the flow of blood. Also, there may be reflex pulmonary vasoconstriction, which further compromises outflow of the right heart.

—The presence of nitrous oxide may increase the risk of significant venous air embolism. Because nitrous oxide is highly soluble in blood and used in high concentrations (50–75%), large amounts are carried in the blood. Nitrogen in air is not very soluble in blood, so that entry of nitrous oxide into an air bubble is not matched with an equal exit of nitrogen (composing about 70% of air). The result is expansion of the air bubble.

Air Embolism Interactions with Anesthesia Drugs
Air embolism and nitrous oxide

—Nitrous oxide can result in rapid expansion of gas- or air-filled cavities in the anesthetized patient. For this reason, it should not be administered to patients with a pneumothorax, acute intestinal obstruction, or to patients at significant risk for air embolism.

—Additionally, for patients having surgery for retinal detachment, where sulfahexafluoride gas, nitrogen, or a combination is injected into the vitreous cavity, use of nitrous oxide could produce unwanted expansion or pressure in the eye. The same is true for patients having tympanoplasty.

—Because nitrous oxide is used in high concentrations (50–70%) and is 35 times more soluble in blood than nitrogen, nitrous oxide will enter an air-containing cavity, causing expansion or increase in pressure. This effect cannot be offset by displacement of nitrogen (composing 78% of air) because of nitrogen's low solubility.

ALCOHOL—ACUTE INTOXICATION

—Acute alcohol (ethanol) intoxication is usually defined as a blood concentration of alcohol greater than 100 mg/dL (100 mL of blood). Patients who are not chronic abusers may demonstrate symptoms of acute alcohol intoxication at much lower blood alcohol levels.

—Patients who are acutely intoxicated with alcohol usually will experience increased respiratory depression from opiates, inhaled anesthetics, benzodiazepines, and barbiturates. Also, intoxicated patients have increased susceptibility to hypoglycemia, hypothermia, and hypotension.

Alcohol (Acute Intoxication) Interactions with Anesthesia Drugs

Alcohol—acute intoxication and narcotics (alfentanil, buprenorphine, butorphanol, fentanyl, meperidine, morphine, nalbuphine, sufentanil)

—Patients who are acutely intoxicated with alcohol (including chronic alcoholics) usually demonstrate increased sensitivity to narcotics.

—Although the precise mechanism of interactions are not agreed on, it appears that alcohol intoxication has additive CNS depression with barbiturates, benzodiazepines, and narcotics, as well as inhalational agents.

Alcohol—acute intoxication and inhalational anesthetics (enflurane, desflurane, halothane, isoflurane, nitrous oxide, sevoflurane)

—Patients with acute alcohol intoxication (including chronic abusers of alcohol) have a lower MAC for inhalational anesthetics.

—The mechanism of this interaction appears to be additive CNS depressant effects between alcohol and inhalational agents.

Alcohol—acute intoxication and intravenous anesthetics (etomidate, sodium pentothal, propofol)

—Patients who are acutely intoxicated with alcohol (including chronic alcoholics) usually demonstrate increased sensitivity to all anesthetics, including intravenous induction agents.

—Although the precise mechanisms of interaction are not agreed on, it appears that alcohol intoxication has additive CNS depression with barbiturates, benzodiazepines, and narcotics, as well as inhalational agents.

Alcohol—acute intoxication and benzodiazepines (chlordiazepoxide, diazepam, lorazepam, midazolam)

—Although the precise mechanisms of interaction are not agreed on, it appears that alcohol intoxication has additive CNS depression with barbiturates, benzodiazepines, and narcotics, as well as inhalational agents.

ALCOHOL—CHRONIC ABUSE

—Chronic alcohol abuse results in complex changes with regard to anesthetic agents. Some of these changes are poorly understood and controversial. For example, thiopental induction doses are believed to be essentially unchanged for most patients with chronic alcoholic liver disease. In some cases, however, patients have been reported to have higher induction dose requirements, supposedly on the basis of cross-tolerance to barbiturates as a result of enzyme induction. This same mechanism is used to explain similar tolerance to benzodiazepines and narcotics.

—The MAC for inhalational agents is usually increased in these patients and is attributed to an increase in cellular tolerance rather than an alteration in metabolism. Exceptions to this increased MAC would be patients with alcohol-induced cardiomyopathy. These patients will usually be more sensitive to the myocardial depression from inhalational anesthetics.

—Some patients with a history of alcohol abuse receive disulfiram, which is used to encourage avoidance of alcohol consumption. Patients taking disulfiram who are exposed to alcohol experience severe systemic reactions including vomiting, diaphoresis, hypotension, hyperventilation, and, in severe reactions, cardiovascular collapse. Disulfiram has been associated with delayed metabolism of some benzodiazepines and may potentiate and prolong effects from benzodiazepine administration.

—Also, hypotension may be accentuated in patients taking disulfiram. This is thought to be a result of inhibition of dopamine beta oxidase, which converts dopamine to norepinephrine.

Alcohol (Chronic Abuse) Interactions with Anesthesia Drugs
*Alcohol-chronic abuse and benzodiazepines, inhalational and intravenous anesthetics, narcotics**

—Chronic abuse of alcohol has complex and incompletely understood effects on a patient's response to anesthetic agents. In general, these patients tend to be more tolerant (in a nonintoxicated state) to barbiturates, benzodiazepines, narcotics, and inhalational agents.

---

* Inhalational anesthetics (desflurane, enflurane, halothane, isoflurane, nitrous oxide, sevoflurane)
Benzodiazepines (chlordiazepoxide, diazepam, lorazepam, midazolam)
Intravenous anesthetics (etomidate, methohexital, propofol, sodium pentothal)
Narcotics (alfentanil, buprenorphine, butorphanol, fentanyl, meperidine, morphine, nalbuphine, sufentanil).

—Exceptions to this generalization include the alcoholic patient with a cardiomyopathy who may demonstrate increased sensitivity to myocardial depression from inhalational agents.

—Also, the patient with severe liver disease may have an impaired ability to metabolize succinylcholine due to decreased levels of plasma pseudocholinesterase.

ALKALOSIS

—Alkalosis exists when the arterial pH is >7.45. Respiratory alkalosis results from increased alveolar ventilation as a result of hypoxemia, CNS disease, pregnancy, salicylate overdose, and some other disorders. Metabolic alkalosis is a result of loss of acid, usually in the form of hydrochloric acid from vomiting of stomach contents. Hypokalemia and hyponatremia from inhibition of renal tubular resorption of these cations secondary to diuretic therapy are also associated with alkalosis.

—Alkalosis, because of the relationship with hypokalemia, may be significant in terms of its effect on digitalis toxicity.

—This interaction is a result of the fact that digitalis glycosides exert their effect on the heart by binding to the Na-K ATPase enzyme in cardiac tissue and inhibit this enzyme.

—Studies have shown that binding of digitalis to the Na-K ATPase enzyme is increased in hypokalemia.

—Potassium infusion to patients with digitalis toxicity who are hypokalemic results in decreased binding of digitalis and may decrease cardiotoxicity.

Alkalosis Interactions with Anesthesia Drugs
Alkalosis and digitalis

—Alkalosis, because of the relationship with hypokalemia, can precipitate or worsen digitalis toxicity.

—This interaction is a result of the fact that digitalis glycosides exert their effect on the heart by binding to the Na-K ATPase enzyme in cardiac tissue and inhibit this enzyme.

—Studies have shown that binding of digitalis to the Na-K ATPase enzyme is increased in hypokalemia.

AMYOTROPHIC LATERAL SCLEROSIS

—Amyotrophic lateral sclerosis (ALS) is characterized by degeneration of motor neurons in the CNS and spinal cord with secondary changes in muscle. It occurs usually in males between

the age of 40 and 60 and in a small percentage of patients may follow an autosomal dominant pattern of inheritance.
—Although the disease can present in different ways, most commonly it begins with weakness of the intrinsic muscles of the hand and then spreads proximally to the arms, shoulders, and cranium. There may be prominent involvement of cranial nerves (except ocular muscles) resulting in choking, regurgitation, and problems with vocalization from laryngeal muscle weakness.
—Some patients survive 10 or more years after onset of the disease, but the life expectancy for most patients is 18 months to 6 years.
—Patients with ALS can respond to succinylcholine with life-threatening hyperkalemia because of involvement of the motor neurons. Nondepolarizing agents tend to have prolonged effects in such patients.

Amyotrophic Lateral Sclerosis Interactions with Anesthesia Drugs

Amyotrophic lateral sclerosis and muscle relaxants (atracurium, doxacurium, gallamine, metocurine, mivacurium, pancuronium, pipercuronium, rocuronium, tubocurarine, vecuronium)

—Patients with a wide variety of neuromuscular disorders may be more resistant than normal patients to the effects of non-depolarizing neuromuscular blockers.
—This includes patients with disuse atrophy of the muscles (such as bedridden patients with chronic disease) as well as patients with upper or lower motor neuron disease (such as from trauma, stroke, or chronic illness like ALS).
—Disuse or denervation of muscle results in production of extrajunctional acetylcholine receptors on the muscle membrane. These receptors are less easily blocked by non-depolarizing agents but are activated by lower concentrations of depolarizing drugs (succinylcholine).
—Despite initial resistance to blockade, such patients may demonstrate prolonged neuromuscular weakness as a result of decreased muscle strength and mass.

Amyotrophic lateral sclerosis and succinylcholine

—Chronic or progressive motor neuron disease places patients at continuous risk for hyperkalemia from succinylcholine. Syringomyelia, amyotrophic lateral sclerosis, multiple sclerosis, acute idiopathic polyneuritis (Guillain–Barre syndrome), and all forms of muscular dystrophy have been associated with this response.

—Patients with neuromuscular disease (upper and lower motor neuron abnormalities) can respond to succinylcholine with a dangerous, sometimes fatal hyperkalemia. This probably occurs because of proliferation of extrajunctional acetylcholine receptors on the muscle membrane. Depolarization of these receptors causes potassium leak through the muscle membrane.

ANGINA

—Disease of the coronary arteries can be manifested in different or combined ways: angina, myocardial infarction, arrhythmias, or sudden cardiac death from ventricular fibrillation or tachycardia that is not associated with prior symptoms or myocardial infarction (MI).

—In patients with no history of previous MI, the risk of perioperative MI (within 72 hours of surgery) for noncardiac surgery is approximately 0.13%.

—For patients with a history of previous MI, the risks for perioperative MI are considerably greater and have been reviewed in a number of studies. Some of the older studies (from 1964 to 1978) indicated that for surgery within 3 months of an MI, the risks for re-infarction could be as high as 37%. More recent studies have shown much lower risks of approximately 6% within 3 months of MI and 2.5% for noncardiac surgery 4–6 months following the MI. After 6 months, the risk appears to decrease to about 1.5%, which is still almost 10 times the risk for perioperative infarction of patients without evidence of prior MI.

—The reduced risk of perioperative MI shown in the more recent investigations has been attributed to more skillful surgical and anesthetic management both intraoperatively and postoperatively. For example, the increased use of invasive monitors such as pulmonary artery catheters has allowed earlier identification and treatment of impending cardiac problems.

—Risk of MI in the perioperative period is also influenced by the type of surgical procedure. For example, whereas the risks appear to be high for patients undergoing vascular procedures, patients having ophthalmic operations have a much lower risk.

Angina Interactions with Anesthesia Drugs
Angina and ketamine

—Ketamine has significant, mostly stimulatory, effects on the cardiovascular system. Cardiovascular stimulation in patients with coronary artery disease can cause an undesirable increase in myocardial oxygen demand.

—Other clinical situations in which ketamine would be contraindicated because of the cardiovascular stimulation are aortic or intracranial aneurysms, thyrotoxicosis, and inadequately controlled hypertension.

—Ketamine causes an increase in heart rate, cardiac output, and arterial pressure (as much as 25%) by stimulation of the CNS and inhibition of neuronal norepinephrine reuptake.

—In severely ill patients, such as those in septic shock or in chronic congestive heart failure, the cardiovascular system is resistant to indirect stimulation. In these cases, the direct myocardial depressant effects of ketamine may be manifested by hypotension.

AORTIC STENOSIS

—Isolated aortic stenosis in adults is usually of non-rheumatic origin. In patients with symptoms prior to the age of 60, the cause of the aortic valvular stenosis is usually a congenitally abnormal valve (bicuspid). Patients who become symptomatic after the age of 60 generally have normal valves that undergo degenerative thickening and calcification.

—Obstruction to the outflow from the left ventricle results in hypertrophy and increased myocardial oxygen demands. With disease progression, symptoms worsen and consist of angina, dyspnea on exertion, and syncope. Further deterioration may result in sudden death, which occurs in up to 20% of patients with the symptom triad above, or ventricular failure.

—Hypertrophy of the myocardium makes it especially vulnerable to ischemia during any situation that compromises coronary artery blood flow. Because coronary filling occurs primarily during diastole, tachycardia is detrimental. Furthermore, tachycardia reduces diastole to a greater extent than the reduction in systole. Subendocardial coronary vessels are also more compressed than in patients with normal hearts because of the increased left ventricular pressure.

—The severity of disease is usually quantitated by measurement of the aortic valve area and the pressure gradient across the valve.

The normal aortic valve orifice area is 2.5–3.5 cm$_2$. Patients with severe aortic stenosis have valve openings of <1 cm$_2$ with pressure gradients of >50 mm Hg.

Aortic stenosis Interactions with Anesthesia Drugs
Aortic stenosis and bretylium

—Patients with severe pulmonary hypertension or aortic stenosis may experience cardiac decompensation with bretylium therapy.

—Within 1 hour following bretylium administration, as much as 65% of patients will have a drop in blood pressure. Patients with severe aortic stenosis or pulmonary hypertension may not be able to compensate adequately for this hypotension.

—If treatment of life-threatening arrhythmias indicates treatment with bretylium in such patients, observation, monitoring, and treatment for the hypotension may be necessary.

ASTHMA

—Asthma is a disorder of the respiratory tract that has certain characteristics that are helpful in distinguishing it from other, similar diseases.

—It is characterized by widespread narrowing of the airways, as opposed to localized narrowing as occurs in epiglottitis, for example.

—Also, asthmatics have an increased responsiveness to irritants compared to patients with normal airway reactivity.

—Finally, reversibility of this bronchospasm either spontaneously or with treatment differentiates most asthmatics from patients with a more fixed obstruction as seen in chronic obstructive pulmonary disease, bronchiectasis, cystic fibrosis, and bronchiolitis.

—Outpatients are treated with two classes of medications: bronchodilators (such as theophylline and beta agonists) or anti-inflammatory medications (such as corticosteroids and cromolyn sodium).

—Whereas stimulation of beta 2 receptors in the lung results in bronchodilation, beta 2 blockade can cause increased airway resistance. For this reason, beta-blocking medications are probably best avoided in these patients if possible. When beta blockers are unavoidable, cardioselective agents (with predominantly beta 1 blocking properties) or labetalol (which has very weak, nonselective beta blocking properties) should be used.

—Suppression of airway reflexes on induction of anesthesia is necessary to avoid bronchospasm after intubation of the trachea. Thiopental, etomidate, and propofol induce unconsciousness but unreliably depress airway reflexes. After induction with any of the above agents, ventilation with a volatile anesthetic will suppress airway responsiveness to allow for a safe intubation in most asthmatics.

Asthma Interactions with Anesthesia Drugs
Asthma and beta blockers (esmolol, labetalol, propranolol)

—Use of beta blockers in patients with reactive airway disease (asthma, chronic obstructive pulmonary disease) can result in significant increases in airway resistance.

—Although noncardioselective beta blockers (labetalol, propranolol) are most likely to precipitate bronchospasm in these patients, even selective beta 1 blockers (esmolol) have enough beta 2 blocking properties to require caution.

ATRIAL FIBRILLATION OR FLUTTER

—Atrial fibrillation is characterized by chaotic atrial activity with rates of 350–500 per minute. The ventricular rate is determined by the number of impulses that can be conducted through the atrioventricular node, which in untreated patients can be from 140 to 170 beats per minute.

—In patients with a new onset of atrial fibrillation who are hypotensive, immediate electrical cardioversion may be the appropriate therapy. In other patients, medications to slow atrioventricular (AV) conduction can be used.

—Medications that delay AV conduction effectively are digitalis, some calcium channel blockers (verapamil and diltiazem), and beta blockers. In 20% of patients, digitalis is also effective in converting the arrhythmia to sinus rhythm.

—In other cases, medications such as quinidine or procainamide are used in an attempt to convert to sinus rhythm. These medications have the ability to increase AV conduction and should be used after AV conduction has been controlled with digitalis, calcium channel blockers, or beta blockers.

—Atrial flutter is characterized by a regular atrial rate of 250–350 per beats/min with a varying AV block. In patients with paroxysmal atrial tachycardia with block (most often a result of digitalis toxicity), the atrial rate is slower (130–200 beats/min).

—In hypotensive patients or paroxysmal cases, electrical cardioversion may be the appropriate initial therapy. Pharmacologic management is similar to that of atrial fibrillation with use of digitalis, verapamil, or beta blockers to slow AV conduction and decrease the ventricular rate.

Atrial Fibrillation or Flutter Interactions with Anesthesia Drugs

Atrial fibrillation or flutter and calcium channel blockers (verapamil, diltiazem)

—Patients who have atrial fibrillation or flutter associated with the Wolf–Parkinson–White syndrome should not be treated with verapamil or diltiazem.

—These medications may cause a worsening tachycardia that is thought to be due to reflex increases in sympathetic activity.

Atrial fibrillation or flutter and procainamide, quinidine

—Quinidine and procainamide (class IA antiarrhythmics) can cause an increased ventricular response in some patients with atrial fibrillation or flutter.

—Although class IA antiarrhythmics depress conduction through the AV node, they can also have a vagolytic effect that offsets this effect and can result in increased conduction through the AV node. This is more pronounced with quinidine than with procainamide.

—In patients with atrial fibrillation, a decreased conduction time (increased rate of conduction) through the AV node would result in a more rapid ventricular rate.

—Because of quinidine's depressant effect on atrial conduction, patients with atrial flutter may experience a decreased atrial rate, but the increased conduction rate through the AV node may offset this effect with a net increase in the ventricular rate.

—Both quinidine and procainamide can be effective for management of these arrhythmias, but prior digitalization or treatment with verapamil or beta blockers is recommended to avoid increased AV conduction.

AUTONOMIC DYSFUNCTION

—The autonomic nervous system helps maintain blood pressure and organ perfusion through innervation of the heart and blood vessels. Specifically, sympathetic stimulation of the cardiovascular system results in increased heart rate, contractility, and cardiac output, whereas increased arteriolar tone increases perfusion pressure.

—Shy–Drager syndrome is a disorder of the autonomic nervous system combined with signs of degeneration of the CNS. Evidence of autonomic dysfunction includes postural hypotension that may be severe enough to cause syncope. Degeneration of areas in the CNS is manifested as signs of Parkinsonism with rigidity, intention tremor, and ataxia.

—The most common cause of autonomic dysfunction is diabetes mellitus. Sympathetic denervation is milder and more slow in onset than in patients with Shy–Drager syndrome.

—In patients with autonomic dysfunction, hypotension induced by certain medications (such as verapamil, nifedipine) or that blocks sympathetic receptors (such as beta blockers) may result in exaggerated hypotension due to inadequate compensatory responses.

Autonomic Dysfunction Interactions with Anesthesia Drugs
Autonomic dysfunction and calcium channel blockers (nicardipine, nifedipine, verapamil)

—Patients whose autonomic nervous system responses are impaired by disease (Shy–Drager) or medications (beta blockers) may be unable to adequately compensate for vasodilation or negative inotropic and chronotropic effects of calcium channel blockers.

—In these patients, exaggerated hypotension or bradycardia may be seen with calcium channel blockers.

BURNS

—Patients with burn injuries are susceptible to a life-threatening hyperkalemic response to succinylcholine and can have marked resistance to non-depolarizing muscle relaxants.

—Both of these altered responses to neuromuscular blocking agents have been attributed to proliferation of extrajunctional acetylcholine receptors, similar to that in the patient with a denervation injury. When these receptors, which can be scattered over a large surface of the muscle, are depolarized by succinylcholine, ion flow takes place through the receptor channel. Large amounts of potassium may exit the muscle cell causing hyperkalemia.

—The cause of onset of the hyperkalemic response to succinylcholine following a burn is not clearly understood. Abnormal responses to succinylcholine may begin 24 hours after the injury, but probably peak between 10 and 50 days later.

—The duration of this response is also unclear. Although evidence indicates return of normal muscle membrane physiology after the burn has healed, skin has regrown, and infection is eliminated, conservative recommendations are to avoid succinylcholine for at least 1 or 2 years after the injury has healed.

—The extent of the hyperkalemic response is not reliably correlated to the extent of the burn. A documented severe hyperkalemic response to succinylcholine occurred in a patient with an 8% surface area burn.

—Resistance to non-depolarizing agents appears to increase with larger area burns and, in fact, may not be significant in patients with less than 30% body surface area burns. In addition to proliferation of extrajunctional acetylcholine receptors, this abnormal response is probably also related to the increased metabolic rate and hepatic and renal clearance seen in burn patients. Doses of non-depolarizing agents may need to be increased by as much as 300%.

—Duration of this resistance usually is 2 months following the injury but has been reported in a patient 463 days after the burn.

Burns Interactions with Anesthesia Drugs

Burns and muscle relaxants (atracurium, doxacurium, gallamine, metocurine, mivacurium, pancuronium, pipercuronium, rocuronium, tubocurarine, vecuronium)

—Patients with burn injuries are susceptible to a life-threatening hyperkalemic response to succinylcholine and can have marked resistance to non-depolarizing muscle relaxants.

—Both of these altered responses to neuromuscular blocking agents have been attributed to proliferation of extrajunctional acetylcholine receptors, similar to that in the patient with a denervation injury.

—Resistance to non-depolarizing agents appears to increase with larger area burns and, in fact, may not be significant in patients with less than 30% body surface area burns. In addition to proliferation of extrajunctional acetylcholine receptors, this abnormal response is probably also related to the increased metabolic rate and hepatic and renal clearance seen in burn patients. Doses of non-depolarizing agents may need to be increased by as much as 300%.

—Duration of this resistance usually is 2 months following the injury but has been reported in a patient 463 days after the burn.

Burns and succinylcholine

—A marked hyperkalemic response to succinylcholine can occur in burn patients. This response does not usually occur until 24–48 hours following the injury but may persist for up to 1 year or more.

—The mechanism involved appears to be related to proliferation of extrajunctional acetylcholine receptors, similar to what occurs after denervation injuries. The extent of the burn is unreliable in predicting the extent of the hyperkalemic response.

CEREBRAL EDEMA

—Cerebral edema is an increase in the water content of the brain and results from disruption of the blood–brain barrier (vasogenic cerebral edema) or from miscellaneous causes in which the blood–brain barrier remains intact (cytotoxic cerebral edema).

—Examples of disorders that disrupt the blood–brain barrier include trauma, tumors, hypertensive encephalopathy, and inflammatory diseases.

—Cytotoxic cerebral edema is characterized by an increased content of water in the brain tissue but without protein. Examples of this form of cerebral edema include metabolic encephalopathy, hypoxia, and pseudotumor cerebri.

—Control of the intracranial hypertension associated with cerebral edema involves management of cerebral blood volume. By increasing cerebral vascular resistance (using hyperventilation to decrease pCO_2) and decreasing cerebral venous pressure (elevation of head, decreasing central venous pressure with elimination of PEEP, using muscle relaxants, and sedation) intracranial pressure (ICP) can usually be reduced.

—Other methods of controlling ICP involve medication (thiopental, lidocaine, propofol, etomidate) and hypothermia.

—Elevation of arterial pressure from mechanical stimulation (laryngoscopy) or pharmacologic stimulation (doxapram) may result in increased ICP and neurologic deterioration.

Cerebral edema Interactions with Anesthesia Drugs
Cerebral edema and adenosine

—Most systemic vasodilators (nitroglycerin, nitroprusside, hydralazine, calcium channel blockers, and adenosine) can produce cerebrovascular vasodilation as well. As a result, cerebral blood volume is either maintained or increased even though systemic blood pressure is decreased.

—Trimethaphan, a ganglionic blocker, usually will not increase cerebral blood volume because ganglionic blockade normally does not cause vasodilation of the cerebral circulation.

*Cerebral edema and benzodiazepines, intravenous anesthetics, narcotics**

—Most intravenous anesthetics cause a reduction in cerebral blood flow and intracranial pressure or have no effect on ICP. Although this effect is primarily from depression of cerebral metabolic rate, in some cases a direct vasoconstriction occurs.

—The exception to the above is ketamine, which causes an increased cerebral metabolic rate and cerebral blood flow with an increase in ICP.

—All of the narcotics, as well as barbiturates, etomidate, benzodiazepines, and propofol, have been associated with a reduction or maintenance of ICP during anesthesia.

Cerebral edema and calcium channel blockers, trimethaphan, and vasodilators†

—Most systemic vasodilators (nitroglycerin, nitroprusside, hydralazine, calcium channel blockers, and adenosine) can produce cerebrovascular vasodilation as well. As a result, cerebral blood volume is either maintained or increased even though systemic blood pressure is decreased.

—Trimethaphan, a ganglionic blocker, usually will not increase cerebral blood volume because ganglionic blockade normally does not cause vasodilation of the cerebral circulation.

---

* Benzodiazepines (chlordiazepoxide, diazepam, lorazepam, midazolam)
Intravenous anesthetics (etomidate, methohexital, propofol, sodium pentothal)
Narcotics (alfentanil, buprenorphine, butorphanol, fentanyl, meperidine, morphine, nalbuphine, sufentanil)
† Calcium channel blockers (diltiazem, nicardipine, nifedipine, verapamil)
Vasodilators (nitroglycerin, nitroprusside, hydralazine, adenosine)

Cerebral edema and doxapram HCl

—Because of its mechanism of action, doxapram is contraindicated in a number of conditions, such as hypertension, convulsive disorders, hyperthyroidism, cerebral edema, and pheochromocytoma.

—Analeptic agents, such as doxapram, are CNS stimulants. Because CNS stimulation can elevate arterial pressure, decrease seizure thresholds, and have additive stimulatory effects in conditions such as the above disorders, doxapram is contraindicated in patients with these underlying conditions.

—Analeptic agents improve ventilation through their effect on the brainstem and, in the case of doxapram, the carotid chemoreceptors.

Cerebral edema and droperidol

—Most intravenous anesthetic agents (except ketamine) can be safely used in patients with elevated intracranial pressure.

—Droperidol appears to have little effect on cerebral blood flow and cerebral metabolic rate.

Cerebral edema and inhalational anesthetics (desflurane, enflurane, halothane, isoflurane, nitrous oxide, sevoflurane)

—All commonly used inhalational volatile anesthetics (halothane > enflurane > isoflurane) cause an increased cerebral flood flow. Less is known about sevoflurane and desflurane, but they are believed to have effects similar to those of isoflurane. Nitrous oxide has minimal effects on cerebral blood flow.

—The volatile anesthetics, although they depress cerebral metabolic rate, cause cerebrovascular dilation which results in increased cerebral blood flow. Hyperventilation to a $PaCO_2$ between 25 and 35 mm Hg will effectively prevent increased cerebral blood flow from isoflurane but not the other volatile anesthetics.

Cerebral edema and ketamine

—Ketamine is contraindicated for use in patients with elevated intracranial pressure or intracranial aneurysm.

—Ketamine stimulates the cardiovascular system indirectly via the CNS and inhibition of neuronal norepinephrine reuptake. The result of these actions is an increase (up to 25%) in heart rate, cardiac output, and arterial pressure. Ketamine also causes an increase in cerebrospinal fluid pressure and intracranial blood flow.

—Some of the cardiovascular effects of ketamine can be blocked with benzodiazepines and/or labetalol.

CIRRHOSIS

—Cirrhosis is a disease of the liver from a variety of different causes that consists of scarring and decreased function of liver cells. In the United States, the most common cause of cirrhosis is chronic alcohol abuse. Other causes include chronic active hepatitis of viral or unknown etiology, primary biliary cirrhosis, Wilson's disease, alpha 1 antitrypsin deficiency, and hemochromatosis.

—The scarring and fibrosis result in alteration in the architecture of the liver and are responsible for increased resistance to blood flow. Because the lower pressure system (the portal venous flow) is compromised earlier, proportionally more liver blood flow is provided by the hepatic artery with disease progression.

—As a result of increased hepatic arterial flow and decreased portal flow, hepatic perfusion is more dependent on arterial perfusion pressures. Decreased arterial pressures as may occur during anesthesia can compromise hepatic oxygenation and result in worsening liver function perioperatively.

—Decreased hepatocellular function can alter metabolism and clearance of anesthetics and other medications. These alterations can be complex and include consideration of changes in volume of distribution as a result of ascites as well as increased tolerance to certain drugs (cross-tolerance) from chronic exposure to alcohol.

—Postoperative mortality in patients with portal hypertension from cirrhosis can be very high (up to 50%) if the serum albumin is lower than 3 g/dL, the serum bilirubin is greater than 3 mg/dL, and the patient has ascites and hepatic encephalopathy.

—Even mildly symptomatic patients with chronic liver disease appear to be at increased risk for worsening of liver function from anesthesia and surgery.

Cirrhosis Interactions with Anesthesia Drugs
Cirrhosis and alfentanil

—Alfentanil is 99% metabolized in the liver. Patients with cirrhosis, therefore, show as much as a 50% reduction in clearance of alfentanil and can have a doubling of its half-life.

—Patients with liver disease therefore may show prolonged effects from alfentanil.

Cirrhosis and aminophylline, theophylline

—Patients with severe liver disease (cirrhosis) or congestive heart failure may require reduced maintenance doses of theophylline (or its more water-soluble derivative, aminophylline). Initial loading doses for untreated patients, however, do not usually require adjustment.

—Reduction in maintenance dosing in the above type of patient is necessary because metabolism of theophylline takes place primarily in the liver.

Cirrhosis and atracurium

—Age, obesity, and liver or renal dysfunction have no significant effect on metabolism of atracurium.

—Atracurium is metabolized by Hoffman elimination as well as ester hydrolysis.

—Hoffman elimination is a nonenzymatic process that occurs at physiologic temperatures and pH. Ester hydrolysis occurs most rapidly in an acid pH and does not require plasma pseudocholinesterase.

Cirrhosis and benzodiazepines (chlordiazepoxide, diazepam, lorazepam, midazolam)

—The benzodiazepines are metabolized extensively in the liver and patients with cirrhosis will demonstrate more prolonged effects of this class of drugs.

Cirrhosis and buprenorphine

—Elimination of buprenorphine is dependent on hepatic metabolism and patients with liver dysfunction will experience prolonged effects from normal doses of buprenorphine.

Cirrhosis and butorphanol

—Butorphanol should be used in reduced dosages in patients with hepatic or renal dysfunction due to the routes of metabolism and excretion of this drug.

Cirrhosis and cimetidine

—Cimetidine is dependent on renal excretion and hepatic metabolism. In patients with renal or hepatic dysfunction, cimetidine accumulation can occur, requiring longer intervals between doses (12 hours versus 6–8 hours).

Cirrhosis and diltiazem

—Elimination of diltiazem depends on hepatic metabolism and urinary excretion. Patients with impaired hepatic or renal function may experience more pronounced effects at usual doses.

Cirrhosis and muscle relaxants (doxacurium, mivacurium, vecuronium, pancuronium, rocuronium, and tubocurarine)

—Prolonged neuromuscular blockade in patients with liver disease can be seen with doxacurium, mivacurium, vecuronium, pancuronium, rocuronium, and tubocurarine.

—This interaction is complex and may be due to decreased clearance, decreased hepatic uptake of the agent, or decreased synthesis of enzymes important for degradation of the neuromuscular blocker. An example of the latter is prolongation of mivacurium's duration of action as a result of decreased plasma cholinesterase from severe liver disease.

—Because of the increased volume of distribution of many drugs seen in patients with liver disease, initial doses of muscle relaxants may need to be larger than in healthy patients. Once neuromuscular blockade is achieved, recovery may be prolonged.

Cirrhosis and meperidine

—Elimination of meperidine depends mainly on hepatic metabolism with some renal excretion. Patients with hepatic dysfunction may have drug accumulation after repeated high doses of meperidine.

Cirrhosis and succinylcholine

—Termination of the effect of succinylcholine is dependent on plasma pseudocholinesterase that is synthesized in the liver. However, even in severe liver disease, plasma pseudocholinesterase levels are not depressed enough to prolong the effects of succinylcholine.

—Mivacurium is also cleared by plasma cholinesterase, but there is evidence that there is significant prolongation of action of mivacurium in patients with severe liver disease.

CONGESTIVE HEART FAILURE

—Congestive heart failure (CHF) describes the inability of the heart to adequately maintain circulation of blood. The causes of CHF may be cardiac disease or noncardiac disease.

—Cardiac causes of CHF may be decreased myocardial contractility (ischemic heart disease, cardiomyopathy, medications) or valvular disease.

—Decreased contractility describes a heart that can do less work for a given volume than a normal heart.

—Improved cardiac contractility results from sympathetic nervous stimulation or treatment with medications such as catecholamines, dopamine, or dobutamine.

—Drugs or anesthetics that are myocardial depressants can precipitate clinical CHF in patients with borderline cardiac function.

—Valvular heart disease can place a volume overload on the heart (as in aortic or mitral insufficiency) or a pressure overload (as in aortic stenosis), which can cause cardiac decompensation and failure.

—Noncardiac causes of congestive heart failure include disorders that cause failure by placing an excessive demand on the heart. Severe volume loss, anemia, hypermetabolic states (thyrotoxicosis), or peripheral shunting (as in septic shock) are some examples.

Congestive Heart Failure Interactions with Anesthesia Drugs
Congestive heart failure and amrinone

—Patients with congestive heart failure and/or compromised renal function may have higher than expected serum concentrations of amrinone during infusion of the drug. This occurs because excretion of amrinone is primarily via the urine.

—Evidence of excessive levels of amrinone may be hypotension or ventricular arrhythmias.

Congestive heart failure and calcium channel blockers (diltiazem, nicardipine, nifedipine, verapamil)

—Some calcium channel blockers have negative inotropic activity (decreased myocardial contractility) and can worsen or precipitate congestive heart failure.

—Verapamil should be avoided in patients with impaired ventricular function. Although diltiazem and nicardipine have less potent negative inotropic effect than verapamil, they should be used cautiously in patients with decreased ventricular function.

—Nifedipine appears to have only slight negative inotropic actions.

Congestive heart failure and aminophylline, theophylline

—Patients with severe liver disease (cirrhosis) or congestive heart failure may require reduced maintenance doses of theophylline (or its more water-soluble derivative, aminophylline). Initial loading doses for untreated patients, however, do not usually require adjustment.

—Reduction in maintenance dosing in the above type of patient is necessary because metabolism of theophylline takes place primarily in the liver.

Congestive heart failure and beta blockers (esmolol, labetalol, propranolol)

—Beta blockers can precipitate congestive heart failure in patients with compromised cardiac function. In patients in congestive heart failure, there may be deterioration in cardiac status. The exception to these consequences might be the situation in which tachyarrhythmias may be precipitating acute cardiac decompensation by increasing the myocardial oxygen demand.

—Beta 1 adrenergic blockade reduces heart rate, myocardial contractility, and, therefore, cardiac ouput. Also, atrioventricular node conduction time is prolonged and sinus node automaticity are decreased.

Congestive heart failure and ketamine

—Ketamine has significant cardiovascular stimulatory effects, which usually contraindicate its use in patients with congestive heart failure from ischemic heart disease.

—Cardiovascular stimulation by ketamine is a result of central nervous stimulation and inhibition of neuronal norepinephrine reuptake. The consequence of these actions is an increase in cardiac output, heart rate, and peripheral vasoconstriction. Additionally, ketamine can cause an increase in pulmonary vascular resistance, placing added strain on the right ventricle.

—Some patients are resistant to indirect cardiovascular stimulation, such as those with septic shock or chronic congestive heart failure. In these patients, the direct myocardial depressant effects of ketamine may be evident.

Congestive heart failure and ketorolac

—Ketorolac (a prostaglandin synthesis inhibitor) can worsen renal function in patients whose compromised renal function is very dependent on the presence of vasodilatory prostaglandins.

—Patients at risk for this interaction are those with renal dysfunction as a result of renal disease or advanced age (>65 years old) or poor renal perfusion from congestive heart failure or hypovolemia.

Congestive heart failure and lidocaine

—Because elimination of lidocaine depends on liver metabolism, conditions that decrease liver blood flow (congestive heart failure) can result in prolonged elimination times.

CORONARY ARTERY DISEASE

—Disease of the coronary arteries can be manifested in different or combined ways: angina, myocardial infarction (MI), arrhythmias, or sudden cardiac death from ventricular fibrillation or tachycardia that is not associated with prior symptoms or MI.

—In patients with no history of previous MI, the risks of perioperative MI (within 72 hours of surgery) for noncardiac surgery are approximately 0.13%.

—For patients with a history of previous MI, the risks for perioperative MI are considerably greater and have been reviewed in a number of studies. Some of the older studies (from 1964 to 1978) indicated that for surgery within 3 months of a MI, the risks for re-infarction could be as high as 37%. More recent studies have shown much lower risks of approximately 6% within 3 months of MI, and 2.5% for noncardiac surgery 4–6 months following the MI. After 6 months, the risk appears to decrease to about 1.5%, which is still almost 10 times the risk for perioperative infarction of patients without evidence of prior MI.

—The reduced risk of perioperative MI shown in the more recent investigations has been attributed to more skillful surgical and anesthetic management both intraoperatively and postoperatively. For example, the increased use of invasive monitors such as pulmonary artery catheters has allowed earlier identification and treatment of impending cardiac problems.

—Risk of MI in the perioperative period is also influenced by the type of surgical procedure. For example, while the risks appear to be high for patients undergoing vascular procedures, patients having ophthalmic operations have a much lower risk.

Coronary Artery Disease Interactions with Anesthesia Drugs

Coronary artery disease and ketamine

—Ketamine has significant, mostly stimulatory, effects on the cardiovascular system. Cardiovascular stimulation in patients with coronary artery disease can cause an undesirable increase in myocardial oxygen demand.

—Other clinical situations in which ketamine would be contraindicated because of the cardiovascular stimulation are aortic or intracranial aneurysms, thyrotoxicosis, and inadequately controlled hypertension.

—Ketamine causes an increase in heart rate, cardiac output, and arterial pressure (as much as 25%) by stimulation of the CNS and inhibition of neuronal norepinephrine reuptake.

—In severely ill patients, such as those in septic shock, or in chronic congestive heart failure, the cardiovascular system is resistant to indirect stimulation. In these cases, the direct myocardial depressant effects of ketamine may be manifested by hypotension.

DIABETES MELLITUS

—Diabetes mellitus is a complex disease whose most obvious characteristic is an abnormality of glucose metabolism resulting in hyperglycemia.

—Type I, or insulin-dependent diabetes, usually begins in childhood or adolescence, whereas type II, or non-insulin-dependent diabetes, begins later in life. Type II diabetics may require insulin therapy but are more resistant to development of ketoacidosis than type I diabetics.

—Insulin therapy for insulin-dependent diabetics can be from bovine, porcine, or human (using recombinant DNA techniques) sources. How these insulin sources are formulated with other substances determines the onset of action and duration.

—The two most frequently used preparations are NPH (neutral protamine Hagedorn) and Lente insulin. NPH insulin is a suspension of insulin containing zinc, protamine, and a phosphate buffer. Lente insulin contains no protamine. The other form of insulin that contains protamine is the slow-onset PZI (protamine zinc insulin).

—The presence of protamine in some of the above preparations has been implicated in allergic reactions to protamine used after cardiopulmonary bypass to reverse heparin. It has been suggested that the protamine in these insulin preparations used chronically in insulin-dependent diabetics may stimulate antibody formation. However, there is some controversy as to whether protamine exposure from insulin increases a patient's risk of such a reaction.

—Patients who are allergic to seafood may be at increased risk for anaphylactic reactions to protamine because protamine is derived from salmon sperm.

—There is no clear documentation that vasectomy or infertility in men is associated with an increased risk of allergic reactions with protamine, even though these patients do have circulating antibodies to spermatozoa.

Diabetes Mellitus Interactions with Anesthesia Drugs
Diabetes mellitus and protamine

—The presence of protamine in some insulin preparations has been implicated in allergic reactions to protamine used after cardiopulmonary bypass to reverse heparin. It has been suggested that the protamine in these insulin preparations used chronically in insulin-dependent diabetics may stimulate antibody formation. However, there is some controversy as to whether protamine exposure from insulin increases a patient's risk of such a reaction.

—The two most frequently used preparations are NPH (neutral protamine Hagedorn) and Lente insulin. NPH insulin is a suspension of insulin containing zinc, protamine, and a phosphate buffer. Lente insulin contains no protamine. The other form of insulin that contains protamine is the slow onset, PZI (protamine zinc insulin).

EATON–LAMBERT SYNDROME

—Eaton–Lambert syndrome is clinically similar to myasthenia gravis. It is a rare disorder that is usually associated with carcinoma (especially small cell carcinoma of the lung), but can occur in patients without cancer.

—Like myasthenia gravis, Eaton–Lambert syndrome may be an autoimmune disease, but one that affects the presynaptic membrane rather than the acetylcholine receptors that are affected in myasthenia gravis.

—Patients with Eaton–Lambert syndrome are very sensitive to both depolarizing and non-depolarizing neuromuscular blocking agents. As a result, patients with this syndrome may have prolonged blockade with normal doses of these agents.

—Sometimes the diagnosis of this syndrome is made at the time of surgical evaluation or removal of pulmonary tumors when there is unexpected, prolonged neuromuscular blockade.

—Anticholinesterases are unreliable in reversing the muscle blockade.

Eaton–Lambert Syndrome Interactions with Anesthesia Drugs

Eaton–Lambert syndrome and muscle relaxants (atracurium, doxacurium, gallamine, metocurine, mivacurium, pancuronium, pipercuronium, rocuronium, succinylcholine, tubocurarine, vecuronium)

—Patients with Eaton–Lambert syndrome are very sensitive to both depolarizing and non-depolarizing neuromuscular blockade.

—This disorder is similar to myasthenia gravis and patients complain of skeletal muscle weakness, but it is usually associated with carcinoma (especially small cell tumors of the lung).

—If the diagnosis is known or suspected prior to surgery, reduced doses of muscle relaxants should be used; however, sometimes the diagnosis is first made when a patient has surgery for a lung tumor and has an unexpected, prolonged neuromuscular block.

—Anticholinesterases are unreliable in reversing muscle weakness.

Eaton–Lambert syndrome and edrophonium, neostigmine, pyridostigmine

—Anticholinesterases are unreliable in reversing the muscle relaxation of non-depolarizing agents in patients with Eaton–Lambert syndrome.

—Patients with this syndrome may experience prolonged neuromuscular blockade with both nondepolarizing and depolarizing agents.

EPILEPSY

—Epilepsy is a disorder of neurons in the brain that is characterized by episodes of brain dysfunction, frequently with alterations in the level of consciousness.

—It is believed that seizures begin as a focal, synchronous discharge of a group of neurons. If the discharge remains localized, a focal seizure results. Wide propagation of the discharge results in generalized seizures.

—Epilepsy that begins in childhood is usually idiopathic, whereas seizures that occur in an adult are more likely to be associated with a focal brain disease such as tumor, trauma, infection, stroke, or withdrawal from alcohol or drugs.

—Although up to 5% of the population may experience a non-febrile seizure at some point during their life, only 0.5–1% of the population has a chronic seizure disorder.

—Drugs or anesthetics used by anesthesiologists or nurse-anesthetists that have been demonstrated to lower the seizure threshold include ethrane, propofol, and doxapram.

Epilepsy Interactions with Anesthesia Drugs

Epilepsy and doxapram HCl

—Because of its mechanism of action, doxapram is contraindicated in a number of conditions, such as hypertension, convulsive disorders, hyperthyroidism, cerebral edema, and pheochromocytoma.

—Analeptic agents, such as doxapram, are CNS stimulants. These agents improve ventilation through their effect on the brainstem and, in the case of doxapram, the carotid chemoreceptors.

Epilepsy and enflurane

—Although there is considerable controversy about the ability of enflurane to elicit clinically significant seizures, most recommendations are to avoid enflurane in patients with such disorders.

—At high concentrations of enflurane (2.5%) and/or low pCO_2 (<25 torr), the likelihood of seizure activity is highest. Facial twitching as well as limb muscle contraction has been associated with electroencephalographic changes in both normal and epileptic patients.

—Characteristic changes in the EEG consist of high frequency and voltage pattern progressing to spike and dome complexes. Electrical seizure activity has been documented, however, not only at high concentrations but at concentrations as low as 1% in normal children.

Epilepsy and propofol

—There are several reports of seizure activity or opisthotonus (tetanic spasm of back and neck) in postoperative patients who had received propofol. The mechanism of this adverse reaction is unknown and is very rare.

—The seizures or opisthotonus have been transient in most patients, but lasted 1–3 weeks in two European patients.

GLAUCOMA

—Glaucoma is a disease of the eyes characterized by increased intraocular pressure that is due to decreased outflow of aqueous humor.

—Angle closure glaucoma is a result of a congenital narrowing of the anterior chamber angle that makes patients more susceptible to angle closure, preventing drainage of aqueous humor. Although acute medical management of this disorder may be required, the definitive management is surgical correction.

—Open angle glaucoma is more common and is a chronic disease requiring medical management. Therapy is designed to reduce formation of aqueous humor (carbonic anhydrase inhibitors, beta blockers) or increase outflow by opening the anterior chamber angle through pupillary constriction (parasympathomimetics).

—Some of the parasympathomimetic agents are also anticholinesterases (echothiophate, isoflurophate, demecarium) and result in reduced plasma pseudocholinesterase. Succinylcholine and ester-type local anesthetics are affected by this interaction.

—Other parasympathomimetics act as miotic agents (causing pupillary constriction). Parasympatholytic agents can produce midriasis (pupillary dilation) and potentially exacerbate glaucoma, mainly in patients with angle closure glaucoma.

—Parasympatholytics used in anesthesia are atropine, scopolamine, and glycopyrrolate. Only scopolamine has been demonstrated to cause significant pupillary dilation in clinically used doses.

—Topically applied, noncardioselective beta blockers used for control of glaucoma can be absorbed systemically. Timolol has been identified as a cause of intraoperative bradycardia and hypotension that may be refractory to treatment with atropine.

—Preoperatively, scopolamine should be avoided because it can cause pupillary dilation, even in the transdermal form at clinical doses. As a result of pupillary dilation, significant increases in intraocular pressures can occur in patients with angle closure glaucoma. Patients with open angle glaucoma rarely experience this interaction.

Glaucoma Interactions with Anesthesia Drugs
Glaucoma and atropine
—Pupillary dilation can result in increased intraocular pressure in patients with angle closure glaucoma. At doses normally used clinically for atropine, this effect is not usually significant.

—Scopolamine, even in the form of transdermal patches, can produce significant increases in intraocular pressure in patients with narrow angle glaucoma.

Glaucoma and general anesthesia
—There are several considerations when anesthetizing a patient with glaucoma. Of the two types of glaucoma (open

angle and angle closure), the open angle form is more common.

—Preoperatively, scopolamine should be avoided because it can cause pupillary dilation, even in the transdermal form at clinical doses. As a result of pupillary dilation, significant increases in intraocular pressures can occur in patients with angle closure glaucoma. Patients with open angle glaucoma rarely experience this interaction.

—Atropine and glycopyrrolate are also parasympathomimetics like scopolamine. At doses used in anesthesia, only scopolamine has significant effects on pupillary size.

—Patients with open angle glaucoma may be treated with beta blockers. Such patients have experienced bradycardia and hypotension during surgery that is refractory to treatment with atropine.

—Other patients with this form of glaucoma may receive parasympathomimetics whose mechanism of action is through inhibition of acetylcholinesterase. Drugs used in anesthesia that depend on plasma cholinesterases for metabolism (succinylcholine, mivacurium, ester-type local anesthetics) may have altered, prolonged effects.

Glaucoma and scopolamine

—Scopolamine, even in the form of transdermal patches, may cause significant increases in intraocular pressure in patients with narrow angle glaucoma. Patients with open angle glaucoma rarely experience a significant increase in intraocular pressure with scopolamine.

Glaucoma and succinylcholine

—Succinylcholine can be used safely in certain patients with glaucoma. Although succinylcholine causes an increase in intraocular pressure, this pressure increase is transient.

—More importantly, certain medications used for treatment of glaucoma are anticholinesterases and can prolong the effect of succinylcholine due to a decrease in plasma cholinesterase. These miotic agents are echothiophate, demecarium bromide, and isoflurophate.

GUILLAIN–BARRÉ SYNDROME

—Guillain–Barré syndrome (acute idiopathic polyneuritis) is an inflammatory disease of the peripheral nervous system.

—It is believed to be a postinfectious complication in most cases with approximately 65% of patients having evidence of viral infection within 8 weeks prior to the onset of symptoms.

—Initially, symptoms of muscle weakness in the legs is then followed by weakness in the trunk and arms. Weakness of intercostal muscles may be severe enough to require ventilatory support. Occasionally, sensory nerves are involved and paresthesias precede symptoms of motor nerve demyelination.

—50% of patients have bulbar involvement with facial weakness and difficulty swallowing.

—Typically, weakness progresses for approximately 1 or 2 weeks and then stabilizes followed by gradual improvement.

—Patients with Guillain–Barré syndrome are at risk for severe hyperkalemia if given succinylcholine. It is believed that patients with upper or lower motor neuron disease develop extrajunctional acetylcholine receptors that result in release of potassium when exposed to the depolarizing neuromuscular blocker.

Guillain–Barré Interactions with Anesthesia Drugs
Guillain–Barré syndrome and succinylcholine

—Chronic or progressive motor neuron disease places patients at continuous risk for hyperkalemia from succinylcholine. Syringomyelia, amyotrophic lateral sclerosis, multiple sclerosis, acute idiopathic polyneuritis (Guillain–Barré syndrome), and all forms of muscular dystrophy have been associated with this response.

—Patients with neuromuscular disease (upper and lower motor neuron abnormalities) can respond to succinylcholine with a dangerous, sometimes fatal, hyperkalemia. This occurs probably because of proliferation of extrajunctional acetylcholine receptors on the muscle membrane. Depolarization of these receptors causes potassium leak through the muscle membrane.

HALOTHANE HEPATITIS

—Halothane anesthesia has been associated with two distinct forms of postanesthetic hepatic toxicity. The more common form is a nonspecific hepatitis characterized by mild elevation of aminotransferases. The fulminant hepatic necrosis associated with halothane occurs in 1 in 22,000–35,000 administrations according to the National Halothane Study, a retrospective study of 850,000 surgical patients.

—Fulminant hepatic necrosis following halothane administration is believed to be an immunologic reaction. Antibodies to hepatocytes are formed from an interaction between halothane metabolites (trifluoroacetyl halide) and liver microsomal proteins.

—Onset of symptoms from fulminant hepatitis usually begins within 7 days and consists of nonspecific signs such as fever, elevated aminotransferases, rash, arthralgias, and eosinophilia. Pathologically, halothane hepatitis produces a nonspecific, centrilobular necrosis.

—Patients identified to be at higher risk for developing hepatic necrosis are those with repeated exposures to halothane, especially within 4 weeks, and middle-aged, obese females.

—Although uncommon, massive hepatic necrosis does occur in pediatric patients.

—Enflurane, isoflurane, nitrous oxide, desflurane, and sevoflurane have not been demonstrated to cause fulminant hepatic necrosis.

Halothane Hepatitis Interactions with Anesthesia Drugs
Halothane hepatitis and halothane

—Mild elevation of liver enzymes may occur in up to 20% of patients who have multiple exposures to halothane and perhaps other anesthetic agents. One in 35,000–40,000 patients exposed to halothane may develop a fulminant and fatal hepatic necrosis.

—Fatal hepatitis associated with halothane may begin 1 day to 2 weeks following halothane administration. The syndrome consists of fever, anorexia, nausea, and, sometimes, rash. Marked eosinophilia, elevated liver enzymes, and hyperbilirubinemia accompanies the severe hepatic necrosis.

—The National Halothane Study was unable to identify a clear-cut histologic lesion associated with hepatitis from halothane and the precise mechanism for this disorder is unknown.

—Use of halothane in pediatric patients, and even repeat use after short intervals, has not been associated with the liver dysfunctions described above.

HEART BLOCK

—Atrioventricular (AV) heart block can be classified in two ways: anatomically based on His bundle electrocardiography and, more common clinically, that based on the standard electrocardiogram.

—First-degree AV block is defined by the clinical method as a P-R interval greater than 0.2 second at a heart rate of 70. It is usually caused by degenerative changes in the AV node from aging but may be associated with digitalis, ischemia from coronary artery disease, or inflammatory conditions such as myocarditis.

—Second-degree AV block can be either Mobitz type I (Wenckebach) or Mobitz type II. Mobitz I block is characterized by progressive P-R prolongation resulting in a dropped QRS. It is considered a more benign disorder than Mobitz II block and is a result of intranodal disease. Mobitz I block rarely progresses to complete (third degree) AV block.

—Mobitz type II block manifests as a sudden interruption of AV conduction resulting in a dropped QRS without the warning seen in Wenckebach block. Type II block frequently progresses to complete heart block and is a result of infranodal disease (below the AV node).

—Third-degree AV block may be nodal or infranodal. Most commonly, the cause of third-degree block is fibrous degenerative changes in the conduction system. Acute myocardial infarction (MI) can cause this type of block. Posterior or inferior MI tends to cause nodal block, while inferior MI is associated with infranodal block. Other causes include infection (myocarditis), inflammatory conditions (rheumatic fever), or medications (digitalis).

—In this disorder, all atrial beats are blocked and ventricular depolarization occurs either in the AV node (if the block is at the nodal level) or below the AV node (if the block is infranodal).

—Third-degree block with a narrow QRS indicates escape beats originating in the AV node, normally at a rate of 45–55 beats/min. Infranodal block will produce a wide QRS with escape rates of 30–40 beats/min.

Heart Block Interactions with Anesthesia Drugs
Heart block and diphenylhydantoin, phenytoin

—The antiarrhythmic properties of diphenylhydantoin involve a decrease in automaticity as well as a decrease in excitability of Purkinje fibers. Because of this effect, phenytoin is contraindicated in patients with sinus bradycardia, sinoatrial block, as well as patients with second- and third-degree heart block, or with Stokes–Adams syndrome.

Heart block and beta blockers (esmolol, labetalol, propranolol)

—Beta blockers are contraindicated in patients with heart block greater than first degree or in patients with severe bradycardia or sick sinus syndrome.

—Blockade of beta 1 receptors results in decreased heart rate and contractility.

HEPATITIS

—Hepatitis is inflammation of the liver. Usually, the cause is viral infection, but toxins such as alcohol and many drugs can also cause hepatitis.

—The presence of hepatitis or any liver disease has been shown to increase the morbidity and mortality in patients receiving anesthesia. The mechanism of this increase in morbidity and mortality is not clear but is most likely related to changes in hepatic blood flow as a result of anesthesia and surgery.

—All forms of anesthesia, including general, regional, and nitrous-narcotic, can cause postoperative changes in liver function tests, although in most cases the changes are transient. Since there is no known method of avoiding exacerbation of preexisting liver disease by anesthesia, most recommendations are to postpone surgery in patients suspected of having acute hepatitis.

—In patients with portal hypertension from chronic liver disease, postoperative mortality can be related to specific laboratory tests; when preoperative serum albumin concentrations are <3 g/dL, bilirubin levels are >3 mg/dL, and there exist ascites and encephalopathy, mortality may reach 50%. When the serum albumin levels are above 3 g/dL, bilirubin is below 3 mg/dL, and there is no ascites or encephalopathy, mortality is about 10 %.

Hepatitis Interactions with Anesthesia Drugs
Hepatitis and inhalational anesthetics (desflurane, enflurane, halothane, isoflurane, nitrous oxide, sevoflurane)

—All forms of anesthesia, including general, regional, and nitrous-narcotic, are associated with postoperative liver function test abnormalities. The exact mechanism of this reaction is not known but is likely related to reduced liver blood flow from anesthesia and surgery.

—The presence of hepatitis or any liver disease has been shown to increase the morbidity and mortality in patients receiving anesthesia. The mechanism of this increase in morbidity and mortality is not clear but is most likely related to changes in hepatic blood flow as a result of anesthesia and surgery.

—Because there is no known method of avoiding exacerbation of preexisting liver disease by anesthesia, most recommendations are to postpone surgery in patients suspected of having acute hepatitis.

—There is no evidence that enflurane, isoflurane, desflurane, or sevoflurane is hepatotoxic. Halothane, however, can occasionally cause fulminant hepatic necrosis in both adults and children. A milder form of hepatotoxicity is also seen with halothane anesthesia.

HERPES SIMPLEX

—The herpesviruses consist of six different human types and several different animal viruses. The human herpesviruses are herpes simplex types 1 and 2, varicella zoster, cytomegalovirus, Epstein–Barr, and herpesvirus type 6.

—The human herpesviruses can cause acute infections followed by latent periods. During these latent periods, the virus remains dormant in different locations, depending on the type of virus. The herpes simplex and varicella zoster viruses persist in neural ganglion cells, whereas Epstein–Barr virus persists in B cells, and cytomegalovirus can persist in several different cells.

—HSV-1 infections are transmitted mainly by direct contact with infected secretions. Primary infection is usually asymptomatic, especially in patients younger than 5 years of age. When symptoms occur in this age patient or older patients, they may be in the form of gingivostomatitis, pharyngitis, or tonsillitis. The pharyngitis consists of small vesicles on the oral mucosa and palate. Primary infection can be associated with systemic symptoms which may be severe.

—HSV-2 is the most common cause (70–90% of cases) of genital herpes. However, a small number of cases are associated with HSV-1 virus. Also, HSV-2 virus can cause oral, pharyngeal, or labial (lip) infection.

—Recurrent disease with either HSV-1 or HS-2 is usually milder than symptomatic primary infections. Oral–labial recurrence is characterized by local pain or tingling and can be associated with exposure to sunlight, emotional stress, or menstruation. Additionally, there have been reports of recurrent herpes labialis from epidural or intrathecal morphine.

Herpes Simplex Interactions with Anesthesia Drugs
Herpes simplex and morphine

—There are several reports of patients receiving epidural morphine who developed reactivation of herpes labialis (oral herpes; herpes simplex virus, type 1).

—In addition, several studies suggested a possible central triggering mechanism for this interaction, though no definite relationship has been proven.

—The original case report involved children who had received subarachnoid morphine.

—There is some controversy about this, since activation of HSV can result from other causes including infections, fever, emotional or physical stress, and surgery.

—Also a high percentage of herpes-infected women experience recurrence in the peripartum period even without having received epidural or intrathecal narcotics.

HYPERTENSION

—Hypertension is classified as primary (essential) or secondary. Primary hypertension has no known cause and accounts for over 90% of patients with high blood pressure. Secondary hypertension has many causes including renal disease, pheochromocytoma, medications, and coarctation.

—Morbidity and mortality increase linearly with increasing levels of either systolic or diastolic hypertension. The levels of blood pressure below are associated with a 50% increase in mortality over normotensive levels (this refers to lifetime statistics, not peri-operative):

—130/90 mm/Hg for men <45 years old
—145/95 mm/Hg for men >45 years old
—160/95 mm/Hg for all women

For children and adolescents, upper limits of normal blood pressure are:

—116/76 mm/Hg for age 3–5
—122/78 mm/Hg for age 6–9
—126/82 mm/Hg for age 10–12
—136/86 mm/Hg for age 13–15
—142/92 mm/Hg for age 16–18

—The question of preoperative treatment of hypertension and its effect on postoperative morbidity has been examined in a number of studies. However, due to the complexity of this problem and deficiencies in the design of these studies, clear conclusions cannot be stated with certainty. (For a complete analysis of the studies, see Ronald D. Miller, *Anesthesia*.)

—Patients with hypertension have been shown to experience greater fluctuations in blood pressure during anesthesia. Though treated patients also experience such fluctuations, they occur less frequently than in nontreated patients.

—Also, the studies did show that patients with hypertension have a significantly increased morbidity compared to nonhypertensive patients.

Hypertension Interaction with Anesthesia Drugs

Hypertension and benzquinamide

—Benzquinamide has been associated with sudden increases in blood pressure when given rapidly intravenously. This may place patients with underlying hypertension at particular risk and should be used cautiously.

Hypertension and doxapram HCl

—Because of its mechanism of action, doxapram is contraindicated in a number of conditions, such as hypertension, convulsive disorders, hyperthyroidism, cerebral edema, and pheochromocytoma.

—Analeptic agents, such as doxapram, are CNS stimulants. Because CNS stimulation can elevate arterial pressure, decrease seizure thresholds, and have additive stimulatory effects in conditions such as the above disorders, doxapram is contraindicated in patients with these underlying conditions.

—Analeptic agents improve ventilation through their effect on the brain stem and, in the case of doxapram, the carotid chemoreceptors.

Hypertension and ketamine

—Ketamine should be used cautiously in patients with hypertension, especially those with inadequate control.

—Ketamine causes hypertension by indirect cardiovascular stimulation, by inhibition of neuronal reuptake of norepinephrine, and by peripheral vasoconstriction.

—Some of the cardiovascular effects can be blunted by administering benzodiazepines and/or labetalol.

Hypertension and methylergonovine

—Patients with hypertension are at highest risk for severe hypertensive reactions to ergot alkaloids such as methylergonovine.

—If stimulation of uterine muscle tone is necessary in these patients, a dilute solution of oxytocin may be preferable.

HYPERTHYROIDISM

—Hyperthyroidism refers to any condition in which a patient is exposed to a supraphysiologic amount of thyroid hormone.

—Most commonly, the cause of hyperthyroidism is Grave's disease. This disorder is felt to be probably of autoimmune origin and occurs more commonly in young adult females. Clinically, these patients experience palpitations, nervousness, insomnia, weight loss, proptosis, and goiter.

—Other causes of hyperthyroidism include pregnancy, thyroiditis, and adenomas of the thyroid or pituitary glands.

—Thyroid hormone affects most tissues in the body by causing an increase in the basal metabolic rate, but of particular concern to the anesthesiologist are its effects on the cardiovascular system and skeletal muscle.

—Increased metabolism in the tissues from thyroid hormone stimulation results in vasodilation because of the requirement for increased blood flow to remove metabolic byproducts. As a result, cardiac output must increase, sometimes by as much as 50% or more.

—Additionally, thyroid hormone may have direct effects on the heart. In some stages, stimulation is evident by an increase in heart rate and contractility in excess of the demands for cardiac output.

—Myocardial failure occurs in some patients from a depressant effect of thyroid hormone on the myocardium. This may be related to excessive protein metabolism induced by thyroid hormone or a result of excessive cardiac demands from the increased metabolic rate.

—Careful use or avoidance of anesthetic agents that cause sympathetic stimulation (ketamine, catecholamines, dopram) is recommended for hyperthyroid patients, even those receiving treatment for the disorder.

—Muscle weakness is commonly seen with hyperthyroidism and affects proximal muscles, usually sparing respiratory function. In some cases, myopathy is the dominant feature of thyroid hormone excess and can resemble myasthenia. Lower doses of muscle relaxants may be indicated.

—Thyroid storm is a life-threatening exacerbation of hyperthyroidism. It results from sudden release of thyroid hormone as a consequence of trauma, illness, or surgery. When caused by surgery, it may occur intraoperatively, but it usually occurs on the first postoperative day.

—Clinically similar to malignant hyperthermia, patients experience hyperpyrexia, tachycardia, altered consciousness, and even cardiac failure. Treatment includes beta blockers (esmolol), antithyroid medications, iodine, and corticosteroids.

Hyperthyroidism Interactions with Anesthesia Drugs
Hyperthyroidism and doxapram HCl
—Because of its mechanism of action, doxapram is contraindicated in a number of conditions, such as hypertension, convulsive disorders, hyperthyroidism, cerebral edema, and pheochromocytoma.

—Analeptic agents, such as doxapram, are CNS stimulants. Because CNS stimulation can elevate arterial pressure, decrease seizure thresholds, and have additive stimulatory effects in conditions such as the above disorders, doxapram is contraindicated in patients with these underlying conditions.

—Analeptic agents improve ventilation through their effect on the brainstem and, in the case of doxapram, the carotid chemoreceptors.

Hyperthyroidism and muscle relaxants (atracurium, doxacurium, gallamine, metocurine, mivacurium, pancuronium, pipercuronium, rocuronium, tubocurarine, vecuronium)
—Muscle weakness is commonly seen with hyperthyroidism and affects proximal muscles, usually sparing respiratory function. In some cases, myopathy is the dominant feature of thyroid hormone excess and can resemble myasthenia. Lower doses of muscle relaxants may be indicated.

Hyperthyroidism and vasopressors (ephedrine, epinephrine, metaraminol, methoxamine, norepinephrine, phenylephrine)
—Agents that stimulate the sympathetic nervous system (catecholamines, ephedrine, phenylephrine, dopram, ketamine) may have exaggerated effects in patients with hyperthyroidism. Although most evident in untreated patients, even patients receiving treatment for excess thyroid hormone may demonstrate this response.

—Excess thyroid hormone causes stimulation of metabolism of most body tissues. As a result, cardiac output increases by 50% or more to remove the extra metabolic byproducts. Also, direct stimulatory effects on the myocardium at even slightly elevated thyroid hormone levels cause tachycardia and increased contractility.

—At higher thyroid hormone levels, myocardial depression may occur as a result of excess demands or a direct myocardial depression.

Hyperthyroidism and ketamine

—Like other medications that stimulate the sympathetic nervous system, ketamine can result in exaggerated effects in patients with hyperthyroidism.

—Although most evident in untreated patients, even patients receiving treatment for excess thyroid hormone may demonstrate this response.

—Excess thyroid hormone causes stimulation of metabolism of most body tissues. As a result, cardiac output increases by 50% or more to remove the extra metabolic byproducts. Also, direct stimulatory effects on the myocardium at even slightly elevated thyroid hormone levels cause tachycardia and increased contractility.

HYPOCALCEMIA

—Normal serum total calcium levels are 9–10 mg/dL. Approximately half of calcium is bound to serum albumin, whereas 40–50% of total calcium exists in ionic form and constitutes the physiologically active form of calcium.

—The most common cause of hypocalcemia is hypoalbuminemia. Other causes include hypoparathyroidism, hypomagnesemia (sepsis, malnutrition), acute pancreatitis, and chronic renal disease. Radiographic contrast media may lower serum calcium through chelation by edetate or citrate.

—Low serum calcium levels are associated with increasing excitability of the nervous system as a result of increased neuronal membrane permeability to sodium ions. Alkalosis resulting from hyperventilation can reduce the ionized calcium level enough to elicit signs of hypocalcemia (tetany, laryngospasm, seizures).

—At the neuromuscular junction, calcium is responsible for release of acetylcholine when the motor nerve is stimulated by a nerve action potential. Decreased levels of ionized calcium may potentiate non-depolarizing neuromuscular blockade and may impair its reversal with anticholinesterases.

—Calcium channel-blocking agents have not been convincingly demonstrated to interfere with the function of the neuromuscular junction. This may be due to the fact that these agents affect calcium transport through different channels than those necessary for acetylcholine release at the neuromuscular junction.

Hypocalcemia Interactions with Anesthesia Drugs
Hypocalcemia and edrophonium, pyridostigmine, neostigmine
—Reversal of neuromuscular blockade can be impaired in the presence of hypocalcemia.
—Stimulation of a motor nerve causes a nerve action potential which allows entry of calcium into the nerve ending. The calcium appears to cause release of acetylcholine from vesicles in the nerve ending into the neuromuscular junction, resulting in endplate depolarization.
—In the presence of inadequate ionized calcium, less acetylcholine is released, impairing the ability of acetylcholinesterase inhibitors to overcome the competitive blockade of acetylcholine receptors by neuromuscular blocking agents.

HYPOKALEMIA

—Hypokalemia is defined as a plasma potassium concentration of less than 3.5 meq/L.
—Potassium is lost from the body through the gastrointestinal tract (vomiting, diarrhea, nasogastric suction) or urinary tract (diuretics, hyperglycemia).
—Since 98% of total body potassium is intracellular, measurements of the extracellular potassium may be an inaccurate indication of potassium levels in some cases. Specifically, acute hypokalemia usually reflects potassium losses from the extracellular compartment, whereas potassium levels intracellularly may be normal or increased.
—Chronic hypokalemia can be associated with total body potassium deficits of more than 600 meq, but due to movement of intracellular potassium to the extracellular compartment, serum potassium levels may be near-normal.
—Reversal of neuromuscular blockade in patients with hypokalemia may be more difficult.
—This is thought to be related to an increase in transmembrane muscle potential at the motor endplate as a result of loss of positive potassium ions from the extracellular compartment. Hyperpolarization of the muscle membrane would make it resistant to depolarization and potentiate the action of neuromuscular blocking agents.

—Acute, rather than chronic, hypokalemia is more likely to cause hyperpolarization of muscle membrane because potassium losses would be more from extracellular, rather than intracellular, compartments. Therefore, chronic hypokalemia is unlikely to potentiate neuromuscular blockade.

—Digitalis toxicity is potentiated by hypokalemia.

—This interaction is a result of the fact that digitalis glycosides exert their effect on the heart by binding to the Na-K ATPase enzyme in cardiac tissue and inhibiting this enzyme.

—Studies have shown that binding of digitalis to the Na-K ATPase enzyme is increased in hypokalemia.

—Potassium infusion to patients with digitalis toxicity who are hypokalemic results in decreased binding of digitalis and may decrease cardiotoxicity.

—Caution with potassium infusions must be used, because in patients who have high potassium and digitalis toxicity further increases in serum potassium may worsen heart block associated with toxicity to digitalis.

Hypokalemia Interactions with Anesthesia Drugs
Hypokalemia and digitalis

—Digitalis toxicity is potentiated by hypokalemia.

—This interaction is a result of the fact that digitalis glycosides exert their effect on the heart by binding to the Na-K ATPase enzyme in cardiac tissue and inhibiting this enzyme.

—Studies have shown that binding of digitalis to the Na-K ATPase enzyme is increased in hypokalemia.

—Potassium infusion to patients with digitalis toxicity who are hypokalemic results in decreased binding of digitalis and may decrease cardiotoxicity.

—Caution with potassium infusions must be used due to the fact that in patients who have high potassium and digitalis toxicity further increases in serum potassium may worsen heart block associated with toxicity to digitalis.

Hypokalemia and edrophonium, pyridostigmine, neostigmine

—Reversal of neuromuscular blockade in patients with hypokalemia may be more difficult. Although this has been demonstrated in animal studies, there is some controversy about the clinical importance of hypokalemia in reversal of muscle blockade in humans.

—Hypokalemia, particularly acute hypokalemia, can potentiate non-depolarizing neuromuscular blockers.

Hypokalemia and muscle relaxants (atracurium, doxacurium, gallamine, metocurine, mivacurium, pancuronium, pipercuronium, rocuronium, tubocurarine, vecuronium)

—Hypokalemia appears to potentiate the effects of neuromuscular blockade from non-depolarizing agents.

—The interaction is probably due to hyperpolarization of the muscle endplate and therefore resistance to depolarization. Hyperpolarization would more likely occur with more acute changes in potassium concentration, because the potassium losses would be from the extracellular compartment rather than from intracellular sites.

—Chronic hypokalemia is more likely to be associated with potassium depletion from both extra- and intracellular compartments with no significant change in transmembrane potential. As a result, significant effects on neuromuscular blockade would be less likely.

HYPOTHERMIA

—Normal body temperature is approximately 37°C. Normally, thermoregulatory responses (vasoconstriction, shivering, non-shivering thermogenesis) begin with core temperature drops of as little as 0.2°.

—In contrast, patients receiving general anesthesia of any kind have an impaired thermoregulatory response. In such patients, thermoregulatory responses may not begin until core temperature has decreased by 3 or 4° (to 34° or less).

—The usual pattern of heat loss is a slow reduction in core temperature for 2–4 hours followed by a plateau at 33–35°C. Heat loss occurs primarily by radiation and somewhat by convection.

—Hypothermia can have significant effects on the duration of action of some anesthetic agents. Specifically, non-depolarizing neuromuscular blockers have a longer duration, whereas infusions of propofol may result in increased plasma levels in patients who are hypothermic.

Hypothermia Interactions with Anesthesia Drugs

Hypothermia and muscle relaxants (atracurium, doxacurium, gallamine, metocurine, mivacurium, pancuronium, pipercuronium, rocuronium, tubocurarine, vecuronium)

—Non-depolarizing muscle blockade is prolonged by hypothermia. This interaction is a result of an effect on the neuromuscular blocking agents themselves rather than on the anticholinesterases used to reverse the neuromuscular blocking agents.

—Hypothermia appears to prolong the effect of the non-depolarizing agents by several mechanisms, including delayed metabolism into inactive metabolites as well as delayed excretion via the urinary and biliary routes.

Hypothermia and edrophonium, neostigmine, pyridostigmine

—Non-depolarizing muscle blockade is prolonged by hypothermia. This interaction is a result of an effect on the neuromuscular blocking agents themselves rather than on the anticholinesterases used to reverse the neuromuscular blocking agents.

—Hypothermia appears to prolong the effect of the non-depolarizing agents by several mechanisms, including delayed metabolism into inactive metabolites as well as delayed excretion via the urinary and biliary routes.

Hypothermia and propofol

—Hypothermia can have significant effects on propofol plasma levels.

—Plasma levels of propofol, when administered as a constant infusion, have been shown to be increased by as much as 30% in patients with hypothermia to 34°C.

INTESTINAL OBSTRUCTION

—Several clinical situations exist in which there is accumulation of gas or air with low blood solubility in enclosed body spaces. These situations include intestinal obstruction, pneumothorax, pulmonary air cysts, and patients undergoing procedures in which air or gas is introduced intentionally (retinal detachment repair, pneumoencephalogram) or unintentionally (air embolism, tympanoplasty, pneumocephalus during neurosurgery).

—Because nitrous oxide is used in high concentrations (50–70%) and is 35 times more soluble in blood than nitrogen, nitrous oxide will enter an air-containing cavity causing expansion or increase in pressure. This effect cannot be offset by displacement of nitrogen (composing 78% of air) because of nitrogen's low solubility.

—Additionally, for patients having surgery for retinal detachment, where sulfahexafluoride gas, nitrogen, or a combination is injected into the vitreous cavity, use of nitrous oxide could produce unwanted expansion or pressure in the eye. The same is true for patients having tympanoplasty.

Intestinal Obstruction Interactions with Anesthesia Drugs
Intestinal obstruction and nitrous oxide

—Nitrous oxide can result in rapid expansion of gas- or air-filled cavities in the anesthetized patient. For this reason, it should not be administered to patients with a pneumothorax, acute intestinal obstruction, or patients at significant risk for air embolism.

—Additionally, for patients having surgery for retinal detachment, where sulfahexafluoride gas, nitrogen, or a combination is injected into the vitreous cavity, use of nitrous oxide could produce unwanted expansion or pressure in the eye. The same is true for patients having tympanoplasty.

—Because nitrous oxide is used in high concentrations (50–70%) and is 35 times more soluble in blood than nitrogen, nitrous oxide will enter an air-containing cavity, causing expansion or increase in pressure. This effect cannot be offset by displacement of nitrogen (composing 78% of air) because of nitrogen's low solubility.

LIVER DISEASE

—Liver disease can result from infection (viral hepatitis), toxins (alcohol), or other causes, including primary biliary cirrhosis, Wilson's disease, alpha 1 antitrypsin deficiency, and hemo-chromatosis.

—Cirrhosis is a disease of the liver from a variety of different causes that consists of scarring and decreased function of liver cells. In the United States, the most common cause of cirrhosis is chronic alcohol abuse.

—The scarring and fibrosis result in alteration in the architecture of the liver and are responsible for increased resistance to blood flow. Since the lower pressure system (the portal venous flow) is compromised earlier, proportionally more liver blood flow is provided by the hepatic artery with disease progression.

—As a result of increased hepatic arterial flow and decreased portal flow, hepatic perfusion is more dependent on arterial perfusion pressures. Decreased arterial pressures, as may occur during anesthesia, can compromise hepatic oxygenation and result in worsening of liver function perioperatively.

—Decreased hepatocellular function can alter metabolism and clearance of anesthetics and other medications. These alterations can be complex and include consideration of changes in volume of distribution as a result of ascites as well as increased tolerance to certain drugs (cross-tolerance) from chronic exposure to alcohol.

—Postoperative mortality in patients with portal hypertension from cirrhosis can be very high (up to 50%) if the serum albumin is <3 g/dL, the serum bilirubin is >3 mg/dL, and the patient has ascites and hepatic encephalopathy.

—Even mildly symptomatic patients with chronic liver disease appear to be at increased risk for worsening of liver function from anesthesia and surgery.

Liver Disease Interactions with Anesthesia Drugs

Liver disease and alfentanil

—Alfentanil is 99% metabolized in the liver. Patients with cirrhosis therefore show as much as a 50% reduction in clearance of alfentanil and can have a doubling of its half-life.

—Patients with liver disease therefore may show prolonged effects from alfentanil.

Liver disease and aminophylline, theophylline

—Patients with severe liver disease (cirrhosis) or congestive heart failure may require reduced maintenance doses of theophylline (or its more water-soluble derivative, aminophylline). Initial loading doses for untreated patients, however, do not usually require adjustment.

—Reduction in maintenance dosing in the above type of patients is necessary because metabolism of theophylline takes place primarily in the liver.

Liver disease and atracurium

—Age, obesity, liver, or renal dysfunction have no significant effect on metabolism of atracurium.

—Atracurium is metabolized by Hoffman elimination as well as ester hydrolysis.

—Hoffman elimination is a nonenzymatic process that occurs at physiologic temperatures and pH. Ester hydrolysis occurs most rapidly in an acid pH and does not require plasma pseudocholinesterase.

Liver disease and benzodiazepines (chlordiazepoxide, diazepam, lorazepam, midazolam)

—Elimination of benzodiazepines is dependent on hepatic metabolism. Patients with liver dysfunction may experience prolonged effects from usual doses.

Liver disease and buprenorphine

—Elimination of buprenorphine is dependent on hepatic metabolism and patients with liver dysfunction will experience prolonged effects from normal doses of buprenorphine.

Liver disease and butorphanol

—Butorphanol should be used in reduced dosages in patients with hepatic or renal dysfunction due to the routes of metabolism and excretion of this drug.

Liver disease and cimetidine

—Cimetidine is dependent on renal excretion and hepatic metabolism. In patients with renal or hepatic dysfunction, cimetidine accumulation can occur requiring longer intervals between doses (12 hours versus 6–8 hours).

Liver disease and diltiazem

—Elimination of diltiazem depends on hepatic metabolism and urinary excretion. Patients with impaired hepatic or renal function may experience more pronounced effects at usual doses. Reduced dosage is recommended.

Liver disease and muscle relaxants (doxacurium, mivacurium, vecuronium, pancuronium, rocuronium, and tubocurarine)

—Prolonged neuromuscular blockade in patients with liver disease can be seen with doxacurium, mivacurium, vecuronium, pancuronium, rocuronium, and tubocurarine.

—This interaction is complex and may be due to decreased clearance, decreased hepatic uptake of the agent, or decreased synthesis of enzymes important for degradation of the neuromuscular blocker. An example of the latter is prolongation of mivacurium's duration of action as a result of decreased plasma cholinesterase from severe liver disease.

—Because of the increased volume of distribution of many drugs seen in patients with liver disease, initial doses of muscle relaxants may need to be larger than in healthy patients. Once neuromuscular blockade is achieved, recovery may be prolonged.

Liver disease and meperidine

—Elimination of meperidine depends mainly on hepatic metabolism with some renal excretion. Patients with hepatic dysfunction may have drug accumulation after repeated high doses of meperidine.

Liver disease and succinylcholine

—Termination of the effect of succinylcholine is dependent on plasma pseudocholinesterase, which is synthesized in the liver. However, even in severe liver disease, plasma pseudo-cholinesterase levels are not depressed enough to prolong the effects of succinylcholine.

—Mivacurium is also cleared by plasma cholinesterase, but there is evidence that there is significant prolongation of action of mivacurium in patients with severe liver disease.

MALIGNANT HYPERTHERMIA

—Malignant hyperthermia (MH) is a clinical syndrome of hypermetabolism that usually occurs during anesthesia. It is characterized by rapidly increasing temperature (up to 1°/5 min), tachycardia, hypoxemia, hypercarbia, acidosis, and skeletal muscle rigidity. MH is inherited as an autosomal dominant, autosomal recessive, or an unclassified form.

—Episodes of MH appear to be triggered in susceptible patients by exposure to succinylcholine and/or volatile anesthetics (halothane, enflurane, isoflurane, desflurane, sevoflurane). There is some evidence suggesting MH episodes may occur in susceptible patients as a result of other stresses, such as exercise or heat stress.

—Also, some susceptible patients may not experience MH even when exposed to triggering agents, whereas other susceptible patients may experience MH with nontriggering anesthetics in spite of pretreatment with dantrolene.

—The underlying defect in patients with malignant hyperthermia appears to be a loss of control of intracellular calcium. Specifically, the site of malfunction is the sarcoplasmic reticulum (SR), where muscle endplate depolarization normally results in release of calcium from the SR, causing muscle contraction.

—In MH susceptible patients, a receptor at the SR, the ryanodine receptor, is abnormal and allows for excessive calcium release. Since ATP is required for both contraction and relaxation of muscle, the result of excess calcium is stimulation of muscle metabolism.

—Patients exposed to triggering agents who develop signs of MH must be differentiated from patients with other disorders, such as hyperthyroidism, pheochromocytoma, and neuroleptic malignant syndrome.

—Treatment with dantrolene should be initiated if fulminant MH is occurring as evidenced by rapidly increasing temperature (>1°/15 min), acidosis (base deficit >5 meq/L and worsening), and $PaCO_2$ >60 mm Hg or mixed venous PCO_2 >90 mm Hg. Discontinuation of triggering agents and supportive measures is also indicated.

—The occurrence of mild trismus (jaw muscle spasm) may be seen in normal patients when exposed to succinylcholine. However, extreme spasm (impossible to open mouth) has a high association with MH susceptibility.

—As many as 50% of children and 25% of adults with extreme jaw muscle spasm may be MH-susceptible, whereas only a small, but unknown, number of children with mild or moderate spasm are MH-susceptible.

—In cases of extreme masseter muscle spasm, cancellation of the procedure is recommended. The presence of total body rigidity is another indication for cancellation of the procedure, regardless of the severity of masseter muscle spasm.

—In cases of mild or moderate jaw muscle spasm, it may be appropriate to continue the surgical procedure. In such cases, all triggering anesthetics should be stopped and there should be close monitoring for signs of MH.

—Several disorders are associated with a high susceptibility to MH. These include the King–Denborough syndrome (short stature, musculoskeletal abnormalities, mental retardation), central core disease (inherited myopathy with weakness and hypotonia), and Duchenne's muscular dystrophy.

—Testing of individuals suspected of susceptibility for MH includes a history and physical examination, family history, creatine phosphokinase (CPK) levels, and muscle contracture tests.

—The resting CPK (also known as creatine kinase, or CK) level is elevated in about 70% of susceptible individuals and is therefore a useful screening tool. If the resting CK is elevated in a person with a close relative who is known to be MH-susceptible, this person can be considered to be MH-susceptible without further testing.

—Because a normal CK level does not exclude the possibility of MH susceptibility, suspected individuals will require muscle contracture testing. The test is performed with a viable muscle specimen placed in a tissue bath and stimulated while exposed to halothane or caffeine. Some testing methods use halothane and caffeine together, but this may yield results that are difficult to interpret.

—MH-susceptible muscle specimens have a lower threshold for contraction when exposed to halothane or caffeine than muscle from nonsusceptible patients. Although accuracy of the tests is difficult to assess, muscle contracture tests are probably about 95% reliable.

—Current recommendations for management of the susceptible patient include the possibility of outpatient surgery. Prolonged flushing of the anesthesia machine is no longer mandatory. Instead, use of disposable circuit, replacement of the fresh gas outlet hose, removal or sealing of the vaporizers, and a flush at 6 L/min for 5 minutes are acceptable.

—Anesthetic agents considered safe for use in patients with known or suspected susceptibility for developing malignant hyperthermia include propofol, barbiturates, etomidate, ketamine, non-depolarizing neuromuscular blocking agents, narcotics, benzodiazepines, droperidol, epinephrine, norepinephrine, and anticholinesterases.

—Nitrous oxide is probably safe in the susceptible patient based on repeated use in MH-susceptible humans and swine.

—Local or regional anesthesia with either amide (such as lidocaine) or ester (such as procaine) anesthetics is now considered safe for MH-susceptible patients.

Malignant Hyperthermia Interactions with Anesthesia Drugs
Malignant hyperthermia and anticholinesterases,
benzodiazepines, local anesthetics, intravenous anesthetics,
non-depolarizing muscle relaxants, and vasopressors *

—Anesthetic agents considered safe for use in patients with known or suspected susceptibility for developing malignant

---

* Anticholinesterases (edrophonium, neostigmine, pyridostigmine).
Benzodiazepines (chlordiazepoxide, diazepam, lorazepam, midazolam).
Local anesthetics (amides, such as lidocaine, bupivacaine, or esters, such as procaine, tetracaine).
Intravenous anesthetics (etomidate, methohexital, propofol, sodium pentothal).
Narcotics (alfentanil, buprenorphine, butorphanol, fentanyl, meperidine, morphine, nalbuphine, sufentanil).
Non-depolarizing muscle relaxants (atracurium, doxacurium, gallamine, metocurine, mivacurium, pancuronium, pipecuronium, rocuronium, vecuronium).

hyperthermia include propofol, barbiturates, etomidate, ketamine, non-depolarizing neuromuscular blocking agents, narcotics, benzodiazepines, droperidol, epinephrine, norepinephrine, and anticholinesterases.

—Nitrous oxide is probably safe in the susceptible patient based on repeated use in MH-susceptible humans and swine.

—Local or regional anesthesia with either amide (such as lidocaine) or ester (such as procaine) anesthetics is now considered safe for MH-susceptible patients.

Malignant hyperthermia and Inhalational anesthetics, Succinylcholine, Tubocurarine*

—Halothane, isoflurane, enflurane, desflurane, sevoflurane, as well as other older inhalational agents are all potent triggering agents of malignant hyperthermia in the susceptible patient.

—Succinylcholine, decamethonium, and possibly tubocurarine are also triggering agents.

—Nitrous oxide is probably safe in the susceptible patient based on repeated use in MH-susceptible humans and swine.

Malignant hyperthermia and Droperidol, Ketamine

—Droperidol and ketamine are considered to be non-triggering agents for malignant hyperthermia and are therefore safe for use in susceptible patients.

MULTIPLE SCLEROSIS

—Multiple sclerosis (MS) is a disorder of the brain and spinal cord characterized pathologically by zones of demyelination and by a clinical course of exacerbations and remissions of neurologic symptoms and signs. The demyelination is confined to the CNS.

—The incidence of the disease is about 10 times greater in temperate (northern) versus tropical latitudes and the etiology is unknown, although a viral cause is suspected. Onset of this disorder prior to age 15 or after age 40 is rare.

—Symptoms of the disease include motor symptoms of weakness, clumsiness, or stiffness, as well as visual symptoms as a result of optic nerve or ocular muscle involvement.

—Anesthetic management of the patient with MS should involve several considerations. First, exacerbation of the disease postop-

---

* Inhalational anesthetics (desflurane, enflurane, halothane, isoflurane, nitrous oxide, sevoflurane).

eratively is likely as a result of surgical stress, regardless of the type of anesthetic.

—Second, spinal anesthesia is thought to worsen clinical symptoms for unclear reasons. Epidural anesthesia, perhaps related to lower dosage requirements of local anesthetics, appears to be safer.

—Depolarizing neuromuscular blocking drugs (succinylcholine) may result in hyperkalemia as a result of extrajunctional acetylcholine receptors that are associated with chronic neuromuscular disorders. These same extrajunctional receptors are more resistant to blockade from non-depolarizing agents. Despite initial resistance to muscle blockade, MS patients may experience prolonged muscle weakness as a result of decreased muscle mass.

Multiple Sclerosis Interactions with Anesthesia Drugs
Multiple sclerosis and muscle relaxants (atracurium, doxacurium, gallamine, metocurine, mivacurium, pancuronium, pipercuronium, rocuronium, tubocurarine, vecuronium)

—Patients with a wide variety of neuromuscular disorders, such as multiple sclerosis, may be more resistant than normal patients to the effects of non-depolarizing neuromuscular blockers.

—Disuse or denervation of muscle results in production of extrajunctional acetylcholine receptors on the muscle membrane. These receptors are less easily blocked by non-depolarizing agents but are activated by lower concentrations of depolarizing drugs (succinylcholine).

—Despite initial resistance to blockade, such patients may demonstrate prolonged neuromuscular weakness as a result of decreased muscle strength and mass.

Multiple sclerosis and succinylcholine

—Chronic or progressive motor neuron disease places patients at continuous risk for hyperkalemia from succinylcholine. Syringomyelia, amyotrophic lateral sclerosis, multiple sclerosis, acute idiopathic polyneuritis (Guillain–Barré syndrome), and all forms of muscular dystrophy have been associated with this response.

—Patients with neuromuscular disease (upper and lower motor neuron abnormalities) can respond to succinylcholine with a dangerous, sometimes fatal, hyperkalemia. This occurs probably because of proliferation of extrajunctional acetylcholine receptors on the muscle membrane. Depolarization of these receptors causes potassium leak through the muscle membrane.

MUSCULAR DYSTROPHY

—Muscular dystrophy is a group of disorders in which there is degeneration of muscle. They are classified on the basis of mode of inheritance, age of onset, rate of progression, and distribution of muscles involved.

—The most common of these disorders is Duchenne's dystrophy (pseudohypertrophic). Usually, it is an X-linked recessive disease that becomes evident by age 2 or 3 years. It is characterized by an abnormal gait, kyphoscoliosis, and cardiac abnormalities (mitral regurgitation, decreased contractility). Death at age 15–25 is from cardiac or respiratory complications. There is a high probability of malignant hyperthermia if these patients are exposed to succinylcholine or halothane (and possibly other volatile anesthetics).

—Other forms of muscular dystrophy include limb-girdle (shoulder or hip muscle weakness), facioscapulohumeral (facial, chest, shoulder muscle wasting), nemaline rod (nonprogressive muscle weakness with facial and skeletal abnormalities), and oculopharyngeal dystrophy (dysphagia and ptosis).

—Although only patients with Duchenne's dystrophy appear to have a high susceptibility to MH, hyperkalemia from succinylcholine may occur in any patient with myopathy.

Muscular Dystrophy Interactions with Anesthesia Drugs
Muscular dystrophy and verapamil
—Use of verapamil in patients with Duchenne's muscular dystrophy has resulted in respiratory failure.

Muscular dystrophy and succinylcholine
—Chronic or progressive motor neuron disease places patients at continuous risk for hyperkalemia from succinylcholine. Syringomyelia, amyotrophic lateral sclerosis, multiple sclerosis, acute idiopathic polyneuritis (Guillain–Barré syndrome), and all forms of muscular dystrophy have been associated with this response.

—Patients with neuromuscular disease (upper and lower motor neuron abnormalities) can respond to succinylcholine with a dangerous, sometimes fatal, hyperkalemia. This occurs probably because of proliferation of extrajunctional acetylcholine receptors on the muscle membrane. Depolarization of these receptors causes potassium leak through the muscle membrane.

MYASTHENIA GRAVIS

—Myasthenia gravis is a disease of the neuromuscular junction that is characterized by muscle weakness. The disease can occur at any age but is most often seen in women between the ages of 20 and 30 or in men after age 60.

—The disease is one of autoimmunity in which antibodies destroy acetylcholine receptors at the neuromuscular junction.

—There are several types of myasthenia, varying from involvement of only ocular muscles to a severe, fulminant disease with rapid progression over 6 months and high mortality.

—The hallmark of myasthenia gravis is rapid exhaustion and weakness of muscles with repetitive use. Cranial nerve involvement is common and presents as diplopia, ptosis, difficulty swallowing, dysphagia, and dysarthria. Myocarditis and cardiomyopathy may be associated with myasthenia.

—Treatment of this disease includes anticholinesterases (neostigmine, pyridostigmine), corticosteroids, plasmapheresis, and thymectomy for drug-resistant patients.

—Management of anesthesia for these patients requires adjustment of doses for neuromuscular blocking drugs. Specifically, myasthenic patients are very sensitive to non-depolarizing agents, probably as a result of the decreased number of acetylcholine receptor sites.

—Reversal of a non-depolarizing blockade is controversial. Because patients are treated chronically with anticholinesterases, anticholinesterase inhibition is already nearly maximized. Conservative recommendations are to not use anticholinesterases for reversal of muscle blockade but rather to allow spontaneous recovery.

—Patients with myasthenia gravis may be resistant to succinylcholine, according to one study. However, there are other considerations: anticholinesterases may significantly prolong the blockade from succinylcholine (from inhibition of plasma cholinesterase), and some patients will have significant clinical muscle weakness, suggesting a lower requirement for muscle relaxant.

—Postoperative ventilation may be necessary for patients with myasthenia gravis. Patients most likely to need ventilation after anesthesia and surgery are those patients with disease of more than 6 years duration, chronic obstructive pulmonary disease, daily pyridostigmine requirements of 750 mg, and patients who have a vital capacity of less than 40 ml/kg.

Myasthenia Gravis Interactions with Anesthesia Drugs
Myasthenia gravis and edrophonium, neostigmine, pyridostigmine
—Reversal of a non-depolarizing blockade in patients with myasthenia gravis is controversial. Because patients are treated chronically with anticholinesterases, anticholinesterase inhibition is already nearly maximized.
—Conservative recommendations are to not use anticholinesterases for reversal of muscle blockade, but rather to allow spontaneous recovery.

Myasthenia gravis and muscle relaxants (atracurium, doxacurium, gallamine, metocurine, mivacurium, pancuronium, pipercuronium, rocuronium, tubocurarine, vecuronium)
—Patients with myasthenia gravis are very sensitive to neuromuscular blockade from non-depolarizing agents.
—This is probably a result of decreased acetylcholine receptors from autoimmune destruction associated with myasthenia gravis.
—Although these patients are treated with the same or similar anticholinesterases used to antagonize muscle blockade, sensitivity (not resistance) to neuromuscular blockade is seen clinically.

Myasthenia gravis and procainamide
—Patients receiving anticholinesterase drugs for myasthenia gravis can have exacerbation of muscle weakness if given procainamide or quinidine.
—This is related to the ability of these drugs to enhance neuromuscular blockade from depolarizing and non-depolarizing agents.
—Lidocaine and propranolol would also be expected to have this interaction but appear to be safe for use in myasthenics.

Myasthenia gravis and succinylcholine
—The response of myasthenics to succinylcholine is usually similar to non-depolarizing agents in that a reduced dose is normally appropriate. However, one study has shown a resistance of myasthenics compared to normal patients. The clinical significance of this finding is not clear and most sources suggest lower doses of succinylcholine for patients with myasthenia gravis.
—Factors affecting patients' response to succinylcholine include treatment with anticholinesterase medications that also

reduce plasma pseudocholinesterase. As a result, duration of neuromuscular blockade from succinylcholine is usually prolonged.

—Also, significant clinical muscle weakness would dictate lower doses than those for normal patients or myasthenic patients with good muscle strength.

MYOTONIA

—Myotonia is a symptom of abnormal slowness in relaxation of muscle after voluntary or induced muscle contraction. It is evident by an inability to relax a handgrip or by tapping a muscle group such as the thenar eminence of the hand.

—Myotonia is seen in different disorders including myotonic dystrophy, the hyperkalemic form of periodic paralysis, myotonia congenita, and glycogen storage diseases.

—Patients with myotonic dystrophy have muscle wasting of primarily face, jaw, and temporalis groups. Mental retardation and cardiomyopathy are usually present. Although onset is usually in adulthood, childhood onset can occur.

—In myotonia congenita, myotonia is present from infancy, muscle wasting is absent, and other organs are not involved.

—Hyperkalemic periodic paralysis is an autosomal dominant trait that is more severe in males. Its onset is usually in childhood and the disease is characterized by periods of muscle paralysis (most severely the legs), usually sparing the respiratory muscles. It is usually precipitated by rest after strong exertion and lasts for several hours. Myotonia persists between episodes. Hyperkalemia occurs during acute episodes, but the exact etiology of this disorder is unclear.

—The glycogen storage diseases are a group of disorders that result in accumulation of glycogen in different tissues. Several types (II, III, V, VII) have prominent muscle involvement and patients may have myotonia. Some of the syndromes can be associated with severe cardiomyopathy.

—Anesthetic management of patients with myotonia includes avoidance of succinylcholine (can produce sustained muscle contraction and hyperkalemia) and careful use of inhaled anesthetics (primarily in patients with cardiomyopathy). Non-depolarizing agents and reversal of these agents with anticholinesterases will not precipitate muscle contraction in patients with myotonia.

Myotonia Interactions with Anesthesia Drugs
Myotonia and inhalational anesthetics (desflurane, enflurane, halothane, isoflurane, sevoflurane)
—Inhalational anesthetics may cause exaggerated cardiac depression in patients with myotonia dystrophica.
—Patients with myotonia dystrophica, but not the other myotonic syndromes, are likely to have some degree of cardiomyopathy even in the absence of clinical symptoms. As a result, these patients may be very sensitive to any myocardial depressant.

Myotonia and succinylcholine
—Myotonic dystrophy includes three forms of the disease; myotonia dystrophica (most common form), myotonia congenita, and paramyotonia.
—All three forms can respond to depolarization from succinylcholine with persistent muscle contraction lasting several minutes. Use of non-depolarizing agents alone does not produce muscle contraction nor does reversal of neuromuscular blockade with anticholinesterases.

NARCOTIC DEPENDENCE

—Drug addiction is the inability to stop or control drug abuse. Narcotic-addicted patients who require anesthesia for surgery should be maintained on methadone (or other narcotic) during the perioperative period.
—The withdrawal syndrome can begin 8–12 hours after the last dose of narcotics, consisting of dilated pupils and common cold symptoms (rhinorrhea, lacrimation, sweating, fever). Later signs are those of sympathetic stimulation (hypertension, insomnia, tachycardia), skeletal muscle spasm, and diarrhea.
—Administration of agonist–antagonist medications (buprenorphine, nalbuphine, butorphanol) or naloxone to the narcotic addict is not recommended unless narcotic antagonism is intended. Agonist–antagonist medications may precipitate acute withdrawal within minutes of administration to some dependent patients.

Narcotic Dependence Interactions with Anesthesia Drugs
Narcotic dependence and buprenorphine
—Buprenorphine has both narcotic agonist and antagonist properties and has been shown to produce withdrawal symptoms in patients receiving morphine-like drugs.

Narcotic dependence and butorphanol
—Butorphanol, a narcotic agonist–antagonist, may precipitate acute withdrawal in patients who are maintained on methadone.
—Patients who are receiving low doses of morphine (60 mg daily) have not been shown to demonstrate withdrawal symptoms with administration of butorphanol.

Narcotic dependence and nalbuphine
—Nalbuphine has both narcotic agonist and antagonist properties. Patients who are dependent on low doses of morphine (60 mg daily) demonstrate withdrawal symptoms when given nalbuphine.
—Patients addicted to other narcotics (such as methadone) may also experience withdrawal symptoms when given a narcotic agonist/antagonist (butorphanol, buprenorphine, nalbuphine).

Narcotic dependence and naloxone
—Naloxone can precipitate withdrawal symptoms in patients who are physically dependent on narcotics.

NEUROMUSCULAR DISEASE

—For the sake of this discussion, neuromuscular disease refers to disorders in which extrajunctional acetylcholine receptors are formed in response to different disease processes. These receptors are formed by muscle cells that have reduced or no activity as a result of chronic illness (resulting in inactivity), burns, or damage to muscle cell innervation (stroke, brain or spinal cord trauma, amyotrophic lateral sclerosis, multiple sclerosis, syringomyelia).
—Disuse or denervation of muscle results in production of extrajunctional acetylcholine receptors on the muscle membrane. These receptors are less easily blocked by non-depolarizing agents but are activated by lower concentrations of depolarizing drugs (succinylcholine).
—Formation of these receptors, as well as their removal, occurs rapidly following the insult. In some cases, extrajunctional receptors begin to form within hours of diminished activity of the muscle.
—Despite initial resistance to blockade, such patients may demonstrate prolonged neuromuscular weakness as a result of decreased muscle strength and mass.

—Hyperkalemia is associated with the presence of extrajunctional receptors when exposed to succinylcholine. When these receptors, which can be scattered over a large surface of the muscle, are depolarized by succinylcholine, ion flow takes place through the receptor channel. Large amounts of potassium may exit the muscle cell, causing hyperkalemia.

Neuromuscular Disease Interactions with Anesthesia Drugs

Neuromuscular disease and muscle relaxants (atracurium, doxacurium, gallamine, metocurine, mivacurium, pancuronium, pipercuronium, rocuronium, tubocurarine, vecuronium)

—Patients with a wide variety of neuromuscular disorders may be more resistant than normal patients to the effects of nondepolarizing neuromuscular blockers.

—This includes patients with disuse atrophy of the muscles (such as bedridden patients with chronic disease) as well as patients with upper or lower motor neuron disease (such as from trauma, stroke, or chronic illness like amyotrophic lateral sclerosis).

—Disuse or denervation of muscle results in production of extrajunctional acetylcholine receptors on the muscle membrane. These receptors are less easily blocked by non-depolarizing agents but are activated by lower concentrations of depolarizing drugs (succinylcholine).

—Despite initial resistance to blockade, such patients may demonstrate prolonged neuromuscular weakness as a result of decreased muscle strength and mass.

Neuromuscular disease and succinylcholine

—Patients with neuromuscular disease (upper and lower motor neuron abnormalities) can respond to succinylcholine with a dangerous, sometimes fatal, hyperkalemia. This occurs probably because of proliferation of extrajunctional acetylcholine receptors on the muscle membrane. Depolarization of these receptors causes potassium leak through the muscle membrane.

—Patients with traumatic spinal cord damage can manifest this hyperkalemic response as early as 24–48 hours after administration. The period of time that such patients remain at risk for this response is not clear. As in burn patients, the potential for hyperkalemia following succinylcholine may persist for over 1 year following the injury.

—Chronic or progressive motor neuron disease places patients at continuous risk for hyperkalemia from succinylcholine.

Syringomyelia, amyotrophic lateral sclerosis, multiple sclerosis, acute idiopathic polyneuritis (Guillain–Barré syndrome), all forms of muscular dystrophy, and familial periodic paralysis (hyperkalemic form) have all been associated with this response.

OBESITY

—Obesity (an excess of body fat) may affect recovery from muscle relaxants and narcotics. Although increased deposition of inhaled volatile anesthetics has been suggested to be greater in obese patients, this has not been shown to be clinically significant.

—Some narcotics (sufentanil and alfentanil) have been shown to have increased volumes of distribution and prolonged elimination time in obese patients. It is not known if other narcotics have similar pharmacodynamics and, therefore, some recommend initiating narcotic dosing on the basis of lean body weight.

—Similar controversy exists on the effect of non-depolarizing muscle relaxants. While obesity can prolong the blockade from vecuronium and metocurine, pancuronium is unaffected. Also unaffected is atracurium. Use of lean body mass may be more appropriate for initial dosage of non-depolarizing muscle relaxants.

Obesity Interactions with Anesthesia Drugs

Obesity and alfentanil

—Obesity doubles the elimination half-life of alfentanil.

—The implications of this for the anesthesiologist are that obese patients may demonstrate prolonged effects from alfentanil. Also, to maintain steady-state levels of alfentanil in an obese patient, the loading dose may need to be increased, but the maintenance dose can remain unchanged.

Obesity and atracurium

—Age, obesity, and liver or renal dysfunction have no significant effect on metabolism of atracurium.

—Atracurium is metabolized by Hoffman elimination as well as ester hydrolysis.

—Hoffman elimination is a nonenzymatic process that occurs at physiologic temperatures and pH. Ester hydrolysis occurs most rapidly in an acid pH and does not require plasma pseudocholinesterase.

Obesity and sufentanil

—The elimination half-life of sufentanil can be significantly prolonged in obese patients.

—A study of obese neurosurgical patients determined that the volume of distribution of sufentanil was increased, thereby delaying its elimination. The amount of increase in the volume of distribution was determined by the extent of obesity.

Obesity and vecuronium

—Vecuronium's duration of action can be significantly prolonged in obese patients.

PARKINSON'S DISEASE

—Parkinson's disease results from degeneration of the basal ganglia. Its onset is usually in middle age (40–60 years) and when fully developed is very distinctive.

—Clinical features of the disease include a resting tremor (which diminishes with intentional movement), limb rigidity, expressionless facies, and an abnormal, shuffling gait with limited arm swing. Depression and dementia (mental decline) are common.

—The disease is a result of decreased dopamine production by the basal ganglia of the brain. Dopamine is believed to inhibit extrapyramidal motor stimulation by acetylcholine and a lack of this neurotransmitter allows unopposed stimulation by acetylcholine.

—Treatment of this disease is with anticholinesterases and levodopa, which crosses the blood–brain barrier and is converted to dopamine. Since the half-life of dopamine is short, symptoms of Parkinsonism may appear within 6–12 hours of the last dose of levodopa, necessitating continuation of this medication in the perioperative period.

—Additionally, avoidance of dopamine antagonists such as butyrophenones (droperidol) is recommended. Other dopamine antagonists are the phenothiazines (prochlorperazine or Compazine), which are also probably best avoided.

Parkinson's Disease Interactions with Anesthesia Drugs
Parkinson's disease and droperidol

—Droperidol antagonizes the effects of dopamine in the basal ganglia and can worsen the condition of patients with Parkinson's disease.

PERIODIC PARALYSIS

—Periodic paralysis (familial periodic paralysis) is an autosomal dominant disorder that can take one of three forms: hypokalemic, normokalemic, or hyperkalemic. The diseases are characterized by episodes of muscle weakness, usually sparing the muscles of respiration.

—During episodes of weakness, which begin in the first or second decade of life, muscle cells are electrically inexcitable. The duration of these episodes is variable, usually hours or days and, rarely, weeks.

—The exact pathophysiology is unknown, but patients with the hypo- or hyperkalemic forms can experience weakness if serum potassium drops below 3 meq/L (hypokalemic form) or exceeds 5.5 meq/L (hyperkalemic form). Patients are usually treated with acetazolamide, which causes potassium diuresis in patients with the hyperkalemic form and mild acidosis in the hypokalemic form (thus increasing serum potassium).

—Anesthetic management of these patients requires careful monitoring of serum potassium during the perioperative period. For patients with the hyperkalemic form, avoidance of succinylcholine is recommended because these patients can have myotonia (sustained muscle contraction) that is present between episodes of muscle weakness. Exposure to succinylcholine could produce severe and prolonged muscle contraction and hyperkalemia.

Periodic Paralysis Interactions with Anesthesia Drugs
Periodic paralysis and succinylcholine

—Succinylcholine should be avoided in patients with the hyperkalemic form of familial periodic paralysis. These patients can respond to succinylcholine with sustained muscle contraction, similar to patients with myotonia.

—Patients with the hypokalemic form have been given succinylcholine without complications.

PHEOCHROMOCYTOMA

—Pheochromocytoma is a tumor that secretes catecholamines and is characterized by paroxysmal hypertension. It is the cause of few cases of hypertension (<0.1%).

—Although 90% are found in the adrenal gland and 95% within the abdominal cavity, pheochromocytomas can occur anywhere, including the ovary, spleen, heart, or along the sympathetic chain.

—Tumors may be found in both adrenals (10% of cases) or multiple locations elsewhere (20% of cases). Less than 10% are malignant.

—Symptoms and signs are episodic lasting from minutes to hours and typically consist of headache, palpitations, sweating, hypertension, and weight loss.

—Diagnosis relies on detection of excessive urine levels of catecholamines or catecholamine metabolites (normetanephrine, metanephrine, vanillylmandelic acid) and localization of the tumor with computed tomography.

—Preoperative preparation is directed initially at blocking the vasoconstriction from excess catecholamines. Alpha-blocking drugs (phenoxybenzamine, or less commonly prazosin) may require 10 days or more to adequately control blood pressure and allow correction of hypovolemia. Beta blockade may be indicated (only after alpha blockade) for persistent arrhythmias or tachycardia.

—Anesthetic management of these patients is based on avoiding sympathetic stimulation. Although no specific induction technique has been shown to be superior and no technique can be expected to eliminate transient tachycardia or hypertension, certain drugs should probably be avoided. These include doxapram (because it is a sympathetic stimulant) and diazoxide (because it can result in catecholamine release).

Pheochromocytoma Interactions with Anesthesia Drugs
Pheochromocytoma and alpha adrenergic blockers (phentolamine)

—Significant interactions with anesthetics can occur with patients who are receiving alpha-blocking agents. Blockade of alpha 1 receptors can result in unresponsiveness to vasopressors, depending on the vasopressor being used.

—In patients receiving alpha 1 blockers, the response to vasopressors that are primarily alpha agonists (phenylephrine and methoxamine) can be suppressed.

—Vasopressors that stimulate both alpha and beta receptors can interact with alpha 1 blockers in different ways, depending on the amount of alpha and beta agonist activity.

—Epinephrine, at lower doses, stimulates beta receptors more than alpha receptors. When epinephrine is used to treat patients receiving alpha blockers, hypotension may occur due to the vasodilating effect from epinephrine's prominent beta 2 stimulation.

—Norepinephrine differs from epinephrine by stimulating mainly beta 1 and alpha receptors rather than beta 2 receptors. When norepinephrine is given to patients on alpha blockers, the beta 1 stimulation may produce some increase in blood pressure. Hypotension is unlikely because of minimal beta 2 agonism. Metaraminol may have similar effects.

—Ephedrine and mephentermine are likely to have interactions similar to epinephrine with patients receiving alpha blockers. These agents have significant beta 2 stimulation along with beta 1 and alpha adrenergic activity.

Pheochromocytoma and diazoxide

—Diazoxide is contraindicated in patients with hypertension from pheochromocytoma because it may stimulate release of epinephrine from the adrenal medulla.

—It is this property of diazoxide that makes it useful in treatment, when given orally, for hypoglycemia.

Pheochromocytoma and doxapram HCl

—Because of its mechanism of action, doxapram is contraindicated in a number of conditions, such as hypertension, convulsive disorders, hyperthyroidism, cerebral edema, and pheochromocytoma.

—Analeptic agents, such as doxapram, are CNS stimulants. Because CNS stimulation can elevate arterial pressure, decrease seizure thresholds, and have additive stimulatory effects in conditions such as the above disorders, doxapram is contraindicated in patients with these underlying conditions.

—Analeptic agents improve ventilation through their effect on the brainstem and, in the case of doxapram, the carotid chemoreceptors.

Pheochromocytoma and vasopressors (ephedrine, epinephrine, metaraminol, methoxamine, norepinephrine, phenylephrine)

—Blockade of alpha 1 receptors can result in unresponsiveness to vasopressors, depending on the vasopressor being used.

—Ephedrine and mephentermine have significant beta 2 stimulation along with beta 1 and alpha adrenergic activity. As a result, it is possible that hypotension could worsen in patients on alpha blockers given ephedrine due to the unopposed vasodilation resulting from beta 2 stimulation.

—Although good documentation of this interaction is scarce, this is similar to the response that can be seen with epinephrine.

—Because norepinephrine has beta 1 activity, it is more likely to be effective in treating hypotension in patients on alpha blockers.

PNEUMOTHORAX

—Several clinical situations exist in which there is accumulation of gas or air with low blood solubility in enclosed body spaces. These situations include intestinal obstruction, pneumothorax, pulmonary air cysts, and patients undergoing procedures in which air or gas is introduced intentionally (retinal detachment repair, pneumoencephalogram) or unintentionally (air embolism, tympanoplasty, pneumocephalus during neurosurgery).

—Because nitrous oxide is used in high concentrations (50–70%) and is 35 times more soluble in blood than is nitrogen, nitrous oxide will enter an air-containing cavity causing expansion or increase in pressure. This effect cannot be offset by displacement of nitrogen (composing 78% of air) because of nitrogen's low solubility.

—Additionally, for patients having surgery for retinal detachment, where sulfahexafluoride gas, nitrogen, or a combination is injected into the vitreous cavity, use of nitrous oxide could produce unwanted expansion or pressure in the eye. The same is true for patients having tympanoplasty.

Pneumothorax Interactions with Anesthesia Drugs
Pneumothorax and nitrous oxide

—Nitrous oxide can result in rapid expansion of gas- or air-filled cavities in the anesthetized patient. For this reason, it should not be administered to patients with a pneumothorax, acute intestinal obstruction, or patients at significant risk for air embolism.

—Additionally, for patients having surgery for retinal detachment, where sulfahexafluoride gas, nitrogen, or a combination is injected into the vitreous cavity, use of nitrous oxide could produce unwanted expansion or pressure in the eye. The same is true for patients having tympanoplasty.

—Because nitrous oxide is used in high concentrations (50–70%) and is 35 times more soluble in blood than is nitrogen, nitrous oxide will enter an air-containing cavity causing expansion or increase in pressure. This effect cannot be offset by displacement of nitrogen (composing 78% of air) because of nitrogen's low solubility.

PORPHYRIA

—Porphyria refers to a group of disorders characterized by abnormal porphyrin metabolism. Porphyrin metabolism begins with glycine and succinyl-CoA and results in the production of heme and important enzymes (such as cytochromes).

—Abnormalities of porphyrin metabolism result from defects in enzymes along the path, resulting in accumulation of heme precursors, which are believed to account for the symptoms of porphyria.

—Certain medications, drugs, or clinical situations result in stimulation of the rate-limiting enzyme [aminolevulinic acid (ALA) synthetase]. Because of defects in enzymes further along the metabolic pathway to heme formation, porphyrin precursors accumulate, depending on the site of the affected enzyme.

—Stimuli for ALA synthetase include barbiturates, phenytoin, sulfonamides, ergot alkaloids, and many others. Menstruation, pregnancy, and malnutrition (severe dieting or carbohydrate depletion) can also be precipitating factors.

—Questionable medications include benzodiazepines, ketamine, and corticosteroids.

—Heme production occurs mainly in the bone marrow (erythrocytes) and the liver. Depending on the site most affected by the enzymatic defect, porphyrias are classified as hepatic, erythropoietic, or both.

—The only disorders that can be induced by medications are three of the four hepatic porphyrias (acute intermittent, variegate porphyrias, and hereditary coproporphyria).

—Symptoms from these disorders are characterized by several of the "five P's":
  —Onset after puberty
  —Psychiatric abnormalities
  —Pain
  —Polyneuropathy
  —Photosensitivity

—Acute episodes can be precipitated by the "four M's":
  —Medicines (barbiturates, etc.)
  —Menstrual periods
  —Malnutrition
  —Medical illness (infection)

—Anesthetic management of these patients requires avoidance of triggering agents such as barbiturates, and possibly benzodiazepines or ketamine. Use of narcotics, muscle relaxants, inhalational agents, or propofol, among others, is considered safe.

—Because of polyneuropathy and psychiatric abnormalities, regional anesthesia is best avoided to eliminate confusion between disease exacerbation and residual nerve blockade from regional anesthetics.

Porphyria Interactions with Anesthesia Drugs

Porphyria and benzodiazepines (chlordiazepoxide, diazepam, lorazepam, midazolam), etomidate, and ketamine

—Benzodiazepines and etomidate are considered questionable triggering agents for porphyria. This is based on their ability to provoke attacks of porphyria in rat models, although use in humans has not been associated with this reaction.

—Ketamine is also considered a questionable triggering agent for porphyria.

—Not all of the porphyrias have significance for the anesthesiologist. Three of the four hepatic porphyrias (acute intermittent, variegate, hereditary coproporphyria) and none of the erythropoietic porphyrias are associated with neurologic symptoms that can be triggered by certain medications: barbiturates, etomidate, and corticosteroids.

—Safe anesthetics are inhalational agents, narcotics, muscle relaxants, anticholinesterases, and propofol.

Porphyria and anticholinesterases, inhalational anesthetics, muscle relaxants, narcotics, propofol*

—Inhalational agents are considered to be safe for use in patients with porphyria, as are narcotics, depolarizing and non-depolarizing muscle relaxants, anticholinesterases, and propofol.

Porphyria and methohexital, sodium pentothal

—Barbiturates are contraindicated in three of the four hepatic porphyrias (acute intermittent porphyria, variegate porphyria, and hereditary coproporphyria). Porphyria cutanea tarda and the erythropoietic porphyrias are not exacerbated by barbiturates.

—It is theorized that barbiturates can provoke an attack of porphyria by inducing the enzyme aminolevulinic acid syn-

---

* Anticholinesterases (edrophonium, neostigmine, pyridostigmine)

Inhalational anesthetics (desflurane, enflurane, halothane, isoflurane, nitrous oxide, sevoflurane)

Muscle relaxants (atracurium, doxacurium, gallamine, metocurine, mivacurium, pancuronium, pipercuronium, rocuronium, succinylcholine, tubocurarine, vecuronium)

Narcotics (alfentanil, buprenorphine, butorphanol, fentanyl, meperidine, morphine, nalbuphine, sufentanil)

thetase, which results in synthesis of more porphyrin compounds and their precursors.

—Anesthesia can be safely administered to these patients using narcotics, depolarizing and non-depolarizing muscle relaxants, anticholinesterases, propofol, and inhalational agents.

—Questionable agents are benzodiazepines, etomidate, and ketamine.

PREECLAMPSIA/ECLAMPSIA

—Preeclampsia/eclampsia is one of the four hypertensive disorders of pregnancy. Other than preeclampsia/eclampsia, pregnant patients may have chronic hypertension without preeclampsia/eclampsia, chronic hypertension with preclamsia/eclampsia, or gestational hypertension (hypertension evident only during pregnancy, without evidence of preeclampsia).

—Preeclampsia is characterized by the triad of hypertension, proteinuria, and generalized edema after the 20th week of pregnancy. If hypertension is present before the 20th week or persists for more than 6 weeks after delivery, it is considered chronic hypertension. When seizures accompany preeclampsia, the disorder is called eclampsia.

—Preeclampsia/eclampsia is seen most often in primigravidas younger than 20 years old, but it can occur in older, multiparous women.

—The onset of disease, even in hospitalized patients, may not be clinically apparent until delivery or the post-partum period.

—The etiology of this disorder is still unknown. It is theorized that poor placental perfusion may result in release of factors from the placenta that cause damage to endothelial cells (cells lining the blood vessels) in the maternal vasculature and myocardium. These damaged endothelial cells release a peptide (fibronectin), which results in further endothelial damage and vasoconstriction, loss of plasma protein (leading to edema), platelet aggregation, and activation of coagulation.

—Pathophysiologic changes involve most organ systems. The cardiovascular system is affected by vasoconstriction and a hyperdynamic state resulting in increased cardiac output. Decreased plasma volume and decreased plasma oncotic pressures are characteristic of preeclamptic patients. Coagulation abnormalities include decreased platelet number and function, as well as increased partial thromboplastin time (probably clinically insignificant). Renal impairment is reflected in decreased glomerular filtration rate and creatinine clearance. Hepatic involvement is usually mild unless complicated by the HELLP (Hemolysis, Elevated Liver enzymes, Low Platelets) syndrome.

—Severe preeclampsia exists when the systolic blood pressure is >160 mm Hg or diastolic pressure is >110 mm Hg, or proteinuria is >5 g/day, or oliguria <500 mL/day, or there is clinical evidence of cerebral disturbance, visual abnormalities, pulmonary edema, or cyanosis.

—HELLP syndrome is another severe complication of preeclampsia. This usually occurs before 36 weeks gestation, with symptoms of malaise, epigastric pain, nausea, and vomiting. Rapid progression of this disorder to disseminated intravascular coagulation, renal, and hepatic failure requires delivery of the fetus, regardless of the gestational age.

—Anesthetic management must include consideration of physiologic abnormalities such as reduced plasma volume and oncotic pressure in the setting of hypertension as well as drug interactions such as between magnesium sulfate and neuromuscular blockers or calcium channel blockers.

Preeclampsia/Eclampsia Interactions with Anesthesia Drugs
Preeclampsia/eclampsia and calcium channel blockers (diltiazem, nicardipine, nifedipine, verapamil)
—Calcium channel blockers should be used cautiously in patients who have pregnancy-induced hypertension (preeclampsia, eclampsia, toxemia).

—Such patients are likely to be treated with magnesium sulfate which, combined with calcium channel blockers, can cause profound hypotension.

Preeclampsia/eclampsia and diazoxide
—Diazoxide is a potent antihypertensive. Although it is not contraindicated, there are a number of side effects that make other agents more useful.

—Diazoxide inhibits uterine contractions and has been used to terminate premature labor.

—Both maternal and neonatal hyperglycemia have been associated with its use in the prepartum period. The hyperglycemia is a result of epinephrine release from the adrenal medulla caused by diazoxide.

Preeclampsia/eclampsia and methylergonovine
—Patients with hypertension are at highest risk for severe hypertensive reactions to ergot alkaloids such as methylergonovine.

—If stimulation of uterine muscle tone is necessary in these patients, a dilute solution of oxytocin may be preferable.

Preeclampsia/eclampsia and muscle relaxants (atracurium, doxacurium, gallamine, metocurine, mivacurium, pancuronium, pipercuronium, rocuronium, succinylcholine, tubocurarine, vecuronium)

—Patients with hypertensive disorders of pregnancy may require treatment with antihypertensives such as trimethaphan or magnesium sulfate (for preeclampsia/eclampsia). These medications can have significant interactions with anesthetic agents such as succinylcholine, non-depolarizing neuromuscular blocking agents, or calcium channel blockers.

—Neuromuscular blockade produced by both depolarizing and non-depolarizing agents can be potentiated in patients receiving magnesium sulfate. The mechanisms involved include a decreased amount of acetylcholine released by the nerve impulse at the motor nerve terminal and a decrease in the depolarizing action of acetylcholine on the muscle.

Preeclampsia/eclampsia and trimethaphan

—Patients with hypertensive disorders of pregnancy may require treatment with antihypertensives such as trimethaphan or magnesium sulfate (for preeclampsia/eclampsia). These medications can have significant interactions with anesthetic agents such as succinylcholine, non-depolarizing neuromuscular blocking agents, or calcium channel blockers.

—Trimethaphan can significantly prolong the effects of succinylcholine but not of non-depolarizing agents.

—This interaction results from inhibition of plasma pseudocholinesterase by trimethaphan. The result is delayed metabolism of succinylcholine.

PREGNANCY

—In the pregnant patient, drugs and anesthetics can have significant effects on both mother and fetus. Specifically, drug selection in the pregnant patient must include considerations of effects on uterine blood flow as well as potential teratogenicity (causing abnormal fetal development).

—During anesthesia for pregnant patients, treatment of hypotension should be with agents or techniques (uterine displacement, Trendelenburg, fluids) that do not compromise uterine blood flow.

—Vasopressors that produce uterine artery vasoconstriction and should be avoided include phenylephrine, norepinephrine, angiotensin, and methoxamine. These agents are primarily alpha adrenergic stimulants causing peripheral vasoconstriction and potentially compromising placental perfusion.

—Ephedrine, mephentermine, and metaraminol are the preferred agents for treatment of hypotension in pregnancy. These agents have both alpha and beta agonist activity and are not associated with reduced placental blood flow.

—Risk of birth defects is a concern of many patients receiving anesthesia during pregnancy. The period of highest risk for teratogenicity is from day 15 to day 90 of gestation, during the period of organ development of the fetus.

—Although there exist a number of well-known teratogens, the only agents administered by anesthesia personnel associated with birth defects are cocaine, ACE (angiotension-converting enzyme) inhibitors, and benzodiazepines.

—Although controversy exists about the teratogenicity of nitrous oxide, it has not been proven to cause fetal abnormalities in humans. Controversy about the use of nitrous oxide comes from animal studies, but retrospective studies in humans have not shown any association with fetal abnormalities.

Pregnancy Interactions with Anesthesia Drugs

Pregnancy and ACE inhibitors [enalapril (enalaprilat)]

—ACE inhibitors are not considered safe for use in pregnant women. Especially in the second and third trimesters, fetal abnormalities have been linked to ACE therapy.

Pregnancy and benzodiazepines (chlordiazepoxide, diazepam, lorazepam, midazolam)

—Benzodiazepines may cause damage to the fetus, especially during the first trimester of pregnancy.

—Retrospective studies of chlordiazepoxide and diazepam have shown an increased risk of congenital malformations when administered to pregnant patients in their first trimester of pregnancy.

—Administration of preoperative benzodiazepines for obstetric procedures (such as caesarean sections) may produce CNS depression in neonates.

Pregnancy and diazoxide

—Diazoxide is a potent antihypertensive. Although it is not contraindicated, there are a number of side effects that make other agents more useful.

—Diazoxide inhibits uterine contractions and has been used to terminate premature labor.

—Both maternal and neonatal hyperglycemia have been associated with its use in the pre-partum period. The hyperglycemia is a result of epinephrine release from the adrenal medulla caused by diazoxide.

Pregnancy and inhalational anesthetics (desflurane enflurane halothane isoflurane, sevoflurane)

—Pregnancy is associated with significant reductions in minimal alveolar concentrations (MAC) for inhalational agents.

—In animal studies and some human studies, decreases in MAC of up to 40% have been documented. However, these studies did not include desflurane.

—The suggested mechanism for this decreased MAC includes increases in progesterone and endorphin levels associated with pregnancy.

Pregnancy and ketamine

—Ketamine appears to be safe for use in pregnancy or for anesthesia for caesarean section if the dose is less than 2 mg/kg. Doses above this appear to be associated with fetal depression.

Pregnancy and ketorolac

—Ketorolac is contraindicated in labor and delivery or for nursing mothers.

—Because it is a prostaglandin synthesis inhibitor, ketorolac can interfere with platelet function and prolong the bleeding time, resulting in bleeding. It may also inhibit uterine contractions.

—Small amounts of ketorolac have been detected in the breast milk of nursing mothers who have been given the drug for postpartum analgesia. Because bleeding complications can potentially occur in the neonate, ketorolac is contraindicated in nursing mothers.

Pregnancy and morphine

—Reactivation of oral herpes simplex virus (HSV-1) in post-caesarean section patients has been associated with administration of epidural or intrathecal morphine. There is apparently no association with recurrence of genital herpes.

—There is some controversy about this because activation of HSV can result from other causes including infections, fever, emotional or physical stress, and surgery. Also a high percentage of herpes-infected women experience recurrence in the peripartum period even without having received epidural or intrathecal narcotics.

Pregnancy and succinylcholine

—Plasma pseudocholinesterase levels in pregnant women have been shown to be significantly lower than in nonpregnant women. However, in a study of 50 women, the response to succinylcholine and recovery of twitch height were not significantly different in pregnant versus nonpregnant patients.

Pregnancy and vasopressors (ephedrine, epinephrine, metaraminol, methoxamine, norepinephrine, phenylephrine)

—Ephedrine, mephentermine, and metaraminol are the preferred agents for treatment of hypotension in pregnancy.

—The above agents have both alpha and beta agonist activity and are not associated with reduced placental blood flow.

—Phenylephrine, norepinephrine, angiotensin, and methoxamine are predominantly alpha adrenergic agents that act peripherally and can cause uterine artery vasoconstriction and placental hypoperfusion.

PREGNANCY-INDUCED HYPERTENSION

—The term "pregnancy-induced hypertension" (PIH) is at times used interchangeably with "preeclampsia/eclampsia" but actually refers to four different disorders in which hypertension is associated with pregnancy. These include hypertension as a result of preeclampsia/eclampsia, chronic hypertension with preeclampsia/eclampsia, chronic hypertension without preeclampsia/eclampsia, and gestational hypertension (hypertension only during pregnancy and not associated with preeclampsia).

—Chronic hypertension refers to hypertension that has its onset before 20 weeks of gestation or that persists for more than 6 weeks after termination of pregnancy.

—Hypertension in the pregnant patient is defined as an increase in systolic blood pressure of 30 mm Hg or above 140 mm Hg, or a diastolic pressure increase of 15 mm Hg or above 90 mm Hg.

—A number of medications used to treat hypertension in the pregnant patient can have important interactions with medications used by anesthesia personnel. Examples of these interactions include those between magnesium sulfate and muscle relaxants, as well as interactions between trimethaphan and succinylcholine.

Both magnesium and trimethaphan can prolong neuromuscular blockade, but through different mechanisms.

PIH Interactions with Anesthesia Drugs

PIH (Pregnancy-Induced Hypertension) and calcium channel blockers (diltiazem, nicardipine, nifedipine, verapamil)

—Calcium channel blockers should be used cautiously in patients who have pregnancy-induced hypertension (preeclampsia, eclampsia, toxemia).

—Such patients are likely to be treated with magnesium sulfate, which when combined with calcium channel blockers can cause profound hypotension.

PIH (Pregnancy-Induced Hypertension) and diazoxide

—Diazoxide is a potent antihypertensive. Although it is not contraindicated, there are a number of side effects that make other agents more useful.

—Diazoxide inhibits uterine contractions and has been used to terminate premature labor.

—Both maternal and neonatal hyperglycemia has been associated with its use in the prepartum period. The hyperglycemia is a result of epinephrine release from the adrenal medulla caused by diazoxide.

PIH (Pregnancy-Induced Hypertension) and methylergonovine

—Patients with hypertension are at highest risk for severe hypertensive reactions to ergot alkaloids such as methylergonovine.

—If stimulation of uterine muscle tone is necessary in these patients, a dilute solution of oxytocin may be preferable.

PIH (Pregnancy-Induced Hypertension) and muscle relaxants (atracurium, doxacurium gallamine, metocurine, mivacurium, pancuronium, pipercuronium, rocuronium, succinylcholine, tubocurarine, vecuronium)

—Patients with hypertensive disorders of pregnancy may require treatment with antihypertensives such as trimethaphan or magnesium sulfate (for preeclampsia/eclampsia). These medications can have significant interactions with anesthetic agents such as succinylcholine, non-depolarizing neuromuscular blocking agents, or calcium channel blockers.

—Neuromuscular blockade produced by both depolarizing and non-depolarizing agents can be potentiated in patients receiving magnesium sulfate. The mechanisms involved include a decreased amount of acetylcholine released by the nerve impulse at the motor nerve terminal and a decrease in the depolarizing action of acetylcholine on the muscle.

PIH (Pregnancy-Induced Hypertension) and trimethaphan

—Patients with hypertensive disorders of pregnancy may require treatment with antihypertensives such as trimethaphan or magnesium sulfate (for preeclampsia/eclampsia). These medications can have significant interactions with anesthetic agents such as succinylcholine, non-depolarizing neuromuscular blocking agents, or calcium channel blockers.

—Trimethaphan can significantly prolong the effects of succinylcholine but not of non-depolarizing agents.

—This interaction results from inhibition of plasma pseudocholinesterase by trimethaphan. The result is delayed metabolism of succinylcholine.

PULMONARY AIR CYSTS

—Several clinical situations exist in which there is accumulation of gas or air with low blood solubility in enclosed body spaces. These situations include intestinal obstruction, pneumothorax, pulmonary air cysts, and patients undergoing procedures in which air or gas is introduced intentionally (retinal detachment repair, pneumoencephalogram) or unintentionally (air embolism, tympanoplasty, pneumocephalus during neurosurgery).

—Because nitrous oxide is used in high concentrations (50–70%) and is 35 times more soluble in blood than is nitrogen, nitrous oxide will enter an air-containing cavity causing expansion or increase in pressure. This effect cannot be offset by displacement of nitrogen (composing 78% of air) because of nitrogen's low solubility.

—Additionally, for patients having surgery for retinal detachment, where sulfahexafluoride gas, nitrogen, or a combination is injected into the vitreous cavity, use of nitrous oxide could produce unwanted expansion or pressure in the eye. The same is true for patients having tympanoplasty.

Pulmonary Air Cysts Interactions with Anesthesia Drugs
Pulmonary air cysts and nitrous oxide

—Nitrous oxide can result in rapid expansion of gas- or air-filled cavities in the anesthetized patient. For this reason, it should not be administered to patients with a pneumothorax, acute intestinal obstruction, pulmonary air cysts, or patients at significant risk for air embolism.

—Additionally, for patients having surgery for retinal detachment, where sulfahexafluoride gas, nitrogen, or a combination is injected into the vitreous cavity, use of nitrous oxide could produce unwanted expansion or pressure in the eye. The same is true for patients having tympanoplasty.

—Because nitrous oxide is used in high concentrations (50–70%) and is 35 times more soluble in blood than is nitrogen, nitrous oxide will enter an air-containing cavity causing expansion or increase in pressure. This effect cannot be offset by displacement of nitrogen (composing 78% of air) because of nitrogen's low solubility.

PULMONARY HYPERTENSION

—Normal pulmonary artery pressures are approximately 25 mm Hg systolic, 8 mm Hg diastolic, and a mean pressure of 15 mm Hg. Pulmonary hypertension exists when the mean pressure is greater than 20 mm Hg and is considered moderate when mean pressures exceed 30 mm Hg.

—Pulmonary hypertension may be either primary (primary pulmonary hypertension) or secondary to some other disorder.

—Primary pulmonary hypertension is a disease of the small pulmonary vessels, seen mostly in young adults. Symptoms begin with dyspnea on exertion and progress to syncope, angina, and, eventually, congestive heart failure.

—Of the secondary causes of pulmonary hypertension, there are five general classes: (1) a loss of some portion of the normal pulmonary vascular bed (lung resection, pulmonary embolus, emphysema), (2) pulmonary vasoconstriction (secondary to hypoxia, acidosis, drugs), (3) increased blood viscosity (polycythemia), (4) secondary to increased left atrial pressures, and (5) communication with systemic circulation [ventricular septal defect, atrial septal defect (ASD), and patent ductus arteriosus (PDA)].

—The most common disorder associated with secondary pulmonary hypertension is chronic obstructive pulmonary disease (COPD). When pulmonary hypertension is mild to moderate, symptoms are mainly those related to lung disease. As in primary pulmonary hypertension, cardiac symptoms may include dyspnea on exertion, exertional syncope, and right heart failure (hepatosplenomegaly, dependent edema, elevated jugular venous pressure).

—Cor pulmonale refers to heart disease that is secondary to pulmonary hypertension (some define cor pulmonale as secondary only to lung disease). Pulmonary hypertension from any cause results in dilatation, hypertrophy, and, sometimes, failure of the right ventricle.

—Anesthetic management of patients with pulmonary hypertension must include consideration of stimuli to pulmonary vasoconstriction (hypoxia, acidosis). Decreases in systemic vascular resistance may result in unexpected hypotension (because of obstruction to right heart outflow). Avoidance of excessive cardiac stimulation (ketamine) is recommended. Use of nitrous oxide is controversial because some studies have indicated that it may worsen pulmonary vasoconstriction.

Pulmonary Hypertension Interactions with Anesthesia Drugs

Pulmonary hypertension and bretylium

—Patients with severe pulmonary hypertension or aortic stenosis may experience cardiac decompensation with bretylium therapy.

—Within 1 hour following bretylium administration, as much as 65% of patients will have a drop in blood pressure. Patients with severe aortic stenosis or pulmonary hypertension may not be able to compensate adequately for this hypotension.

—If treatment of life-threatening arrhythmias indicates treatment with bretylium in such patients, observation, monitoring, and treatment for the hypotension may be necessary.

Pulmonary hypertension and ketamine

—Ketamine can cause an increase in pulmonary vascular resistance and should be used cautiously in patients with pulmonary hypertension.

—Cardiovascular stimulation by ketamine is a result of central nervous stimulation and inhibition of neuronal norepinephrine reuptake. The consequence of these actions is an increase in cardiac output, heart rate, and peripheral vasoconstriction.

—Some patients are resistant to indirect cardiovascular stimulation, such as those with septic shock or chronic congestive heart failure. In these patients, the direct myocardial depressant effects of ketamine may be evident.

Pulmonary hypertension and nitrous oxide
—Use of nitrous oxide is controversial in patients with elevated pulmonary vascular pressure.
—Although some studies have shown no significant effect of nitrous oxide in patients with pulmonary hypertension, others demonstrate that nitrous oxide is capable of producing pulmonary vasoconstriction.

RAYNAUD'S PHENOMENON

—Raynaud's phenomenon is a disease of the arteries of the extremities. It is characterized by digital vasospasm, frequently induced by cold, and is almost always associated with an underlying immunologic disorder (scleroderma, systemic lupus erythematosus, primary pulmonary hypertension).
—Raynaud's disease refers to a primary disorder, more frequent in women, not associated with another disease, and is often bilateral (unlike Raynaud's phenomenon).
—Beta blockers must be used with extreme caution in patients with Raynaud's phenomenon because of the ability of these drugs to worsen or precipitate digital vasospasm.
—Arteriovenous shunts exist in the fingertips and dilate with beta adrenergic stimulation. Beta 1 blockade can result in vasoconstriction. Labetalol, because of its ability to block alpha receptors, would be less likely to cause this problem.

Raynaud's Phenomenon Interactions with Anesthesia Drugs
Raynaud's phenomenon and beta blockers (esmolol, labetalol, propranolol)
—Beta blockers must be used with extreme caution in patients with Raynaud's phenomenon because of the ability of these drugs to worsen or precipitate digital vasospasm.
—Arteriovenous shunts exist in the fingertips and dilate with beta adrenergic stimulation. Beta 1 blockade can result in vasoconstriction. Labetalol, because of its ability to block alpha receptors, would be less likely to cause this problem.

RENAL DYSFUNCTION

—Renal dysfunction or failure refers to a decline in glomerular filtration as well as tubular functions (reabsorption and secretion of ions, primarily hydrogen and potassium). As a result, there is accumulation of urea, creatinine, uric acid, and hydrogen ions, among other substances.

—Two basic types of renal failure are (1) acute (usually reversible failure as a result of some insult such as ischemia) and (2) chronic (usually irreversible decline resulting from hypertension, diabetic nephropathy, polycystic kidney disease, etc.).

—Signs and symptoms of patients with chronic renal failure include weight loss, brownish skin pigmentation, hypertension, peripheral neuropathy, and osteodystrophy (hypocalcemia is partly related to decreased vitamin D activation, which normally occurs in the kidney). Also seen are normochromic, normocytic anemia (from decreased erythropoietin) and bleeding disorders (partly related to platelet abnormalities).

—Excretion of many drugs and some anesthetics is significantly affected by renal failure. Several muscle relaxants, for example, have a prolonged duration of action in patients with renal dysfunction. The excretion of some drugs, such as narcotics and benzodiazepines, are not significantly affected, although their effects seem to be potentiated in some patients with renal failure. This interaction may be due to the systemic effects of renal disease, which for unclear reasons increases the CNS effects of these medications.

Renal Dysfunction Interactions with Anesthesia Drugs

Renal dysfunction and amrinone

—Patients with congestive heart failure and/or compromised renal function may have higher-than-expected serum concentrations of amrinone during infusion of the drug. This occurs because excretion of amrinone is primarily via the urine.

—Evidence of excessive levels of amrinone may be hypotension or ventricular arrhythmias.

Renal dysfunction and atracurium

—Age, obesity, liver or renal dysfunction have no significant effect on metabolism of atracurium.

—Atracurium is metabolized by Hoffman elimination as well as ester hydrolysis.

—Hoffman elimination is a nonenzymatic process that occurs at physiologic temperatures and pH. Ester hydrolysis occurs most rapidly in an acid pH and does not require plasma pseudocholinesterase.

Renal dysfunction and barbiturates, benzodiazepines, narcotics, propofol*

—Renal dysfunction has not been demonstrated to cause significant changes in pharmacokinetics or pharmacodynamics of benzodiazepines, narcotics (with the possible exception of butorphanol), barbiturates, or propofol.

—In patients with renal dysfunction, the above drugs may appear to have an increase in duration or intensity. This has been explained as a response to the systemic effects of renal dysfunction rather than specific effects on the metabolism of theses drugs.

—Some muscle relaxants are significantly affected by renal failure.

Renal dysfunction and butorphanol

—Butorphanol should be used in reduced dosages in patients with hepatic or renal dysfunction due to the routes of metabolism and excretion of this drug.

Renal dysfunction and calcium chloride

—Since calcium chloride administration may worsen acidosis, patients who have both hypokalemia and acidosis (such as renal failure patients) may be best treated with other forms of calcium replacement (such as calcium gluconate or gluceptate).

—This interaction is probably only significant when large doses of calcium are required.

Renal dysfunction and cimetidine

—Cimetidine is dependent on renal excretion and hepatic metabolism. In patients with renal or hepatic dysfunction, accumulation of cimetidine can occur, requiring longer intervals between doses (12 hours versus 6–8 hours).

Renal dysfunction and inhalational anesthetics (desflurane, enflurane, halothane, isoflurane, sevoflurane)

—Enflurane, isoflurane, halothane, and desflurane are considered safe for administration to patients with renal dysfunction.

—Although enflurane undergoes biotransformation with the formation of inorganic fluoride to a greater extent than other agents (with the exception of methoxyflurane, which is very nephrotoxic), even 4 hours of anesthesia with enflurane pro-

---

* Barbiturates (methohexital, sodium pentothal)
Benzodiazepines (chlordiazepoxide, diazepam, lorazepam, midazolam)
Narcotics (alfentanil, buprenorphine, fentanyl, meperidine, morphine, nalbuphine, sufentanil)

duces nontoxic fluoride levels. There is some question, however, of renal toxicity after prolonged (9 hours) anesthesia with enflurane.

—Sevoflurane is also biotransformed to inorganic fluoride, but at potentially nephrotoxic levels (50 μmol/L), according to some studies. However, there is no clinical evidence of renal toxicity from sevoflurane use.

—All inhaled anesthetic agents can cause a transient, reversible decrease in renal function as reflected in lowered glomerular filtration rate (GFR), urine output, and urinary sodium excretion.

—The mechanism for this action may include alterations in antidiuretic hormone, vasopressin, or renin, as well as decreases in renal blood flow.

Renal dysfunction and diltiazem

—Elimination of diltiazem depends on hepatic metabolism and urinary excretion. Patients with impaired hepatic or renal function may experience more pronounced effects at usual doses.

Renal dysfunction and ketorolac

—Ketorolac (a prostaglandin synthesis inhibitor) can worsen renal function in patients whose compromised renal function is very dependent on the presence of vasodilatory prostaglandins.

—Patients at risk for this interaction are those with renal dysfunction as a result of renal disease or advanced age (>65 years old) or poor renal perfusion from congestive heart failure or hypovolemia.

—Nonsteroidal agents may also cause interstitial nephritis, glomerulonephritis, or renal papillary necrosis.

—In these patients, reduced doses of ketorolac should be used.

Renal dysfunction and muscle relaxants (atracurium, doxacurium, gallamine, metocurine, mivacurium, pancuronium, pipecuronium, rocuronium, tubocurarine, vecuronium)

—Neuromuscular blocking agents that are highly dependent on the kidneys for their elimination include gallamine (100%), metocurine (80–100%), pancuronium (80–100%), doxacurium, rocuronium, and pipecuronium.

—Agents that are less or nondependent on renal function for elimination include *d*-tubocurarine (40–60%), vecuronium (10–20%), atracurium (<5%), and succinylcholine.

—Mivacurium is prolonged in renal failure primarily because of a decrease in plasma cholinesterase that is responsible for degradation of mivacurium. Infusions of mivacurium should be decreased as much as 40% in renal failure patients.

Renal dysfunction and procainamide

—Elimination of procainamide is very dependent on adequate renal function and patients with renal disease can show toxicity from procainamide earlier than normal patients.

—Up to 70% of a procainamide dose can be eliminated unchanged in the urine. Hepatic metabolism converts procainamide into *N*-acetylprocainamide, which has slightly different properties from the parent compound but can cause toxicity at high levels.

—In patients with renal disease, more procainamide is converted to *N*-acetylprocainamide, which can accumulate to toxic levels.

Renal dysfunction and succinylcholine

—Succinylcholine does not appear to result in significantly prolonged neuromuscular blockade in patients with renal failure unless given by infusion.

—Because one of the metabolites of succinylcholine is highly dependent on renal clearance, use of succinylcholine by infusion can result in prolonged neuromuscular blockade.

—Although there is controversy about decreased levels of plasma cholinesterase in patients with renal failure, recent studies have indicated that mivacurium elimination is prolonged in such patients because of decreased plasma cholinesterase.

RETINAL DETACHMENT

—Several clinical situations exist in which there is accumulation of gas or air with low blood solubility in enclosed body spaces. These situations include intestinal obstruction, pneumothorax, pulmonary air cysts, and patients undergoing procedures in which air or gas is introduced intentionally (retinal detachment repair, pneumoencephalogram) or unintentionally (air embolism, tympanoplasty, pneumocephalus during neurosurgery).

—Because nitrous oxide is used in high concentrations (50–70%) and is 35 times more soluble in blood than is nitrogen, nitrous oxide will enter an air-containing cavity causing expansion or increase in pressure. This effect cannot be offset by displacement of nitrogen (composing 78% of air) because of nitrogen's low solubility.

—Additionally, for patients having surgery for retinal detachment, where sulfahexafluoride gas, nitrogen, or a combination is injected into the vitreous cavity, use of nitrous oxide could produce unwanted expansion or pressure in the eye. The same is true for patients having tympanoplasty.

Retinal Detachment Interactions with Anesthesia Drugs
Retinal detachment and nitrous oxide
- —Nitrous oxide can result in rapid expansion of gas- or air-filled cavities in the anesthetized patient. For this reason, it should not be administered to patients with pneumothorax, acute intestinal obstruction, or patients at significant risk for air embolism.
- —Additionally, for patients having surgery for retinal detachment, where sulfahexafluoride gas, nitrogen, or a combination is injected into the vitreous cavity, use of nitrous oxide could produce unwanted expansion or pressure in the eye. The same is true for patients having tympanoplasty.
- —Because nitrous oxide is used in high concentrations (50–70%) and is 35 times more soluble in blood than is nitrogen, nitrous oxide will enter an air-containing cavity causing expansion or increase in pressure. This effect cannot be offset by displacement of nitrogen (composing 78% of air) because of nitrogen's low solubility.

SHY–DRAGER SYNDROME

- —Shy–Drager syndrome is a disorder of the autonomic nervous system combined with signs of degeneration of the CNS. Evidence of autonomic dysfunction includes postural hypotension that may be severe enough to cause syncope. Degeneration of areas in the CNS is manifested as signs of Parkinsonism with rigidity, intention tremor, and ataxia.
- —The autonomic nervous system helps maintain blood pressure and organ perfusion through innervation of the heart and blood vessels. Specifically, sympathetic stimulation of the cardiovascular system results in increased heart rate, contractility, and cardiac output whereas increased arteriolar tone increases perfusion pressure.
- —The most common cause of autonomic dysfunction is diabetes mellitus. Sympathetic denervation is milder and more slow in onset than in patients with Shy–Drager syndrome.
- —In patients with autonomic dysfunction, hypotension induced by certain medications (such as verapamil, nifedipine) or that

block sympathetic receptors (such as beta blockers) may result in exaggerated hypotension due to inadequate compensatory responses.

Shy–Drager Syndrome Interactions with Anesthesia Drugs
Shy–Drager syndrome and calcium channel blockers (diltiazem, nicardipine, nifedipine, verapamil)

—Patients whose autonomic nervous system responses are impaired by disease (Shy–Drager) or medications (beta blockers) may be unable to adequately compensate for vasodilation or negative inotropic and chronotropic effects of calcium channel blockers.

—In these patients, exaggerated hypotension or bradycardia may be seen with calcium channel blockers.

—Nifedipine and nicardipine would be more likely to be associated with hypotension than either bradycardia or myocardial depression, which would be more often seen with verapamil or diltiazem.

SICK SINUS SYNDROME

—Sick sinus syndrome is characterized by periods of inappropriate sinus bradycardia and even sinus arrest. Episodes of supraventricular tachycardia are commonly seen during periods of bradycardia.

—The disorder is a result of disease in the sinus node, caused by different pathologic processes that produce fibrosis and degenerative changes in the sinus node. It is seen mostly in elderly patients, about 50% of whom also have disorders of the atrioventricular and intraventricular conduction tissues (first-, second-, third-degree block, bundle branch block, etc.).

—Symptoms include syncope, palpitations, and congestive heart failure. Treatment of choice for recurrent bradycardia is electrical pacing, whereas digitalis is usually effective for recurrent tachycardias.

—Extreme caution should be used with certain drugs in patients with sick sinus syndrome. The diseased sinus nodes of these patients appear to be very sensitive to depression by, among other things, class IA antiarrhythmics (quinidine, procainamide, disopyramide), and treatment of arrhythmias in patients with sick sinus syndrome can result in severe sinus bradycardia or asystole.

—Beta blockers and some calcium channel blockers (diltiazem, verapamil) are also potent depressants of the sinus node and must be used with caution unless a pacemaker is in place.

Sick Sinus Syndrome Interactions with Anesthesia Drugs

Sick sinus syndrome and beta blockers (esmolol, labetalol, propranolol) and calcium channel blockers (diltiazem, verapamil)

—Diltiazem, verapamil, and beta blockers should be avoided or used with extreme caution in patients with sick sinus syndrome.

—Use of these drugs, which depress sinus node automaticity, may cause severe bradycardia even in patients with sick sinus syndrome who are experiencing supraventricular tachycardia.

—Digitalis may be effective in controlling supraventricular tachycardias.

Sick sinus syndrome and procainamide

—Patients with sick sinus syndrome can experience supraventricular tachyarrhythmias. The diseased sinus nodes of these patients appear to be very sensitive to depression by, among other things, class IA antiarrhythmics (quinidine, procainamide, disopyramide) and treatment of arrhythmias in patients with sick sinus syndrome can result in severe sinus bradycardia or asystole.

STOKES–ADAMS SYNDROME

—Stokes–Adams syndrome is one of several different causes of cardiac syncope. Patients with this syndrome experience loss of consciousness (syncope) due to a sudden decrease in cardiac output that results from an atrioventricular conduction block.

—The atrioventricular block that causes the syncope may be persistent but is commonly intermittent. In such cases, an electrocardiogram taken following the episode may be normal.

—Although most patients recover consciousness promptly, cerebral ischemia may result in some cases, with a resultant transient or permanent neurologic deficit. Also, in some patients, ventricular standstill may be followed by a life-threatening arrhythmia, such as ventricular tachycardia or fibrillation.

—Treatment for Stokes–Adams syndrome is an implantable pacemaker.

—Because phenytoin reduces automaticity in the His-Purkinje conduction system, this medication is contraindicated in patients with known Stokes–Adams syndrome who do not have a pacemaker.

—Other causes of cardiac syncope include tachyarrhythmias (supraventricular and ventricular), disorders of sinus node automaticity, and aortic stenosis.

Stokes-Adams Interactions with Anesthesia Drugs
Stokes-Adams and diphenylhydantoin

—The antiarrhythmic properties of diphenylhydantoin involve a decrease in automaticity as well as a decrease in excitability of Purkinje fibers. Because of this effect, phenytoin is contraindicated in patients with sinus bradycardia, sinoatrial block, as well as patients with second- and third-degree heart block, or with Stokes–Adams syndrome.

SYRINGOMYELIA

—Syringomyelia is a disorder in which there is cavitation of the spinal cord. Usually, it results from the Arnold–Chiari malformation (downward displacement of the cerebellar tonsils and medulla), but can result from trauma.

—The disease usually presents in patients 20–30 years old with symptoms of sensory impairment in the upper extremities. Progression of the disease results in motor nerve impairment with skeletal muscle weakness and atrophy.

—As in other disorders associated with abnormalities of muscle cell innervation, patients with syringogmyelia may be at risk of severe hyperkalemia with succinylcholine. Also, resistance to non-depolarizing agents and/or prolonged neuromuscular blockade can also be seen.

—Disuse or denervation of muscle results in production of extrajunctional acetylcholine receptors on the muscle membrane. These receptors are less easily blocked by non-depolarizing agents but are activated by lower concentrations of depolarizing drugs (succinylcholine).

—Despite initial resistance to blockade, such patients may demonstrate prolonged neuromuscular weakness as a result of decreased muscle strength and mass.

—Hyperkalemia is associated with the presence of extrajunctional receptors when exposed to succinylcholine. When these receptors, which can be scattered over a large surface of the muscle, are depolarized by succinylcholine, ion flow takes place through the receptor channel. Large amounts of potassium may exit the muscle cell, causing hyperkalemia.

Syringomyelia Interactions with Anesthesia Drugs

Syringomyelia and non-depolarizing muscle relaxants (atracurium, doxacurium, gallamine, metocurine, mivacurium, pancuronium, pipercuronium, rocuronium, tubocurarine, vecuronium)

—As in other disorders associated with abnormalities of muscle cell innervation, patients with syringomyelia may be at risk of severe hyperkalemia with succinylcholine. In addition, resistance to non-depolarizing agents and/or prolonged neuromuscular blockade can also be seen.

—Disuse or denervation of muscle results in production of extrajunctional acetylcholine receptors on the muscle membrane. These receptors are less easily blocked by non-depolarizing agents but are activated by lower concentrations of depolarizing drugs (succinylcholine).

—Despite initial resistance to blockade, such patients may demonstrate prolonged neuromuscular weakness as a result of decreased muscle strength and mass.

—Hyperkalemia is associated with the presence of extrajunctional receptors when exposed to succinylcholine. When these receptors, which can be scattered over a large surface of the muscle, are depolarized by succinylcholine, ion flow takes place through the receptor channel. Large amounts of potassium may exit the muscle cell, causing hyperkalemia.

Syringomyelia and succinylcholine

—Chronic or progressive motor neuron disease places patients at continuous risk for hyperkalemia from succinylcholine. Syringomyelia, amyotrophic lateral sclerosis, multiple sclerosis, acute idiopathic polyneuritis (Guillain–Barré syndrome), and all forms of muscular dystrophy have been associated with this response.

—Patients with neuromuscular disease (upper and lower motor neuron abnormalities) can respond to succinylcholine with a dangerous, sometimes fatal, hyperkalemia. This probably occurs because of proliferation of extrajunctional acetylcholine receptors on the muscle membrane. Depolarization of these receptors causes potassium leak through the muscle membrane.

WOLF–PARKINSON–WHITE SYNDROME

—Wolf–Parkinson–White (WPW) syndrome is the most common of the preexcitation syndromes. It is a result of the presence of bypass tracts (Kent fibers) that conduct atrial impulses to the ventricles, bypassing the atrioventricular node. The other preexcitation syndromes are a result of different bypass tracts: James fibers (Lown–Ganong–Levine syndrome) or Mahaim fibers.

—Electrocardiograms of patients with WPW show a short PR interval because atrial contraction is conducted rapidly to the ventricles by the bypass tracts. A delta wave results from activation of ventricular tissue by the impulse carried over the bypass tract, whereas the remainder of the QRS is partly a result of ventricular depolarization from an impulse carried by normal conduction tissues.

—Patients with WPW syndrome can have cardiac arrhythmias, the most common of which is paroxysmal supraventricular tachycardia. Atrial fibrillation or flutter can also occur.

—Reciprocal tachycardia is usually initiated by a premature atrial contraction. This impulse is then most likely to be conducted by the AV node because the bypass tracts have a longer refractory period than normal conduction tissue. By the time ventricular depolarization is accomplished, the bypass tracts are no longer refractory and retrograde conduction to the atria can take place, resulting in atrial depolarization and a self-propagating tachycardia.

—In the above situation, the electrocardiographic pattern will be usually a narrow QRS complex. If antegrade conduction occurs via the bypass tracts, wide QRS complex tachycardia will be seen on the ECG because ventricular depolarization does not proceed through normal conduction tissue.

—Acute treatment of tachyarrhythmias in patients with WPW depends on the pathophysiology. If the QRS complex is narrow, indicating antegrade conduction via normal conduction paths, treatment can be with agents that slow conduction through the AV node: verapamil, propranolol, digitalis, procainamide, or diltiazem.

—In tachyarrhythmias with wide QRS complexes, antegrade conduction must be assumed to be taking place via accessory paths. Conduction through these paths can be accelerated by verapamil, diltiazem, digitalis, lidocaine, or propranolol. Intravenous procainamide is the treatment of choice.

Wolf–Parkinson–White Syndrome Interactions with Anesthesia Drugs

*Wolf–Parkinson–White syndrome and beta blockers, calcium channel blockers, digitalis, lidocaine**

—Verapamil, diltiazem, digitalis, beta blockers, and lidocaine should not be used to acutely treat wide complex tachyarrhythmias associated with the Wolf–Parkinson–White syndrome.

—In tachyarrhythmias with wide QRS complexes, antegrade conduction must be assumed to be taking place via accessory paths. Conduction through these paths can be accelerated by verapamil, diltiazem, digitalis, lidocaine, or propranolol. Intravenous procainamide is the treatment of choice.

—If the QRS complex is narrow, indicating antegrade conduction via normal conduction paths, treatment can be with agents that slow conduction through the AV node: verapamil, propranolol, digitalis, procainamide, or diltiazem.

Wolf–Parkinson–White syndrome and procainamide

—In situations of wide complex tachyarrhythmias in patients with Wolf–Parkinson–White syndrome, intravenous procainamide is the preferred treatment.

—In tachyarrhythmias with wide QRS complexes, antegrade conduction must be assumed to be taking place via accessory paths. Conduction through these paths can be accelerated by verapamil, diltiazem, digitalis, lidocaine, or propranolol.

---

* Beta blockers (esmolol, labetalol, propranolol)
  Calcium channel blockers (diltiazem, verapamil)

3

ANESTHETIC AGENTS

ADENOSINE (Adenocard)

Classification and indications

—Adenosine is a nucleoside that exists endogenously in all body tissues.

—It is indicated for conversion of paroxysmal supraventricular tachycardias (PSVT) to sinus rhythm. This includes PSVT caused by Wolf–Parkinson–White syndrome and other syndromes with bypass tracts.

—Although ventricular slowing may occur in patients with rapid ventricular response to atrial fibrillation or flutter, adenosine is unlikely to convert these arrhythmias to sinus rhythm.

Pharmacology

—Adenosine slows conduction through the atrioventricular node.

—It is cleared very rapidly from the circulation, with a half-life of approximately 10 seconds.

—Usual doses of adenosine (6–12 mg) will not cause hypotension.

Dose

—Initial dose should be 6 mg given intravenously over 1 or 2 seconds. A repeat dose of 12 mg may be given twice after 1 or 2 minutes if necessary.

Adenosine Interactions with Anesthesia Drugs
Adenosine and aminophylline, theophylline

—Adenosine is a nucleoside that slows conduction through the atrioventricular node. Xanthines such as theophylline, aminophylline, and caffeine can reverse or block the physiologic effects of adenosine.

Adenosine Interactions with Diseases
Adenosine and cerebral edema, intracranial hypertension

—Most systemic vasodilators (nitroglycerin, nitroprusside, hydralazine, calcium channel blockers, and adenosine) can produce cerebrovascular vasodilation as well. As a result, cerebral blood volume is either maintained or increased even though systemic blood pressure is decreased.

—Trimethaphan, a ganglionic blocker, usually will not increase cerebral blood volume because ganglionic blockade normally does not cause vasodilation of the cerebral circulation.

Adenosine Interactions with Patient Drugs
Adenosine and aminophylline, theophylline

—Adenosine is a nucleoside that slows conduction through the atrioventricular node. Xanthines such as theophylline, aminophylline, and caffeine can reverse or block the physiologic effects of adenosine.

Adenosine and carbamazepine

—Adenosine when used in patients taking carbamazepine may produce a greater blockade than anticipated. A decrease in adenosine dosage may be appropriate in such patients.

Adenosine and dipyridamole

—Dipyridamole blocks the uptake and metabolism of adenosine by erythrocytes and some other cells. As a result, the dose necessary to produce hemodynamic changes from adenosine may be significantly decreased.

—In one study, pretreatment of patients with dipyridamole decreased the required dose of adenosine by 75–90%.

ALBUTEROL (Airet, Proventil, Ventolin, Volmax)

Classification and indications

—Albuterol is a beta agonist that is mainly selective for beta 2 receptors.

—It is indicated for the treatment or prevention of bronchospasm in patients 2 years or older.

Pharmacology

—Albuterol causes relaxation of bronchial and uterine smooth muscle by stimulation of beta 2 receptors which stimulate adenyl cyclase.

—Although in most patients effects are mainly confined to the respiratory tract, some patients experience significant cardiovascular stimulation (tachycardia, hypertension).

—Systemic levels are low when albuterol is administered by inhalation due to slow absorption from the respiratory tract.

—Onset of improvement in pulmonary function can occur within 15 minutes after inhalation and may last 4 hours or more.

Dose

—Inhalation aerosol: This formulation is intended for patients 4 years or older and should be administered as 2 inhalations every 4 hours.

—Inhalation solution: Intended for administration by nebulization, this formulation is recommended for patients 12 or older at a dose of 2.5 mg in 2.5 mL of saline every 6–8 hours.

—Albuterol is also available as a syrup or tablets for oral administration.

Albuterol Interactions with Anesthesia Drugs
Albuterol and digitalis
—Acute administration of albuterol either intravenously or orally resulted in a 16% reduction of digoxin concentration within 30 minutes in a number of patients with stable digoxin levels. Additionally, serum potassium concentrations also declined approximately 15% within 10 minutes of the albuterol dose.

Albuterol Interactions with Patient Drugs
Albuterol and digitalis
—Acute administration of albuterol either intravenously or orally resulted in a 16% reduction of digoxin concentration within 30 minutes in a number of patients with stable digoxin levels. Additionally, serum potassium concentrations also declined approximately 15% within 10 minutes of the albuterol dose.

ALFENTANIL (Alfenta)

Classification and indications
—Alfentanil is an opioid analgesic.
—It is indicated for use in patients being anesthetized for surgery. It can be used as part of a technique for general anesthesia (such as nitrous/narcotic) or as part of a regimen for intravenous sedation (such as with propofol or midazolam).

Pharmacology
—Alfentanil, like other narcotics, exerts its analgesic effects through opioid receptors in the CNS (brain and spinal cord).
—Although narcotics used in anesthesia are potent analgesics, there is controversy about the level of amnesia induced with even large doses of narcotics. To avoid awareness during anesthesia, use of other anesthetic agents (benzodiazepines, inhalation agents, etc.) is recommended.
—Somatosensory evoked potentials (SEPs) are not significantly affected by narcotics.
—Although there is some controversy about increases in intracranial pressure from opioids, in general opioids cause slight decreases in cerebral blood flow, metabolic rate, and intracranial pressure.
—Cardiovascular effects of alfentanil, sufentanil, and fentanyl include variable degrees of bradycardia and hypotension. This is thought to be mostly from decreased central sympa-

thetic outflow, although some direct effects have been suggested.
— Like other narcotics, alfentanil causes respiratory depression and reduced hypoxic ventilatory drive.
— Muscle rigidity, particularly of the chest wall, has been associated with rapid administration of narcotics. The mechanism of this action is not clear, but older patients seem more prone to this response. It has also been associated most frequently with alfentanil.
— Muscle rigidity can occur not only during induction but also on emergence from anesthesia or, rarely, hours after the last opioid dose.
— Alfentanil has a very rapid onset of action and a duration of action less than that of sufentanil or fentanyl. The half-life of alfentanil is about 4–17 minutes.
— For comparison, the elimination half-lives of fentanyl, sufentanil, and alfentanil are 219, 164, and 90 minutes, respectively.
— Elimination of alfentanil, sufentanil, and fentanyl is a result of hepatic metabolism.
— Continuous infusion or repeated dosing results in accumulation of alfentanil and prolonged effect.
— Older patients and those with liver disease may demonstrate prolonged effects from alfentanil due to decreased clearance of the drug.

Dose
— Although there may be significant patient variability, induction doses as part of a general anesthetic technique with sodium pentothal or propofol should be 8–20 µg/kg body weight. Larger doses can be used for procedures of longer duration or to reduce cardiovascular responses to intubation.
— Continuous infusions doses: 0.5–3 µg/kg/min.

Alfentanil Interactions with Anesthesia Drugs
Alfentanil and clonidine
— Clonidine has been shown to potentiate narcotics and reduce the minimal alveolar concentration (MAC) of inhaled anesthetics.
— This effect may be related to clonidine's inhibition of the sympathetic outflow from the vasomotor center in the medulla (clonidine is a central alpha 2 receptor agonist, which results in inhibition of CNS sympathetic centers).

Alfentanil and naloxone

—Cases of pulmonary edema, hypertension, and ventricular arrhythmias have occurred in postoperative patients receiving naloxone for reversal of respiratory depression induced by narcotics. The precise etiology of these reactions is not known.

Alfentanil Interactions with Diseases

Alfentanil and advanced age

—Alfentanil is primarily metabolized in the liver (>99%).

—In elderly patients, clearance of alfentanil may be significantly reduced, increasing the half-life and causing prolongation of effects.

—Also, elderly patients demonstrate an increased CNS sensitivity to alfentanil, reducing dosing requirements for this age group.

Alfentanil and alcohol—acute intoxication

—Patients who are acutely intoxicated with alcohol (including chronic alcoholics) usually demonstrate increased sensitivity to general anesthesia.

—Although the precise mechanism of interactions is not agreed upon, it appears that alcohol intoxication has additive CNS depression with barbiturates, benzodiazepines, and narcotics, as well as inhalational agents.

Alfentanil and alcohol—chronic abuse

—Chronic abuse of alcohol has complex and incompletely understood effects on a patient's response to anesthetic agents. In general, these patients tend to be more tolerant (in a nonintoxicated state) to barbiturates, benzodiazepines, narcotics, and inhalational agents.

—Exceptions to this generalization include the alcoholic patient with a cardiomyopathy who may demonstrate increased sensitivity to myocardial depression from inhalational agents.

—Also, the patient with severe liver disease may have impaired ability to metabolize succinylcholine due to decreased levels of plasma pseudocholinesterase.

Alfentanil and cerebral edema, intracranial hypertension

—Most intravenous anesthetics cause a reduction in cerebral blood flow and intracranial pressure or have no effect on intracranial hypertension (ICP). Although this effect is primarily from depression of cerebral metabolic rate, in some cases a direct vasoconstriction occurs.

—The exception to the above is ketamine, which causes an increased cerebral metabolic rate and cerebral blood flow with an increase in ICP.

—All the narcotics, as well as barbiturates, etomidate, benzodiazepines, and propofol, have been associated with a reduction or maintenance of ICP during anesthesia.

Alfentanil and cirrhosis, liver disease

—Alfentanil is 99% metabolized in the liver. Patients with cirrhosis, therefore, show as much as a 50% reduction in clearance of alfentanil and it can have a doubling of its half-life.

—Patients with liver disease, therefore, may show prolonged effects from alfentanil.

Alfentanil and malignant hyperthermia

—Anesthetic agents considered safe for use in patients with known or suspected susceptibility for developing malignant hyperthermia (MH) include propofol, barbiturates, etomidate, ketamine, non-depolarizing neuromuscular blocking agents, narcotics, benzodiazepines, droperidol, epinephrine, norepinephrine, and anticholinesterases.

—Nitrous oxide is probably safe in the susceptible patient, based on repeated use in MH-susceptible humans and swine.

—Local or regional anesthesia with either amide (such as lidocaine) or ester (such as procaine) anesthetics is now considered safe for MH-susceptible patients.

Alfentanil and obesity

—Obesity doubles the elimination half-life of alfentanil.

—The implications of this for the anesthesiologist are that obese patients may demonstrate prolonged effects from alfentanil. Also, to maintain steady-state levels of alfentanil in an obese patient, the loading dose may need to be increased, but the maintenance dose can remain unchanged.

Alfentanil and porphyria

—Narcotics are considered safe anesthetics for use in porphyrias.

—Not all of the porphyrias have significance for the anesthesiologist. Three of the four hepatic porphyrias (acute intermittent, variegate, hereditary coproporphyria) and none of the erythropoietic porphyrias are associated with neurologic symptoms that can be triggered by certain medications: barbiturates, etomidate, and corticosteroids.

—Benzodiazepines and etomidate are considered to be questionable triggering agents, whereas safe anesthetics are inhalational agents, narcotics, muscle relaxants, anticholinesterases, and propofol.

Alfentanil Interactions with Patient Drugs
Alfentanil and cimetidine

—Cimetidine may potentiate narcotics, causing greater respiratory depression and sedation than expected. This may be related to the alteration of hepatic metabolism of narcotics produced by cimetidine.

—This effect is seen less with morphine than other narcotics and is probably related to the fact that morphine undergoes a different metabolic process than some other narcotics such as fentanyl or meperidine.

—Ranitidine is not associated with this interaction.

Alfentanil and clonidine

—Clonidine has been shown to potentiate narcotics and reduce the MAC of inhaled anesthetics.

—This effect may be related to clonidine's inhibition of the sympathetic outflow from the vasomotor center in the medulla (clonidine is a central alpha 2 receptor agonist, which results in inhibition of CNS sympathetic centers).

Alfentanil and erythromycin

—Patients who are receiving erythromycin may demonstrate prolonged, unexpected respiratory depression following alfentanil. Single doses of erythromycin do not appear to have this interaction with alfentanil.

—The proposed mechanism of this interaction is that several doses of erythromycin are necessary to produce a metabolite that delays alfentanil metabolism.

AMINOPHYLLINE (Aerolate Aminophylline, Bronkodyl, Choledyl, Dilor, Elixophyllin, Lufyllin, Slo-Bid, Slo-Phyllin, Theo-Dur, Theobid, Theolair, Truphylline)

Classification and indications

—Aminophylline is a xanthine derivative.

—It is used as a bronchodilator and also to treat apnea in infants and patients with Cheyne–Stokes respiration.

Pharmacology

—Aminophylline is a compound of theophylline with ethylenediamine, which makes theophylline more water-soluble.

—Theophylline competitively inhibits phosphodiesterase and increases intracellular cyclic AMP, resulting in bronchodilation and pulmonary arteriolar dilation.

—Theophylline is a CNS and cardiovascular stimulant. Partially offsetting the stimulating effect on the cardiovascular system is systemic arteriolar and venous dilation (as well as coronary artery dilation).

—Optimal bronchodilation usually requires serum theophylline levels between 10 and 20 µg/mL. Above 20 µg/mL, adverse effects of theophylline are likely to manifest (tachycardia, nausea, delirium, seizures, etc.).

—Elimination of theophylline is impaired in patients with congestive heart failure, chronic obstructive pulmonary disease, liver disease, or in geriatric patients.

Dose

—Intravenous therapy for acute bronchospasm in patients not receiving theophylline (aminophylline) requires a loading dose of approximately 6 mg/kg of aminophylline (which is the equivalent of 4.7 mg of theophylline).

—Maintenance doses vary according to age or presence of other medical conditions:

  —Children and healthy, young adult smokers: 1–1.2 mg/kg/hr

  —Healthy, nonsmoking adults: 0.7 mg/kg/hr

  —Older patients or those with liver disease, lung, or heart disease: 0.5–0.6 mg/kg/hr

Aminophylline Interactions with Anesthesia Drugs

Aminophylline and adenosine

—Adenosine is a nucleoside that slows conduction through the atrioventricular node. Xanthines such as theophylline, aminophylline, and caffeine can reverse or block the physiologic effects of adenosine.

Aminophylline and cimetidine

—Cimetidine can significantly reduce hepatic metabolism of theophylline or aminophylline. This effect on theophylline metabolism is seen as soon as therapeutic levels of cimetidine are achieved.

Aminophylline Interactions with Diseases

Aminophylline and cirrhosis, liver disease, congestive heart failure

—Patients with severe liver disease (cirrhosis) or congestive heart failure may require reduced maintenance doses of theophylline (or its more water-soluble derivative, amino-phylline). Initial loading doses for untreated patients, how-ever, do not usually require adjustment.

—Reduction in maintenance dosing in the above type of patients is necessary because metabolism of theophylline takes place primarily in the liver.

AMRINONE (Inocor)

Classification and indications

—Amrinone is a cardiac inotropic agent unrelated to catechol-amines or cardiac glycosides. It is a bipyridine derivative.

—It is indicated for management of patients with congestive heart failure or patients undergoing coronary artery bypass.

Pharmacology

—The mechanism by which amrinone increases myocardial contractility is not completely understood, but it does inhibit myocardial cyclic AMP phosphodiesterase.

—In addition to inotropism, amrinone also produces periph-eral and coronary vasodilation.

—Because the primary route of excretion is through the urinary tract, reduced infusion doses may be needed in patients with severe congestive heart failure (with resulting poor renal per-fusion) and patients with renal disease.

—Thrombocytopenia has resulted from infusion of amrinone, primarily to patients receiving prolonged infusions. It is believed to be due to decreased platelet survival.

Dose

—Loading dose: 0.75 mg/kg of undiluted amrinone intra-venously over 2 or 3 minutes

—Following the loading dose, an infusion of amrinone diluted in normal saline (1 mg/mL): 5–10 μg/kg/min. Higher doses have been used in some centers.

Amrinone Interactions with Diseases

Amrinone and congestive heart failure, renal dysfunction

—Patients with congestive heart failure and/or compromised renal function may have higher-than-expected serum con-centrations of amrinone during infusion of the drug. This occurs because excretion of amrinone is primarily via the urine.

—Evidence of excessive levels of amrinone may be hypoten-sion or ventricular arrhythmias.

Amrinone and renal dysfunction

—Patients with congestive heart failure and/or compromised renal function may have higher than expected serum concentrations of amrinone during infusion of the drug. This occurs because excretion of amrinone is primarily via the urine.

—Evidence of excessive levels of amrinone may be hypotension or ventricular arrhythmias.

ATRACURIUM (Tracrium)

Classification and indications

—Atracurium is a non-depolarizing neuromuscular blocker.

—It is used for skeletal muscle relaxation during intubation and for maintenance of muscle relaxation during general anesthesia and surgery.

Pharmacology

—Atracurium competes with acetylcholine at the neuromuscular junction of skeletal muscle by binding to acetylcholine receptors.

—Onset and duration of neuromuscular blockade is dose dependent. At a dose of 0.4–0.5 mg/kg, maximal muscle relaxation occurs within 3–5 minutes and has a duration of approximately 20–35 minutes (25% recovery of twitch height). Within 1 hour, 95% of muscle strength has usually returned.

—The duration of neuromuscular blockade is 30–50% of that from pancuronium and approximately equal to vecuronium.

—Repeated doses or infusion of atracurium does not have a cumulative effect.

—Histamine release does occur but is less than that produced by tubocurarine or metocurine. At doses higher than 0.5 mg/kg, histamine release may be significantly greater.

—Other than changes resulting from histamine release, atracurium has no significant cardiovascular or hemodynamic effects.

—Elimination of atracurium occurs by Hoffman elimination and ester hydrolysis and is minimally affected by renal and/or hepatic failure.

Dose

—Intubating dose: 0.4–0.5 mg/kg.

—Maintenance dosing may be maintained by intermittent boluses or infusion:

   —Intermittent boluses: Approximately 0.1 mg/kg as necessary

   —Infusion: Approximately 5–9 µg/kg/min

—Lower doses are recommended when given in the presence of inhalational anesthetics due to their ability to potentiate neuromuscular blockade.

Atracurium Interactions with Anesthesia Drugs

Atracurium and calcium channel blockers (diltiazem, nicardipine, nifedipine, verapamil)

—Calcium channel blockers have been associated with prolongation of neuromuscular blockade from non-depolarizing agents.

—This interaction is probably related to the depletion of intracellular calcium associated with chronic therapy. This can result in a decrease in acetylcholine release at the neuromuscular junction.

Atracurium and desflurane

—Desflurane can potentiate neuromuscular blockade from non-depolarizing agents. A similar interaction is seen with the other volatile anesthetics (enflurane, isoflurane, halothane).

—Muscle relaxation from succinylcholine is also potentiated by desflurane.

Atracurium and diphenylhydantoin, phenytoin

—Patients on chronic phenytoin therapy may be resistant to non-depolarizing muscle blockade. The studies involved metocurine and vecuronium but may involve other non-depolarizing agents.

—The mechanism of this interaction is not known.

—Acute infusions of phenytoin may prolong non-depolarizing blockade. This was studied prospectively in a small number of patients who received a 10 mg/kg loading dose of phenytoin during steady-state muscle blockade with vecuronium. They had significant potentiation of their neuromuscular block compared to control patients.

Atracurium and enflurane, halothane, isoflurane

—Halothane, isoflurane, and ethrane can significantly potentiate neuromuscular blockade, depending on the neuromuscular blocker used. Nitrous oxide has minimal effects.

—Tubocurarine and pancuronium are potentiated the most by inhalational agents, whereas atracurium and vecuronium are intensified significantly less.

—Potentiation by inhalational agents occurs through depression of spinal cord reflexes as well as effects at or distal to the neuromuscular junction.

Atracurium and furosemide

—Furosemide may potentiate neuromuscular blockade from tubocurarine and succinylcholine. This is based on a case report of several patients given furosemide and tubocurarine during surgery and on animal studies.

—The implication for this interaction for other neuromuscular blocking drugs is uncertain and the mechanism is not known.

Atracurium and lidocaine

—Most local anesthetics can block neuromuscular transmission from non-depolarizing agents as well as depolarizing muscle relaxants. Of clinical significance to the anesthesiologist, lidocaine, given as a 50- to 100-mg bolus or even by infusion, can significantly increase a non-depolarizer block or a phase II block from succinylcholine.

Atracurium and procainamide

—Procainamide can potentiate muscle relaxation from non-depolarizing agents. This is probably a result of decreased acetylcholine release at the neuromuscular junction caused by procainamide.

Atracurium and quinidine

—Quinidine, procainamide, propranolol, and most local anesthetics have been shown to enhance the neuromuscular blockade from depolarizing and non-depolarizing agents.

—A number of well-documented cases have illustrated the ability of these agents, when given in the immediate post-operative period, to convert subclinical muscle weakness from neuromuscular blocking drugs into significant muscle weakness requiring reintubation.

Atracurium and succinylcholine

—Prior administration of succinylcholine has been shown to potentiate neuromuscular blockade of some non-depolarizing agents.

—Although this interaction has been documented with pancuronium, it was not seen with doxacurium and may not be a consistent finding with non-depolarizing agents.

Atracurium Interactions with Diseases

Atracurium and advanced age

—Age, obesity, liver or renal dysfunction have no significant effect on metabolism of atracurium.

—Atracurium is metabolized by Hoffman elimination as well as ester hydrolysis.

—Hoffman elimination is a non-enzymatic process that occurs at physiologic temperatures and pH. Ester hydrolysis occurs most rapidly in an acid pH and does not require plasma pseudocholinesterase.

Atracurium and amyotrophic lateral sclerosis

—Patients with a wide variety of neuromuscular disorders may be more resistant than normal patients to the effects of non-depolarizing neuromuscular blockers.

—This includes patients with disuse atrophy of the muscles (such as bedridden patients with chronic disease) as well as patients with upper or lower motor neuron disease (such as from trauma, stroke, or chronic illness like amyotrophic lateral sclerosis).

—Disuse or denervation of muscle results in production of extrajunctional acetylcholine receptors on the muscle membrane. These receptors are less easily blocked by non-depolarizing agents but are activated by lower concentrations of depolarizing drugs (succinylcholine).

—Despite initial resistance to blockade, such patients may demonstrate prolonged neuromuscular weakness as a result of decreased muscle strength and mass.

Atracurium and burns

—Patients with burn injuries are susceptible to a life-threatening hyperkalemic response to succinylcholine and can have marked resistance to non-depolarizing muscle relaxants.

—Both of these altered responses to neuromuscular blocking agents have been attributed to proliferation of extrajunctional acetylcholine receptors, similar to the response of a patient with a denervation injury.

—Resistance to non-depolarizing agents appears to increase with larger area burns and, in fact, may not be significant in patients with <30% body surface area burns. In addition to proliferation of extrajunctional acetylcholine receptors, this abnormal response is probably also related to the increased metabolic rate and hepatic and renal clearance seen in burn patients. Doses of non-depolarizing agents may need to be increased by as much as 300%.

—Duration of this resistance usually is 2 months following the injury but has been reported in a patient 463 days after the burn.

Atracurium and cirrhosis, liver disease

—Age, obesity, liver or renal dysfunction have no significant effect on metabolism of atracurium.

—Atracurium is metabolized by Hoffman elimination as well as ester hydrolysis.

—Hoffman elimination is a nonenzymatic process that occurs at physiologic temperatures and pH. Ester hydrolysis occurs most rapidly in an acid pH and does not require plasma pseudocholinesterase.

Atracurium and Eaton–Lambert syndrome

—Patients with Eaton–Lambert syndrome are very sensitive to both depolarizing and non-depolarizing neuromuscular blockade.

—This disorder is similar to myasthenia gravis and patients complain of skeletal muscle weakness, but it is usually associated with carcinoma (especially small cell tumors of the lung).

—If the diagnosis is known or suspected prior to surgery, reduced doses of muscle relaxants should be used, but sometimes the diagnosis is first made when a patient has surgery for a lung tumor and has an unexpected, prolonged neuromuscular block.

—Anticholinesterases are unreliable in reversing muscle weakness.

Atracurium and hyperthyroidism, thyrotoxicosis

—Muscle weakness is commonly seen with hyperthyroidism and affects proximal muscles, usually sparing respiratory function. In some cases, myopathy is the dominant feature of thyroid hormone excess and can resemble myasthenia. Lower doses of muscle relaxants may be indicated.

Atracurium and hypokalemia

—Hypokalemia appears to potentiate the effects of neuromuscular blockade from non-depolarizing agents.

—The interaction is probably due to hyperpolarization of the muscle endplate and, therefore, resistance to depolarization. Hyperpolarization would more likely occur with more acute changes in potassium concentration because the potassium losses would be from the extracellular compartment rather than from intracellular sites.

—Chronic hypokalemia is more likely to be associated with potassium depletion from both extra- and intracellular compartments with no significant change in transmembrane potential. As a result, significant effects on neuromuscular blockade would be less likely.

Atracurium and hypothermia

—Non-depolarizing muscle blockade is prolonged by hypothermia. This interaction is a result of an effect on the neuromuscular blocking agents themselves rather than on the anticholinesterases used to reverse the neuromuscular blocking agents.

—Hypothermia appears to prolong the effect of the non-depolarizing agents by several mechanisms, including delayed metabolism into inactive metabolites as well as delayed excretion via the urinary and biliary routes.

Atracurium and malignant hyperthermia

—Anesthetic agents considered safe for use in patients with known or suspected susceptibility for developing malignant hyperthermia include propofol, barbiturates, etomidate, ketamine, non-depolarizing neuromuscular blocking agents, narcotics, benzodiazepines, droperidol, epinephrine, norepinephrine, and anticholinesterases.

—Nitrous oxide is probably safe in the susceptible patient based on repeated use in MH-susceptible humans and swine.

—Local or regional anesthesia with either amide (such as lidocaine) or ester (such as procaine) anesthetics is now considered safe for MH-susceptible patients.

Atracurium and myasthenia gravis

—Patients with myasthenia gravis are very sensitive to neuromuscular blockade from non-depolarizing agents.

—This is probably a result of decreased acetylcholine receptors from autoimmune destruction associated with myasthenia gravis.

—Although these patients are treated with the same or similar anticholinesterases used to antagonize muscle blockade, sensitivity (not resistance) to neuromuscular blockade is seen clinically.

Atracurium and neuromuscular disease (amyotrophic lateral sclerosis, multiple sclerosis, syringomyelia)

—Patients with a wide variety of neuromuscular disorders may be more resistant than normal patients to the effects of non-depolarizing neuromuscular blockers.

—This includes patients with disuse atrophy of the muscles (such as bedridden patients with chronic disease) as well as patients with upper or lower motor neuron disease (such as from trauma, stroke, or chronic illness like amyotrophic lateral sclerosis).

—Disuse or denervation of muscle results in production of extrajunctional acetylcholine receptors on the muscle membrane. These receptors are less easily blocked by non-depolarizing agents but are activated by lower concentrations of depolarizing drugs (succinylcholine).

—When these receptors, which can be scattered over a large surface of the muscle, are depolarized by succinylcholine, ion flow takes place through the receptor channel. Large amounts of potassium may exit the muscle cell, causing hyperkalemia.

—Despite initial resistance to blockade, such patients may demonstrate prolonged neuromuscular weakness as a result of decreased muscle strength and mass.

Atracurium and obesity

—Age, obesity, liver or renal dysfunction have no significant effect on metabolism of atracurium.

—Atracurium is metabolized by Hoffman elimination as well as ester hydrolysis.

—Hoffman elimination is a nonenzymatic process that occurs at physiologic temperatures and pH. Ester hydrolysis occurs most rapidly in an acid pH and does not require plasma pseudocholinesterase.

Atracurium and PIH (pregnancy-induced hypertension), preeclampsia/eclampsia, toxemia

—Patients with hypertensive disorders of pregnancy may require treatment with antihypertensives such as trimethaphan or magnesium sulfate (for preeclampsia/eclampsia). These medications can have significant interactions with anesthetic agents such as succinylcholine, non-depolarizing neuromuscular blocking agents, or calcium channel blockers.

—Neuromuscular blockade produced by both depolarizing and non-depolarizing agents can be potentiated in patients receiving magnesium sulfate. The mechanisms involved include a decreased amount of acetylcholine released by the nerve impulse at the motor nerve terminal and a decrease in the depolarizing action of acetylcholine on the muscle.

Atracurium and renal dysfunction

—Age, obesity, liver or renal dysfunction have no significant effect on metabolism of atracurium.

—Atracurium is metabolized by Hoffman elimination as well as ester hydrolysis.

—Hoffman elimination is a nonenzymatic process that occurs at physiologic temperatures and pH. Ester hydrolysis occurs most rapidly in an acid pH and does not require plasma pseudocholinesterase.

Atracurium Interactions with Patient Drugs

Atracurium and antibiotics

—A number of antibiotics have significant interactions with neuromuscular blocking agents. These include the aminoglycosides (amikacin, gentamicin, kanamycin, neomycin, paromomycin, netilmicin, neomycin, streptomycin, tobramycin), as well as polymyxin B, colistin, amphotericin B, clindamycin, bacitracin, and lincomycin.

—All of the above antibiotics may potentiate non-depolarizing agents, but some (aminoglycosides, amphotericin B, clindamycin, colistin) can also potentiate succinylcholine blockade.

—These antibiotics potentiate neuromuscular blockade by different mechanisms, making management of these problems difficult. Although treatment with anticholinesterases or calcium has been recommended, results are inconsistent.

Atracurium and amphotericin B

—Prolonged neuromuscular blockade can occur with depolarizing and non-depolarizing agents in patients receiving amphotericin B.

—The mechanism for this interaction is thought to be associated with the hypokalemia that can be caused by amphotericin B therapy.

Atracurium and beta blockers, propranolol

—Beta blockers may potentiate non-depolarizing neuromuscular blocking agents. This interaction has been reported between propranolol and tubocurarine.

—Other beta blockers are also capable of causing weakness in patients with myasthenia gravis, but the mechanism or significance of these interactions is unclear.

Atracurium and calcium channel blockers (amlodipine, bepridil, diltiazem, felodipine, isradipine, lidoflazine, nicardipine, nimodipine, nisoldipine, nitrendipine, verapamil)

—Calcium channel blockers have been associated with prolongation of neuromuscular blockade from non-depolarizing agents.

—This interaction is probably related to the depletion of intracellular calcium associated with chronic therapy. This can result in a decrease in acetylcholine release at the neuromuscular junction.

Atracurium and diphenylhydantoin, phenytoin

—Patients on chronic phenytoin therapy may be resistant to non-depolarizing muscle blockade. The studies involved metocurine and vecuronium but may involve other non-depolarizing agents.

—The mechanism of this interaction is not known.

—Acute infusions of phenytoin may prolong non-depolarizing blockade. This was studied prospectively in a small number of patients who received a 10 mg/kg loading dose of phenytoin during steady-state muscle blockade with vecuronium. They had significant potentiation of their neuromuscular block compared to control patients.

Atracurium and lidocaine

—Most local anesthetics can block neuromuscular transmission from non-depolarizing agents as well as depolarizing muscle relaxants. Of clinical significance to the anesthesiologist, lidocaine, given as a 50- to 100-mg bolus or even by infusion, can significantly increase a non-depolarizer block or a phase II block from succinylcholine.

Atracurium and lithium

—Lithium has been reported to increase the duration of both non-depolarizing and depolarizing neuromuscular blocking drugs.

—The mechanism of this interaction is unknown and the clinical significance of this interaction is uncertain.

Atracurium and magnesium sulfate

—Neuromuscular blockade produced by both depolarizing and non-depolarizing agents can be potentiated in patients receiving magnesium sulfate. The mechanisms involved include a decreased amount of acetylcholine released by the nerve impulse at the motor nerve terminal and a decrease in the depolarizing action of acetylcholine on the muscle.

Atracurium and mexilitene
—Mexilitene, like lidocaine and most local anesthetics, can potentiate neuromuscular blockade from depolarizing and non-depolarizing agents.

Atracurium and procainamide
—Procainamide can potentiate muscle relaxation from non-depolarizing agents. This is probably a result of decreased acetylcholine release at the neuromuscular junction caused by procainamide.

Atracurium and quinidine
—Quinidine and quinine can potentiate muscle relaxation from both depolarizing and non-depolarizing agents.
—The mechanism of this interaction is a curare-like action at the myoneural junction. Also, plasma pseudocholinesterase is inhibited by quinidine (and quinine), resulting in possible prolongation of muscle relaxation from succinylcholine.

Atracurium and tocainide
—Tocainide, an orally active form of lidocaine, can potentiate both depolarizing and non-depolarizing neuromuscular blockade. This is a property of most local anesthetics as well as a number of other medications.

ATROPINE

Classification and indications
—Atropine is an anticholinergic agent prepared synthetically or from plant species.
—It is indicated for treatment of different clinical disorders including cardiac arrhythmias (sinus bradycardia), gastrointestinal disorders (peptic ulcer or motility disorders), and as a drying agent for excessive secretions.

Pharmacology
—Atropine is a competitive inhibitor of acetylcholine and has cardiovascular, gastrointestinal, genitourinary, respiratory, CNS, and ophthalmic effects.
—Cardiovascular effects are a result of inhibition of vagal tone and result in increased heart rate. Sinus node automaticity and atrioventricular (AV) pacemaker activity are increased, as well as an increase in AV conduction and a decrease in AV node refractoriness.

—However, adults may respond to atropine doses of <0.5 mg with a slowing of heart rate rather than an increase. Higher doses (1 mg or more) have not been associated with this response.

—Gastrointestinal effects of atropine include decreased intestinal motility as well as antisecretory effects (decreased saliva, gastric acid, and volume).

—Pupillary dilation can occur, but at doses used for decreasing secretions (see below) ophthalmic effects and increased intraocular pressure are unlikely.

—Respiratory effects include decreased volume of secretions in the nose, mouth, and bronchi. Additionally, vagal blockade results in bronchodilation.

Dose

—Adults:

—Preoperative antisialogogue (antisecretory) dose: 0.4–0.6 mg IV, IM, or SC.

—Bradycardia: 0.5–1.0 mg IV, up to 2 mg.

—Children:

—For prevention (when using succinylcholine) or treatment of bradycardia: 0.01–0.03 mg/kg IV or IM, up to 0.4 mg/kg.

Atropine Interactions with Diseases

Atropine and glaucoma

—Pupillary dilation can result in increased intraocular pressure in patients with angle closure glaucoma. At doses normally used clinically for atropine, this effect is not usually significant.

—Scopolamine, even in the form of transdermal patches, can produce significant increases in intraocular pressure in patients with narrow angle glaucoma.

Atropine and heart block (second, third degree)

—Atropine, an acetylcholine inhibitor, is sometimes used to temporarily increase heart rate in patients with symptomatic bradycardia. At doses less than 0.5 mg in adults, a paradoxical decrease in heart rate can occur.

—This is thought to result from central vagal stimulation at low doses of atropine; higher doses cause peripheral anticholinergic effects to predominate.

Atropine Interactions with Patient Drugs

Atropine and ritodrine

—Atropine, a sympatholytic drug, may produce unexpected hypertension in patients receiving ritodrine.

BENZQUINAMIDE (Emete-Con)

Classification and indications

—Benzquinamide is an antiemetic and is a benzoquinolizine derivative. It is unrelated to phenothiazines or antihistamines.

—It is indicated for treatment or prevention of nausea and vomiting associated with surgery or anesthesia.

Pharmacology

—Benzquinamide is believed to cause depression of the chemoreceptor trigger zone for emesis.

—When administered intravenously, it may produce significant cardiovascular stimulation. Hypertension and arrhythmias may result. Intramuscular administration rarely is associated with this response.

—The onset of antiemetic effect begins within 15 minutes following parenteral administration and lasts for 3–4 hours.

Dose

—Intramuscular administration: 50 mg IM for adults or 0.5–1.0 mg/kg every 3–4 hours.

—Intravenous administration: 25 mg slowly IV or 0.2–0.4 mg/kg.

Benzquinamide Interactions with Diseases

Benzquinamide and hypertension

—Benzquinamide has been associated with sudden increases in blood pressure when given rapidly intravenously. This may place patients with underlying hypertension at particular risk and should be used cautiously.

BRETYLIUM (Bretylol)

Classification and indications

—Bretylium is considered an adrenergic blocking agent and a class III antiarrhythmic.

—It is indicated as a second line drug for the treatment or prevention of ventricular fibrillation or tachycardia that is not responsive to lidocaine or procainamide.

Pharmacology

—The mechanism of antiarrhythmic action is not completely understood. Bretylium appears to have two effects: a direct depressant effect on the myocardium that opposes ventricular fibrillation as well as an antiadrenergic action.

—Initially, bretylium causes release of norepinephrine for sympathetic ganglia resulting in elevation of blood pressure. Subsequently, there is blockade of norepinephrine release as well as blockade of reuptake of norepinephrine.

—Hypotension frequently occurs within the first hour after administration and is the result of adrenergic blockade and vasodilation.

—Though antifibrillatory effects begin within several minutes after intravenous administration, maximal effects may not be seen for several hours. The duration of arrhythmia suppression may be 6–24 hours, depending on the dose.

—Bretylium is not metabolized and is excreted unchanged in the urine. In patients with renal failure, the half-life will be prolonged.

Dose

—For treatment of ventricular fibrillation or tachycardia: 5 mg/kg intravenously over 1 minute. If necessary, repeat doses of 10 mg/kg may be given up to a total dose of 30 mg/kg.

—Infusions of bretylium may be used at a rate of 1–2 mg/min for continued arrhythmia suppression.

—Bretylium may also be given intramuscularly in an undiluted form at a dose of 5 mg/kg.

—For pediatric usage, doses recommended are 5 mg/kg IV or 2–5 mg/kg IM.

Bretylium Interactions with Anesthesia Drugs

Bretylium and digitalis

—Digitalis-induced arrhythmias generally should not be treated with bretylium. This is because bretylium initially releases catecholamines, which may potentiate the arrhythmias seen with digitalis toxicity.

Bretylium Interactions with Diseases

Bretylium and aortic stenosis

—Patients with severe pulmonary hypertension or aortic stenosis may experience cardiac decompensation with bretylium therapy.

—Within 1 hour following bretylium administration, as many as 65% of patients will have a drop in blood pressure. Patients with severe aortic stenosis or pulmonary hypertension may not be able to compensate adequately for this hypotension.

—If treatment of life-threatening arrhythmias indicates treatment with bretylium in such patients, observation, monitoring, and treatment for the hypotension may be necessary.

Bretylium and pulmonary hypertension
—Patients with severe pulmonary hypertension or aortic stenosis may experience cardiac decompensation with bretylium therapy.
—Within 1 hour following bretylium administration, as many as 65% of patients will have a drop in blood pressure. Patients with severe aortic stenosis or pulmonary hypertension may not be able to compensate adequately for this hypotension.
—If treatment of life-threatening arrhythmias indicates treatment with bretylium in such patients, observation, monitoring, and treatment for the hypotension may be necessary.

Bretylium Interactions with Patient Drugs
Bretylium and digitalis
—Digitalis-induced arrhythmias generally should not be treated with bretylium. This is because bretylium initially releases catecholamines, which may potentiate the arrhythmias seen with digitalis toxicity.

BUPRENORPHINE (Buprenex)

Classification and indications
—Buprenorphine is a synthetic opioid with partial antagonist properties.
—It is indicated for management of pain of many etiologies, but is used mainly in the postoperative setting. It has also been administered in the epidural space for analgesia.
—Buprenorphine is also used as a preoperative medication and as part of a general anesthetic.

Pharmacology
—Buprenorphine has both agonist and antagonist properties, the predominance of which are dose-related. At intramuscular doses <0.8 mg, opiate agonist properties predominate. Above this dose, opiate antagonist properties appear.
—Analgesia is thought to result from buprenorphine affinity for mu and possibly kappa receptors in the CNS.
—Few significant effects are seen on the cardiovascular system at usual doses.
—Unlike pure opioid agonist drugs (such as fentanyl), increasing doses of buprenorphine do not cause proportionate respiratory depression. This is probably due to antagonist prop-

erties, creating a plateau or decrease in respiratory depression with increasing dose.

—To reverse respiratory depression from buprenorphine, larger than normal doses of naloxone may be necessary.

—Onset of analgesia following parenteral administration (IM or IV) is within minutes and lasts for approximately 6 hours.

—Elimination is dependent on hepatic metabolism and patients with liver dysfunction will experience prolonged effects from normal doses of buprenorphine.

Dose

—Buprenorphine can be administered IV, IM, epidurally, or by continuous IV infusion.

—IV dose: for patients 13 years and older, 0.3–0.6 mg initially followed by 0.3 mg every 4–6 hours. For pediatric use, 3 μg/kg doses have been used.

—IM dose: same as above.

—Continuous IV infusion: A solution of 15 μg/mL infused at a rate of 25–250 μg/hr.

Buprenorphine Interactions with Diseases

Buprenorphine and advanced age

—Elderly patients may require lower doses of narcotics than younger adults.

—This may be a result of reduced metabolism of this class of drugs or represent an increased brains sensitivity to narcotics as a result of aging.

Buprenorphine and alcohol—acute intoxication

—Patients who are acutely intoxicated with alcohol (including chronic alcoholics) usually demonstrate increased sensitivity to general anesthesia.

—Although the precise mechanism of interactions is not agreed on, it appears that alcohol intoxication has additive CNS depression with barbiturates, benzodiazepines, and narcotics, as well as inhalational agents.

Buprenorphine and cerebral edema, intracranial hypertension

—Most intravenous anesthetics cause a reduction in cerebral blood flow (CBF) and intracranial pressure (ICP) or have no effect on ICP. Although this effect is primarily from depression of cerebral metabolic rate (CMR), in some cases a direct vasoconstriction occurs.

—The exception to the above is ketamine, which causes an increased CMR and CBF with an increase in ICP.

—All the narcotics, as well as barbiturates, etomidate, benzodiazepines, and propofol have been associated with a reduction or maintenance of ICP during anesthesia.

Buprenorphine and cirrhosis, liver disease

—Elimination of buprenorphine is dependent on hepatic metabolism and patients with liver dysfunction will experience prolonged effects from normal doses of buprenorphine.

Buprenorphine and malignant hyperthermia

—Narcotics such as buprenorphine, butorphanol, and nalbuphine are considered to be nontriggering agents for malignant hyperthermia.

Buprenorphine and narcotic dependence

—Buprenorphine has both narcotic agonist and antagonist properties and has been shown to produce withdrawal symptoms in patients receiving morphine-like drugs.

Buprenorphine and renal dysfunction

—Renal dysfunction has not been demonstrated to cause significant changes in pharmacokinetics or pharmacodynamics of benzodiazepines, narcotics (with the possible exception of butorphanol), barbiturates, or propofol.

—In patients with renal dysfunction, the above drugs may appear to have an increase in duration or intensity. This has been explained as a response to the systemic effects of renal dysfunction rather than specific effects on the metabolism of theses drugs.

—Some muscle relaxants are significantly affected by renal failure.

Buprenorphine Interactions with Patient Drugs
Buprenorphine and methadone

—Patients who are physically dependent on methadone or other narcotics may experience withdrawal symptoms when given a narcotic with agonist/antagonist properties. This includes buprenorphine, butorphenol, and nalbuphine.

BUTORPHANOL (Stadol)

Classification and indications

—Butorphanol is a synthetic opioid with partial antagonist properties.

—It is indicated for management of pain of many etiologies but is used mainly in the postoperative setting and as an obstetric analgesic during labor.

—Butorphanol is also used as a preoperative medication and as part of a general anesthetic.

Pharmacology

—Butorphanol is thought to be an agonist at the kappa opioid receptors and mixed agonist–antagonist at the mu receptors.

—A single 2-mg dose of butorphanol has equivalent respiratory depression effects to 10 mg of morphine, but greater doses do not result in further respiratory depression.

—Unlike buprenorphine, butorphanol has minimal effects on the biliary tract.

—Onset of analgesia following intravenous administration occurs within 1 minute and lasts for about 2–4 hours.

—Elimination of butorphanol is dependent on hepatic metabolism and renal excretion.

Dose

—Intravenous dose: For use as part of a general anesthetic: 2 mg at the time of induction followed by 0.5–1.0 mg to a total of 4 mg/70 kg (0.04 mg/kg). Higher doses may be necessary, depending on the patient.

—Patients with renal or hepatic disease should receive about half of recommended doses with increased time between doses depending on the individual patient response.

—Intramuscular and nasal administration is also possible.

Butorphanol Interactions with Diseases

Butorphanol and advanced age

—Elderly patients may require lower doses of narcotics than younger adults.

—This may be a result of reduced metabolism of this class of drugs or it may represent an increased brain sensitivity to narcotics as a result of aging.

Butorphanol and alcohol—acute intoxication

—Patients who are acutely intoxicated with alcohol (including chronic alcoholics) usually demonstrate increased sensitivity to general anesthesia.

—Although the precise mechanism of interactions are not agreed on, it appears that alcohol intoxication has additive CNS depression with barbiturates, benzodiazepines, and narcotics, as well as inhalational agents.

Butorphanol and cerebral edema, intracranial hypertension

—Most intravenous anesthetics cause a reduction in cerebral blood flow (CBF) and intracranial pressure (ICP) or have no effect on ICP. Although this effect is primarily from depression of cerebral metabolic rate (CMR), in some cases a direct vasoconstriction occurs.

—The exception to the above is ketamine, which causes an increased CMR and CBF with an increase in ICP.

—All the narcotics, as well as barbiturates, etomidate, benzodiazepines, and propofol, have been associated with a reduction or maintenance of ICP during anesthesia.

Butorphanol and cirrhosis, liver disease

—Butorphanol should be used in reduced dosages in patients with hepatic or renal dysfunction due to the routes of metabolism and excretion of this drug.

Butorphanol and malignant hyperthermia

—Narcotics such as buprenorphine, butorphanol, and nalbuphine are considered to be nontriggering agents for malignant hyperthermia.

Butorphanol and narcotic dependence

—Butorphanol, a narcotic agonist–antagonist, may precipitate acute withdrawal in patients who are maintained on methadone.

—Patients who are receiving low doses of morphine (60 mg daily) have not been shown to demonstrate withdrawal symptoms with administration of butorphanol.

Butorphanol and renal dysfunction

—Butorphanol should be used in reduced dosages in patients with hepatic or renal dysfunction due to the routes of metabolism and excretion of this drug.

Butorphanol Interactions with Patient Drugs

Butorphanol and methadone

—Because butorphanol is a narcotic agonist–antagonist, it may induce withdrawal symptoms when given to patients with narcotic dependence.

CALCIUM CHLORIDE AND CALCIUM GLUCONATE

Classification and indications

—Calcium salts are used in anesthesia, usually in the intravenous form (calcium chloride, calcium gluconate, calcium gluceptate).

—Indications for intravenous calcium for patients receiving anesthesia include treatment of cardiac failure following cardiac bypass or poor myocardial contractility resulting from beta blockers, calcium channel blockers, lidocaine, procaine, or halothane. Calcium is also used occasionally to aid reversal of neuromuscular blockade resulting from interaction of aminoglycosides and non-depolarizing agents. Citrate toxicity resulting from rapid or massive blood transfusion is also treated with calcium.

Pharmacology

—Following IV administration, calcium serum levels increase almost immediately. After 30 minutes to 2 hours, levels return to pretreatment values.

—Calcium is important in many physiologic functions including excitation–contraction of both cardiac and skeletal muscle, excitability of neuronal tissue, and homeostasis, as well as other functions.

—Although calcium chloride is the most concentrated form of calcium for intravenous administration, it can be irritating and cause tissue sloughing if injected extravascularly. Calcium gluconate and calcium gluceptate are less concentrated and less irritating.

Dose

—For emergency elevation of serum calcium, the dose is 0.1–0.2 meq/kg of calcium.

—The above dose will be provided by the following volumes, depending on the formulation:

—Calcium chloride 10%: 0.08–0.15 mL/kg (5–10 mL CaCl per 70-kg adult).

—Calcium gluconate 10%: 0.2–0.4 ml/kg (14–28 mL Ca gluconate per 70-kg adult).

—Because CaCl may produce acidosis, patients who may have both hypocalcemia and acidosis (such as renal failure patients) may be best treated with other forms of calcium.

Calcium Chloride or Gluconate Interactions with Anesthesia Drugs

Calcium chloride or gluconate and calcium channel blockers (diltiazem, nicardipine, nifedipine, verapamil)

—Calcium may antagonize some effects of calcium channel blockers.

—In some patients, intravenous calcium has reduced the hypotensive effects of nifedipine but not its ability to prevent angina. In other cases, calcium has caused a return of an arrhythmia that had been controlled with a calcium channel blocker.

—Because the response to calcium may not be completely predictable in patients treated with calcium channel blockers, caution should be used when using intravenous calcium in such patients.

Calcium chloride or gluconate and digitalis

—Intravenous calcium has been reported to precipitate severe arrhythmias in patients taking digitalis glycosides. If such arrhythmias should occur, lowering of calcium levels may be effective.

Calcium Chloride or Gluconate Interactions with Diseases

Calcium chloride or gluconate and renal dysfunction

—Because calcium chloride administration may worsen acidosis, patients who have both hypokalemia and acidosis (such as renal failure patients) may be best treated with other forms of calcium replacement (such as calcium gluconate or gluceptate).

—This interaction is probably only significant when large doses of calcium are required.

Calcium Chloride or Gluconate Interactions with Patient Drugs

Calcium chloride or gluconate and calcium channel blockers (amlodipine, bepridil, diltiazem, felodipine, isradipine, lidoflazine, nicardipine, nifedipine, nimodipine, nisoldipine, nitrendipine, verapamil)

—Calcium may antagonize some effects of calcium channel blockers.

—In some patients, intravenous calcium has reduced the hypotensive effects of nifedipine but not its ability to prevent angina. In other cases, calcium has caused a return of an arrhythmia that had been controlled with a calcium channel blocker.

—Since the response to calcium may not be completely predictable in patients treated with calcium channel blockers, caution should be used when using intravenous calcium in such patients.

Calcium chloride or gluconate and digitalis

—Intravenous calcium has been reported to precipitate severe arrhythmias in patients taking digitalis glycosides. If such arrhythmias should occur, lowering of calcium levels may be effective.

Calcium chloride or gluconate and magnesium sulfate

—Calcium opposes the neuromuscular depressant effects of magnesium sulfate at the neuromuscular junction.

CHLORDIAZEPOXIDE (Clindex, Clinibrax, Clipoxide, Librax, Libritabs, Librium, Lidoxide, Limbitrol, Menrium, Sereen)

Classification and indications
—Chlordiazepoxide is a benzodiazepine.
—It is indicated for management of anxiety as well as for alcohol withdrawal symptoms.

Pharmacology
—Benzodiazepines apparently exert some of their effects through GABA (gamma aminobutyric acid), but the exact mechanism of action is not known.
—Absorption after intramuscular injection is reliable and rapid with lorazepam and midazolam, but not with other benzodiazepines.
—Onset of sedative, anxiolytic, and anticonvulsant action is from 1 to 5 minutes after intravenous administration. Duration varies from 15 minutes to 1 hour for chlordiazepoxide and diazepam, <2 hours for midazolam, and 12–24 hours after IV lorazepam.
—Since benzodiazepines are metabolized in the liver, patients with liver disease can experience prolonged effects from usual doses. Also, geriatric patients may have prolonged elimination times.

Dose
—For preoperative sedation: 50–100 mg IM 1 hour prior to surgery.
—For intravenous control of acute anxiety initial doses may be 50–100 mg followed by 25–50 mg every 4–6 hours.
—Geriatric patients or those with liver disease should receive lower doses.
—Total 24-hour dosage should not exceed 300 mg.

Chlordiazepoxide Interactions with Diseases
Chlordiazepoxide and advanced age
—Elderly patients may have decreased requirements for benzodiazepines.
—The exact mechanism for this response is controversial but may be related to decreased metabolism of this class of drugs. Alternatively, some elderly patients may be more sensitive to the CNS effects of these medications.

Chlordiazepoxide and alcohol—acute intoxication
—Patients who are acutely intoxicated with alcohol (including chronic alcoholics) usually demonstrate increased sensitivity to general anesthesia.

—Although the precise mechanism of interactions is not agreed on, it appears that alcohol intoxication has additive CNS depression with barbiturates, benzodiazepines, and narcotics, as well as inhalational agents.

Chlordiazepoxide and alcohol—chronic abuse

—Chronic abuse of alcohol has complex and incompletely understood effects on a patient's response to anesthetic agents. In general, these patients tend to be more tolerant (in a nonintoxicated state) to barbiturates, benzodiazepines, narcotics, and inhalational agents.

—Exceptions to this generalization include the alcoholic patient with a cardiomyopathy who may demonstrate increased sensitivity to myocardial depression from inhalational agents.

—Also, the patient with severe liver disease may have impaired ability to metabolize succinylcholine due to decreased levels of plasma pseudocholinesterase.

Chlordiazepoxide and cerebral edema, intracranial hypertension

—Most intravenous anesthetics cause a reduction in cerebral blood flow (CBF) and intracranial pressure (ICP) or have no effect on ICP. Although this effect is primarily from depression of cerebral metabolic rate (CMR), in some cases a direct vasoconstriction occurs.

—The exception to the above is ketamine, which causes an increased CMR and CBF with an increase in ICP.

—All of the narcotics, as well as barbiturates, etomidate, benzodiazepines, and propofol, have been associated with a reduction or maintenance of ICP during anesthesia.

Chlordiazepoxide and cirrhosis

—The benzodiazepines are metabolized extensively in the liver and patients with cirrhosis will demonstrate more prolonged effects of this class of drugs.

Chlordiazepoxide and liver disease

—Elimination of benzodiazepines is dependent on hepatic metabolism. Patients with liver dysfunction may experience prolonged effects from usual doses.

Chlordiazepoxide and malignant hyperthermia

—Anesthetic agents considered safe for use in patients with known or suspected susceptibility for developing malignant hyperthermia (MH) include propofol, barbiturates, etomidate, ketamine, non-depolarizing neuromuscular blocking

agents, narcotics, benzodiazepines, droperidol, epinephrine, norepinephrine, and anticholinesterases.

—Nitrous oxide is probably safe in the susceptible patient, based on repeated use in MH-susceptible humans and swine.

—Local or regional anesthesia with either amide (such as lidocaine) or ester (such as procaine) anesthetics is now considered safe for MH-susceptible patients.

Chlordiazepoxide and porphyria

—Benzodiazepines are considered to be questionable triggering agents for porphyria. This is based on their ability to provoke attacks of porphyria in rat models, though use in humans has not been associated with this reaction.

—Not all of the porphyrias have significance for the anesthesiologist. Three of the four hepatic porphyrias (acute intermittent, variegate, hereditary coproporphyria) and none of the erythropoietic porphyrias are associated with neurologic symptoms that can be triggered by certain medications: barbiturates, etomidate, and corticosteroids.

—Benzodiazepines and etomidate are considered to be questionable triggering agents, whereas safe anesthetics are inhalational agents, narcotics, muscle relaxants, anticholinesterases, and propofol.

Chlordiazepoxide and pregnancy

—Benzodiazepines may cause damage to the fetus, especially during the first trimester of pregnancy.

—Retrospective studies of chlordiazepoxide and diazepam have shown an increased risk of congenital malformations when administered to pregnant patients in their first trimester of pregnancy.

—Administration of preoperative benzodiazepines for obstetric procedures (such as caesarean sections) may produce CNS depression in neonates.

Chlordiazepoxide and renal dysfunction

—Renal dysfunction has not been demonstrated to cause significant changes in pharmacokinetics or pharmacodynamics of benzodiazepines, narcotics, barbiturates, or propofol.

—In patients with renal dysfunction, the above drugs may appear to have an increase in duration or intensity. This has been explained as a response to the systemic effects of renal dysfunction rather than specific effects on the metabolism of these drugs.

—Some muscle relaxants are significantly affected by renal failure.

Chlordiazepoxide Interactions with Patient Drugs
Chlordiazepoxide and diphenylhydantoin, phenytoin

—Benzodiazepines, when given to a patient on chronic diphenylhydantoin therapy, may cause an increased serum level of diphenylhydantoin. This may be due to a decrease in the metabolism of diphenylhydantoin caused by benzodiazepines.

—The half-life of benzodiazepines can be decreased in patients on chronic diphenylhydantoin therapy.

CHLOROPROCAINE (Nesacaine)

Classification and indications
—Chloroprocaine is an ester-type local anesthetic.
—It is indicated for use in peripheral and sympathetic nerve block and epidural and caudal anesthesia (without preservative).
—It is not to be used as a spinal (subarachnoid) anesthetic.
—Solutions that are preservative-free should be used for any caudal or epidural anesthetic because the safety of the preservative (methylparaben) has not been determined in case of intrathecal administration.

Pharmacology
—All local anesthetics block generation and propagation of nerve impulses by decreasing nerve cell membrane permeability to sodium ions, resulting in an increased threshold for depolarization.
—Onset of action depends to some extent on route of administration and dose, but is generally fast (6–12 minutes) and duration is 30–60 minutes. with epinephrine, the duration of blockade may be 60–90 minutes.
—Elimination of chloroprocaine is through rapid hydrolysis by plasma pseudocholinesterases resulting in a plasma half-life of <1 minute.

Dose
—For lumbar epidural anesthesia: 15–25 mL of a 2% or 3% solution. This dose corresponds to approximately 2 or 2.5 mL per spinal segment to be anesthetized. A recommended maximum dose is 800 mg chloroprocaine or 1000 mg with epinephrine (1:200,000 concentration).
—For caudal anesthesia: same as above.

Chloroprocaine Interactions with Diseases
Chloroprocaine and malignant hyperthermia
—Anesthetic agents considered safe for use in patients with known or suspected susceptibility for developing malignant hyperthermia (MH) include propofol, barbiturates, etomidate, ketamine, non-depolarizing neuromuscular blocking agents, narcotics, benzodiazepines, droperidol, epinephrine, norepinephrine, and anticholinesterases.
—Nitrous oxide is probably safe in the susceptible patient based on repeated use in MH-susceptible humans and swine.
—Local or regional anesthesia with either amide (such as lidocaine) or ester (such as procaine) anesthetics is now considered safe for MH-susceptible patients.

CHLORPROMAZINE (Ormazine, Thorazine)
Classification and indications
—Chlorpromazine is a phenothiazine.
—It is indicated for use as an antiemetic, anxiolytic (such as for preoperative anxiolysis), in the treatment of intractable hiccups, and as an antipsychotic agent, among other uses.
Pharmacology
—The exact mechanism of action of phenothiazines is not known, but is suspected to be related to antidopaminergic activity. Phenothiazines have other, complex effects including alpha blockade, antiserotonin, and antihistamine properties.
—Phenothiazines are neuroleptic agents and can produce a characteristic syndrome of flat affect, decreased impulsivity, aggressiveness, spontaneous movement, and decreased psychosis.
—Additionally, chlorpromazine and phenothiazines have antiemetic properties for which they are used in the perioperative setting.
—Because of alpha blocking properties, administration of chlorpromazine can result in hypotension.
—Elimination of phenothiazines is a result of hepatic metabolism and excretion of metabolites in urine and feces.
Dose
—Administration may be oral, rectal, or parenteral (IM or IV).
—For nausea and vomiting:
—Adults:
—Rectal: 50–100 mg every 6–8 hours.

—IM: 25–50 mg every 3–4 hours.
—IV: 2-mg doses every 2 minutes up to 25 mg for acute control of emesis, then IM or rectal treatment.
—Children 6 months and older:
—Rectal: 1.1 mg/kg every 6–8 hours.
—IM: 0.55 mg/kg every 6–8 hours.
—IV: 1-mg doses up to 0.275 mg/kg. If hypotension does not occur, a repeat dose may be given.

Chlorpromazine Interactions with Anesthesia Drugs
Chlorpromazine and epinephrine
—Neuroleptic drugs, particularly chlorpromazine, thioridazine, and clozapine, may produce an unexpected hypotensive response with epinephrine.
—The mechanism for this interaction involves the alpha receptor blockade associated with neuroleptic drugs, leaving the vasodilating beta receptors unopposed.
—Hypotension is possibly better treated with more selective alpha adrenergic agents such as phenylephrine.
—This interaction is not likely to be seen with neuroleptic agents other than the three listed above.
Chlorpromazine and propranolol
—Large doses of propranolol given with chlorpromazine can increase the serum levels of both medications.

Chlorpromazine Interactions with Patient Drugs
Chlorpromazine and guanethidine
—Chlorpromazine can reverse the antihypertensive effects of guanethidine if given in doses larger than 100 mg/day.

CIMETIDINE (Tagamet)
Classification and indications
—Cimetidine is a histamine H2 receptor antagonist.
—It is indicated in the perioperative setting for reduction of the volume and acidity of stomach contents. It is also used for the management of acute and chronic gastric and duodenal ulcer as well as gastroesophageal reflux.
Pharmacology
—Cimetidine, ranitidine, and famotidine compete with histamine for the H2 receptor. Because histamine stimulates secretion of acid and mucus from glands in the stomach, competitive inhibition results in decreased volume and acidity of stomach secretions.

—Cimetidine is associated with numerous drug interactions because it interferes with the cytochrome P450 enzyme system. This system normally is responsible for metabolism of many drugs.

—Additionally, cimetidine decreases liver blood flow, which also can interfere with drug metabolism.

—Ranitidine and famotidine do not interfere with the cytochrome P450 system and are not associated with significant drug interactions.

—After oral administration, 1–2 hours is required to significantly reduce gastric volume and acidity. The effects last for about 4–8 hours after a 300-mg dose.

—Following IV administration, 45–60 minutes is required to reduce gastric volume and acidity.

—Elimination of cimetidine is dependent on hepatic metabolism and renal excretion. In patients with renal dysfunction, the half-life is increased.

Dose

—*Intravenous*

—Adults:

—Bolus: 300 mg in 20-mL normal saline IV over 5 minutes. For preoperative use administer at least 45–60 minutes prior to induction.

—Infusion: 900 mg infused over a 24-hour period.

—Children: 5–10 mg/kg IV (may be administered every 6 hours).

—*Oral*

—Adults: 300–400 mg PO at least 1–2 hours prior to induction of anesthesia.

—Children: 5–10 mg/kg PO (may be administered every 6 hours).

Cimetidine Interactions with Anesthesia Drugs

Cimetidine and aminophylline, theophylline

—Cimetidine can significantly reduce hepatic metabolism of theophylline or aminophylline. This effect on theophylline metabolism is seen as soon as therapeutic levels of cimetidine are achieved.

Cimetidine and lidocaine

—In patients receiving oral but not intravenous cimetidine, acute intravenous infusion of lidocaine may result in early signs of toxicity. This is due to the decrease in hepatic clearance of lidocaine caused by cimetidine.

—This interaction has been documented after single oral doses of cimetidine and may decrease lidocaine clearance by up to 30%.

—This interaction is not seen with other H2 receptor antagonists.

Cimetidine Interactions with Diseases
Cimetidine and cirrhosis

—Cimetidine is dependent on renal excretion and hepatic metabolism. In patients with renal or hepatic dysfunction, cimetidine accumulation can occur, requiring longer intervals between doses (12 hours versus 6–8 hours).

Cimetidine and renal dysfunction

—Cimetidine is dependent on renal excretion and hepatic metabolism. In patients with renal or hepatic dysfunction, accumulation of cimetidine can occur, requiring longer intervals between doses (12 hours versus 6–8 hours).

CLONIDINE (Catapres)

Classification and indications

—Clonidine is an antihypertensive agent.

—It is indicated for the management of hypertension alone or in combination with other agents for hypertension.

Pharmacology

—Clonidine is an alpha 2 adrenergic receptor stimulant. Alpha 2 receptors are located mainly in the medulla oblongata where they modify sympathetic vasomotor centers; stimulation of these receptors causes inhibition of the central sympathetic centers, resulting in lower blood pressure and heart rate. Cardiovascular effects include a decline in cardiac output.

—Sedation may be seen with administration of clonidine and is thought to be related to the central alpha 2 receptor agonism.

—Clonidine has been shown to decrease minimal alveolar concentration (MAC) of inhaled and opioid anesthetics, also attributed to its effect on alpha 2 receptors. Use of naloxone (Narcan) may result in reversal of the antihypertensive effects of clonidine and may precipitate the exaggerated hypertension associated with sudden clonidine withdrawal

—Clonidine is well absorbed via the gastrointestinal tract and is also administered transdermally. After an oral dose, declines in blood pressure occur usually within 30–60 minutes.

—Transdermal blood levels require more time to achieve therapeutic levels and are used for outpatient management of hypertension.

—Elimination depends on hepatic metabolism and renal excretion. Patients with renal dysfunction may have prolonged elimination times because the majority of the drug is excreted via the kidneys.

Dose

—Acute management of hypertension: 0.1–0.2 mg orally. Repeat doses may be given each hour to a total dose of 0.5–0.7 mg.

Clonidine Interactions with Anesthesia Drugs

Clonidine and inhalational anesthetics (desflurane, enflurane, halothane, isoflurane, nitrous oxide, sevoflurane)

—Clonidine has been shown to reduce the MAC of inhaled and opioid anesthetics.

—This effect may be related to clonidine's inhibition of the sympathetic outflow from the vasomotor center in the medulla (clonidine is a central alpha 2 receptor agonist, which results in inhibition of CNS sympathetic centers).

Clonidine and narcotics (alfentanil, fentanyl, meperidine, morphine, sufentanil)

—Clonidine has been shown to potentiate narcotics and reduce the MAC of inhaled anesthetics.

—This effect may be related to clonidine's inhibition of the sympathetic outflow from the vasomotor center in the medulla (clonidine is a central alpha 2 receptor agonist, which results in inhibition of CNS sympathetic centers).

Clonidine and naloxone

—Naloxone can reverse the antihypertensive effects of clonidine. Also, it may precipitate the exaggerated hypertensive response seen from sudden withdrawal of clonidine in patients on chronic therapy with the drug.

Clonidine and nitroprusside

—Severe hypotension developed in several patients who had been receiving nitroprusside and immediately after were given clonidine.

—Apparently, the mechanism involved is one of additive hypotensive effects of the two medications.

COCAINE

Classification and indications
—Cocaine is a local anesthetic derived from the leaves of the plant species *Erythroxylon.*

—It is used as a local anesthetic for topical application to the mucous membranes of the nose and oral and laryngeal cavities. It has also been used as part of a mixture of other substances (tetracaine, adrenalin) to anesthetize skin.

—Cocaine is also an abused drug. It can be abused by the intranasal route (snorting), by smoking it mixed with tobacco or marijuana, or by intravenous administration.

Pharmacology
—Cocaine is a local anesthetic and therefore blocks initiation and conduction of nerve impulses.

—It is a stimulant to the CNS initially, but with increasing doses there may be vomiting, muscle tremors that sometimes lead to convulsions, and, eventually, respiratory depression and death.

—Cocaine also stimulates the sympathetic nervous system by inhibiting the reuptake of norepinephrine resulting in potentiation of catecholamines. This property probably accounts for the vasoconstriction caused by cocaine use.

—Cardiovascular symptoms of hypertension, arrhythmias, and tachycardia are related to both central and sympathetic nervous system effects.

—Cocaine is pyrogenic as a result of increased metabolism combined with vasoconstriction, which limits heat loss.

—Onset of anesthesia after topical nasal application is within 1 minute and lasts about 30 minutes. Peak blood levels occur in 15–20 minutes.

—Elimination of cocaine is a result of metabolism by plasma esterases followed by urinary excretion. The half-life is about 1 hour.

Dose
—Topical solutions of cocaine are typically 4% or 10%, but any concentration can be prepared.

—The solution is applied to the area of mucosa to be anesthetized.

Cocaine Interactions with Anesthesia Drugs
Cocaine and beta blockers (esmolol, labetalol, propranolol)
—Beta blockers have been demonstrated to potentiate coronary vasoconstriction caused by cocaine.

—This interaction was documented in the cardiac catheterization lab using intranasal cocaine followed by administration of propranolol.

—Although the significance of this interaction to clinical practice is not clear, patients who develop hypertension, tachycardia, and angina from cocaine may be best treated by an agent such as labetalol, which has alpha blocking properties.

Cocaine and vasopressors (ephedrine, epinephrine, metaraminol, methoxamine, phenylephrine)

—Cocaine may potentiate the vasopressor responses to sympathomimetic agents.

—The mechanism of this interaction involves the inhibition of reuptake of catecholamines by cocaine. This property probably accounts for the vasoconstriction caused by cocaine use.

—Cardiovascular symptoms of hypertension, arrhythmias, and tachycardia from cocaine use are related to both central and sympathetic nervous system effects of cocaine.

Cocaine Interactions with Patient Drugs

Cocaine and beta blockers (acebutolol, atenolol, betaxolol, carteolol, labetalol, levobunolol, metoprolol, nadolol, penbutolol, pindolol, propranolol, timolol)

—Coronary vasoconstriction has been demonstrated in patients receiving infusions of a beta blocker (propranolol) after intranasal cocaine. The significance of this to clinical practice and particularly for patients on chronic beta blocker therapy is not clear.

—Patients who develop hypertension, tachycardia, and angina from cocaine may be best treated by an agent such as labetalol, which has alpha blocking properties.

DANTROLENE (Dantrium)

Classification and indications

—Dantrolene is a derivative of hydantoin.

—It is an important part of the treatment for malignant hyperthermia and is also used to treat muscle spasm resulting from upper motor neuron disease (cerebral palsy, spinal cord damage, multiple sclerosis, stroke).

Pharmacology

—The mechanism of action of dantrolene appears to be an interference with release of calcium from the sarcoplasmic reticulum of the muscle cells. Calcium is essential for excitation–contraction coupling and excessive calcium release is felt to be the basis of the increased metabolism of malignant hyperthermia.

—Dantrolene does not effect the release of acetylcholine or interfere with activity at the myoneural junction.

—Dantrolene is metabolized in the liver and the metabolites are excreted in the urine.

Dose

—For treatment of malignant hyperthermia: 1 mg/kg doses, repeated as necessary up to 10 mg (usual dose necessary is 2.5 mg/kg). Following resolution of the acute episode, oral therapy should be maintained for 3 days (1–2 mg/kg 4 times daily).

—For prevention in susceptible patients:

　—Oral therapy: 1–2 mg/kg 4 times daily for 2 days prior to surgery.

　—IV therapy: 2.5 mg/kg infused slowly approximately 1.5 hours prior to surgery.

Dantrolene Interactions with Anesthesia Drugs

Dantrolene and verapamil

—There has been a report of hyperkalemia and cardiac decompensation in a patient receiving verapamil who was given prophylactic intravenous dantrolene on the basis of a history of malignant hyperthermia.

—This has not been reported with any other calcium channel blockers and the same patient did not have this response when again given dantrolene for another anesthetic while taking nifedipine.

Dantrolene Interactions with Patient Drugs

Dantrolene and verapamil

—There has been a report of hyperkalemia and cardiac decompensation in a patient receiving verapamil who was given prophylactic intravenous dantrolene on the basis of a history of malignant hyperthermia.

—This has not been reported with any other calcium channel blockers and the same patient did not have this response when again given dantrolene for another anesthetic while taking nifedipine.

DESFLURANE (Suprane)

Classification and indications

—Desflurane is a halogenated ether. It differs from isoflurane by the substitution of a fluorine atom instead of a chlorine atom.

—It is indicated for use as an inhalational anesthetic. Because it is somewhat irritating to the airway, it is not recommended for inhalational induction in children.

Pharmacology

—Desflurane is relatively insoluble in blood compared to other volatile anesthetics, with a blood/gas partition coefficient of 0.42 (about one-third of isoflurane).

—Because of this low solubility, induction and emergence from desflurane anesthesia are faster than from more blood-soluble agents such as isoflurane or enflurane.

—It is poorly soluble in tissues and because of its stability it is minimally metabolized. For this reason, it appears to have minimal potential for toxicity to liver or kidneys.

—The minimal alveolar concentration (MAC) for desflurane is 6–7.25%.

—Desflurane can cause vasodilation, resulting in decreased peripheral vascular resistance and decreased blood pressure.

—Cardiac contractility is mildly depressed but probably less than from other halogenated anesthetics. Because of an increase in heart rate produced by desflurane, cardiac output is less depressed than other agents (enflurane, halothane).

—Desflurane anesthesia results in cerebral vascular dilation and a decrease in cerebral metabolic rate. As with isoflurane, hypocapnia prior to desflurane administration attenuates the increase in cerebral blood flow.

Dose

—Induction:

—Halothane and nitrous oxide can be used for induction through inhalation because they are minimally irritating to the airways.

—Sevoflurane may also be suitable for inhalational induction.

—Isoflurane, enflurane, and desflurane are irritating to the airways and are generally not recommended for inhalational induction.

—Maintenance: Use of other anesthetic agents (opioids, benzodiazepines, barbiturates, propofol, etc.) can reduce the MAC of inhalational anesthetics. As a result, depending on the anesthetic technique used, the type of operation, and variability of patient response, maintenance requirements for inhalational agents are highly variable.

Desflurane Interactions with Anesthesia Drugs

Desflurane and muscle relaxants (atracurium, doxacurium, gallamine, metocurine, mivacurium, pancuronium, pipercuronium, rocuronium, succinylcholine, tubocurarine, vecuronium)

—Desflurane can potentiate neuromuscular blockade from non-depolarizing agents. A similar interaction is seen with the other volatile anesthetics (enflurane, isoflurane, halothane).

—Muscle relaxation from succinylcholine is also potentiated by desflurane.

Desflurane and clonidine

—Clonidine has been shown to reduce the MAC of inhaled and opioid anesthetics.

—This effect may be related to clonidine's inhibition of the sympathetic outflow from the vasomotor center in the medulla (clonidine is a central alpha 2 receptor agonist, which results in inhibition of CNS sympathetic centers).

Desflurane Interactions with Diseases

Desflurane and alcohol—acute intoxication

—Patients who are acutely intoxicated with alcohol (including chronic alcoholics) usually demonstrate increased sensitivity to general anesthesia.

—Although the precise mechanism of interactions is not agreed on, it appears that alcohol intoxication has additive CNS depression with barbiturates, benzodiazepines, and narcotics, as well as inhalational agents.

Desflurane and alcohol—chronic abuse

—Chronic abuse of alcohol has complex and incompletely understood effects on a patient's response to anesthetic agents. In general, these patients tend to be more tolerant (in a nonintoxicated state) to barbiturates, benzodiazepines, narcotics, and inhalational agents.

—Exceptions to this generalization include the alcoholic patient with a cardiomyopathy who may demonstrate increased sensitivity to myocardial depression from inhalational agents.

—Also, the patient with severe liver disease may have impaired ability to metabolize succinylcholine due to decreased levels of plasma pseudocholinesterase.

Desflurane and cerebral edema, intracranial hypertension

—All commonly used inhalational volatile anesthetics (halothane > enflurane > isoflurane) cause an increased cerebral blood flow (CBF). Less is known about sevoflurane and desflurane, but they are believed to have effects similar to isoflurane. Nitrous oxide has minimal effects on CBF.

—The volatile anesthetics, although they depress cerebral metabolic rate, cause cerebrovascular dilation, which results in increased CBF. Hyperventilation to a $PaCO_2$ between 25 and 35 mm Hg will effectively prevent increased CBF from isoflurane, but not the other volatile anesthetics.

Desflurane and hepatitis

—All forms of anesthesia, including general, regional, and nitrous-narcotic, are associated with postoperative liver function test abnormalities. The exact mechanism of this reaction is not known but is likely related to reduced liver blood flow from anesthesia and surgery.

—The presence of hepatitis or any liver disease has been shown to increase the morbidity and mortality in patients receiving anesthesia. The mechanism of this increase in morbidity and mortality is not clear but is most likely related to changes in hepatic blood flow as a result of anesthesia and surgery.

—Because there is no known method of avoiding exacerbation of preexisting liver disease by anesthesia, most recommendations are to postpone surgery in patients suspected of having acute hepatitis.

—There is no evidence that enflurane, isoflurane, desflurane, or sevoflurane is hepatotoxic. Halothane, however, can occasionally cause fulminant hepatic necrosis in both adults and children. A milder form of hepatotoxicity is also seen with halothane anesthesia.

Desflurane and malignant hyperthermia

—Halothane, isoflurane, enflurane, desflurane, sevoflurane, and other, older inhalational agents all are potent triggering agents of malignant hyperthermia (MH) in the susceptible patient.

—Succinylcholine, decamethonium, and possibly tubocurarine are also triggering agents.

—Anesthetic agents considered safe for use in patients with known or suspected susceptibility for developing malignant hyperthermia include propofol, barbiturates, etomidate, ketamine, non-depolarizing neuromuscular blocking agents, narcotics, benzodiazepines, droperidol, epinephrine, norepinephrine, and anticholinesterases.

—Nitrous oxide is probably safe in the susceptible patient based on repeated use in MH-susceptible humans and swine.

—Local or regional anesthesia with either amide (such as lidocaine) or ester (such as procaine) anesthetics is now considered safe for MH-susceptible patients.

Desflurane and myotonia

—Inhalational anesthetics may cause exaggerated cardiac depression in patients with myotonia dystrophica.

—Patients with myotonia dystrophica, but not the other myotonic syndromes, are likely to have some degree of cardiomyopathy even in the absence of clinical symptoms. As a result, these patients may be very sensitive to any myocardial depressant.

Desflurane and porphyria

—Inhalational agents are considered to be safe for use in patients with porphyria, as are narcotics, depolarizing and non-depolarizing muscle relaxants, etomidate, anticholinesterases, and propofol.

—Barbiturates are contraindicated in three of the four hepatic porphyrias (acute intermittent porphyria, variegate porphyria, and hereditary coproporphyria). Porphyria cutanea tarda and the erythropoietic porphyrias are not exacerbated by barbiturates.

—It is theorized that barbiturates can provoke an attack of porphyria by inducing the enzyme aminolevulinic acid synthetase, which results in synthesis of more porphyrin compounds and their precursors.

Desflurane and pregnancy

—Pregnancy is associated with significant reductions in minimal alveolar concentrations (MAC) for inhalational agents.

—In animal studies and some human studies, decreases in MAC of up to 40% have been documented. However, these studies did not include desflurane.

—The suggested mechanism for this decreased MAC includes increases in progesterone and endorphin levels associated with pregnancy.

Desflurane and renal dysfunction

—Enflurane, isoflurane, halothane, and desflurane are considered safe for administration to patients with renal dysfunction.

—Although enflurane undergoes biotransformation with the formation of inorganic fluoride to a greater extent than other agents (with the exception of methoxyflurane, which is very nephrotoxic), even 4 hours of anesthesia with enflurane produces nontoxic fluoride levels. There is some question, however, of renal toxicity after prolonged (9 hours) anesthesia with enflurane.

—Sevoflurane is also biotransformed to inorganic fluoride, but at potentially nephrotoxic levels (50 μmol/L), according to some studies.

—All inhaled anesthetic agents can cause a transient, reversible decrease in renal function as reflected in lowered glomerular filtration rate, urine output, and urinary sodium excretion.

—The mechanism for this action may include alterations in antidiuretic hormone, vasopressin, or renin, as well as decreases in renal blood flow.

Desflurane Interactions with Patient Drugs
Desflurane and amiodarone

—Amiodarone, an antiarrhythmic agent that increases refractoriness and slows conduction in most cardiac tissue, has been associated with severe cardiac complications, including arrhythmias, low cardiac output, and decreased systemic vascular resistance in patients having general anesthesia with inhalational agents.

—The mechanism of these interactions is not known.

Desflurane and clonidine

—Clonidine has been shown to reduce the MAC of inhaled and opioid anesthetics.

—This effect may be related to clonidine's inhibition of the sympathetic outflow from the vasomotor center in the medulla (clonidine is a central alpha 2 receptor agonist, which results in inhibition of CNS sympathetic centers).

Desflurane and disulfiram

—Profound hypotension may occur when patients taking disulfiram are exposed to halogenated anesthetics (enflurane, isoflurane, and halothane).

DIAZEPAM (Valium, Valrelease, Zetran)

Classification and indications

—Diazepam is a benzodiazepine.

—It is used as an anxiolytic for management of anxiety, for preoperative or intraoperative sedation, as part of a general anesthetic, for treatment of muscle spasm, and as an anticonvulsant.

Pharmacology

—Benzodiazepines apparently exert some of their effects through GABA (gamma aminobutyric acid), but the exact mechanism of action is not known.

—Absorption after intramuscular injection is reliable and rapid with lorazepam and midazolam, but not with other benzodiazepines.

—Onset of sedative, anxiolytic, and anticonvulsant action is from 1 to 5 minutes after intravenous administration. Duration varies from 15 minutes to 1 hour for chlordiazepoxide and diazepam, <2 hours for midazolam, and 12–24 hours after IV lorazepam.

—Because benzodiazepines are metabolized in the liver, patients with liver disease can experience prolonged effects from usual doses. Also, geriatric patients may have prolonged elimination times.

Dose

—For management of anxiety: 2–10 mg IV, depending on the level of anxiety, with repeat doses as often as every hour. Limitations of 30 mg/8 hours has been suggested.

—For intravenous sedation: 5–10 mg IV. Higher doses may be necessary.

—For acute alcohol withdrawal: 10 mg IV followed by 5–10 mg as often as every hour as necessary.

Diazepam Interactions with Anesthesia Drugs
Diazepam and heparin

—The administration of heparin to patients given diazepam prior to cardiac bypass may cause a transient but very significant period of hypotension.

—The mechanism of this interaction may be related to a large increase in the concentration of unbound diazepam that has been documented after heparin administration.

Diazepam Interactions with Diseases
Diazepam and advanced age

—Elderly patients may have decreased requirements for benzodiazepines.

—The exact mechanism for this response is controversial but may be related to decreased metabolism of this class of drugs. Alternatively, some elderly patients may be more sensitive to the CNS effects of these medications.

Diazepam and alcohol—acute intoxication

—Patients who are acutely intoxicated with alcohol (including chronic alcoholics) usually demonstrate increased sensitivity to general anesthesia.

—Although the precise mechanism of interactions is not agreed on, it appears that alcohol intoxication has additive CNS depression with barbiturates, benzodiazepines, and narcotics, as well as inhalational agents.

Diazepam and alcohol—chronic abuse

—Chronic abuse of alcohol has complex and incompletely understood effects on a patient's response to anesthetic agents. In general, these patients tend to be more tolerant (in a nonintoxicated state) to barbiturates, benzodiazepines, narcotics, and inhalational agents.

—Exceptions to this generalization include the alcoholic patient with a cardiomyopathy who may demonstrate increased sensitivity to myocardial depression from inhalational agents.

—Also, the patient with severe liver disease may have impaired ability to metabolize succinylcholine due to decreased levels of plasma pseudocholinesterase.

Diazepam and cerebral edema, intracranial hypertension

—Most intravenous anesthetics cause a reduction in cerebral blood flow (CBF) and intracranial pressure (ICP) or have no effect on ICP. Although this effect is primarily from depression of cerebral metabolic rate (CMR), in some cases a direct vasoconstriction occurs.

—The exception to the above is ketamine, which causes an increased CMR and CBF with an increase in ICP.

—All of the narcotics, as well as barbiturates, etomidate, benzodiazepines, and propofol, have been associated with a reduction or maintenance of ICP during anesthesia.

Diazepam and cirrhosis

—The benzodiazepines are metabolized extensively in the liver and patients with cirrhosis will demonstrate more prolonged effects of this class of drugs.

Diazepam and liver disease

—Elimination of benzodiazepines is dependent on hepatic metabolism. Patients with liver dysfunction may experience prolonged effects from usual doses.

Diazepam and malignant hyperthermia

—Anesthetic agents considered safe for use in patients with known or suspected susceptibility for developing malignant hyperthermia (MH) include propofol, barbiturates, etomidate, ketamine, non-depolarizing neuromuscular blocking agents, narcotics, benzodiazepines, droperidol, epinephrine, norepinephrine, and anticholinesterases.

—Nitrous oxide is probably safe in the susceptible patient based on repeated use in MH-susceptible humans and swine.

—Local or regional anesthesia with either amide (such as lidocaine) or ester (such as procaine) anesthetics is now considered safe for MH-susceptible patients.

Diazepam and porphyria

—Benzodiazepines are considered to be questionable triggering agents for porphyria. This is based on their ability to provoke attacks of porphyria in rat models, though use in humans has not been associated with this reaction.

—Not all of the porphyrias have significance for the anesthesiologist. Three of the four hepatic porphyrias (acute intermittent, variegate, hereditary coproporphyria) and none of the erythropoietic porphyrias are associated with neurologic symptoms that can be triggered by certain medications: barbiturates, etomidate, and corticosteroids.

—Benzodiazepines and etomidate are considered to be questionable triggering agents, whereas safe anesthetics are inhalational agents, narcotics, muscle relaxants, anticholinesterases, and propofol.

Diazepam and pregnancy

—Benzodiazepines may cause damage to the fetus, especially during the first trimester of pregnancy.

—Retrospective studies of chlordiazepoxide and diazepam have shown an increased risk of congenital malformations when administered to pregnant patients in their first trimester of pregnancy.

—Administration of preoperative benzodiazepines for obstetric procedures (such as caesarean sections) may produce CNS depression in neonates.

Diazepam and renal dysfunction

—Renal dysfunction has not been demonstrated to cause significant changes in pharmacokinetics or pharmacodynamics of benzodiazepines, narcotics (with the possible exception of butorphanol), barbiturates, or propofol.

—In patients with renal dysfunction, the above drugs may appear to have an increase in duration or intensity. This has been explained as a response to the systemic effects of renal dysfunction rather than specific effects on the metabolism of theses drugs.

—Some muscle relaxants are significantly affected by renal failure.

Diazepam Interactions with Patient Drugs
Diazepam and diphenylhydantoin, phenytoin

—Benzodiazepines, when given to a patient on chronic diphenylhydantoin therapy, may cause an increased serum level of diphenylhydantoin. This may be due to a decrease in the metabolism of diphenylhydantoin caused by benzodiazepines.

—The half-life of benzodiazepines can be decreased in patients on chronic diphenylhydantoin therapy.

DIAZOXIDE (Hyperstat, Proglycem)
Classification and indications

—Diazoxide is a nondiuretic antihypertensive related to the thiazides.

—It is indicated for use as in the treatment of severe hypertension and in this setting is most commonly used intravenously. It can also be used orally for the treatment of hypoglycemia from hyperinsulinism.

Pharmacology

—Diazoxide causes peripheral vasodilation, which is the basis for its antihypertensive action.

—Because it does not block sympathetic responses to vasodilation, administration of diazoxide results in catecholamine release and is therefore contraindicated in patients with pheochromocytoma.

—It is useful in treatment of hypoglycemia from hyperinsulin states because of its ability to stimulate catecholamine release, inhibit pancreatic insulin release, and stimulate glucose release from the liver.

—Following rapid IV administration, blood pressure reduction begins almost immediately and is maximized in 5 minutes.

—The duration of the hypotensive effect is usually 3–12 hours, but may be as short as 30 minutes and as long as 72 hours.

—Most of the drug administered is excreted by the kidneys, resulting in prolonged elimination times in patients with renal dysfunction.

—Diazoxide also relaxes uterine smooth muscle and may result in arrest of labor if given to patients in labor.

Dose

—For severe hypertension: 1–3 mg/kg IV (maximum of 150 mg) every 5–15 minutes until the hypertension is controlled. Use of 300-mg boluses is no longer recommended.

Diazoxide Interactions with Anesthesia Drugs

Diazoxide and beta blockers (esmolol, labetalol, propranolol)

—The hypotensive response to diazoxide may be accentuated in patients taking beta blockers. This is probably due to blunting of the normal sympathetic response that would otherwise occur.

Diazoxide and thiazide diuretics

—Thiazide diuretics work to treat hypertension by causing vasodilation, among other mechanisms. Other drugs that produce vasodilation, such as calcium channel blockers and angiotensin-converting enzyme (ACE) inhibitors, may potentiate this effect and may require a decrease in dosage.

Diazoxide Interactions with Diseases

Diazoxide and PIH (pregnancy-induced hypertension), preeclampsia/eclampsia, toxemia

—Diazoxide is a potent antihypertensive. Although it is not contraindicated, there are a number of side effects that make other agents more useful.

—Diazoxide inhibits uterine contractions and has been used to terminate premature labor.

—Both maternal and neonatal hyperglycemia have been associated with its use in the prepartum period. The hyperglycemia is a result of epinephrine release from the adrenal medulla caused by diazoxide.

Diazoxide and pheochromocytoma

—Diazoxide is contraindicated in patients with hypertension from pheochromocytoma because it may stimulate release of epinephrine from the adrenal medulla.

—It is this property of diazoxide that makes it useful in treatment, when given orally, for hypoglycemia.

Diazoxide and pregnancy

—Diazoxide is a potent antihypertensive. Although it is not contraindicated, there are a number of side effects that make other agents more useful.

—Diazoxide inhibits uterine contractions and has been used to terminate premature labor.

—Both maternal and neonatal hyperglycemia have been associated with its use in the prepartum period. The hyperglycemia is a result of epinephrine release from the adrenal medulla caused by diazoxide.

Diazoxide Interactions with Patient Drugs
Diazoxide and beta blockers (acebutolol, atenolol, betaxolol, carteolol, labetalol, levobunolol, metoprolol, nadolol, penbutolol, pindolol, propranolol, timolol)

—The hypotensive response to diazoxide may be accentuated in patients taking beta blockers.

This may be due to the blunting of the normal sympathetic response that would otherwise occur.

DIGITALIS (Crystodigin, Digitoxin, Lanoxicaps, Lanoxin)

Classification and indications
—Digitalis can be a term used to refer to the entire class of cardiac glycosides, which includes digoxin, digitoxin, deslanoside, and digitalis.

—All of the cardiac glycosides have a positive inotropic action and slow conduction through the atrioventricular node. They are used for treatment of heart failure and to control ventricular rate in patients with atrial fibrillation or flutter or paroxysmal supraventricular tachycardia.

Pharmacology
—The increased contractility of the myocardium appears to be related to inhibition of the Na-K pump by digitalis. The net result of this action is an accumulation of intracellular calcium, which improves contractility.

—Slowed conduction through the atrioventricular (AV) node is a result of a direct action, as well as an increase in vagal tone and a decrease in sympathetic stimulation.

—Digitalis also lengthens the effective refractory period of the AV node. However, in patients with Wolf–Parkinson–White syndrome, digitalis reduces the refractory period of the bypass tracts and may result in a worsening of tachycardia.

—Digitalis toxicity affects several organ systems but most seriously the cardiovascular system. Excessive vagal tone from digitalis may cause severe sinus bradycardia. Tachyarrhythmias and premature atrial or ventricular contractions can be seen and may be explained partly by increased automaticity from excess digitalis.

—Hypokalemia is a frequent causative factor in digitalis toxicity. Potassium reduces the binding of digitalis to the Na-K ATPase enzyme in the myocardium and reduces toxicity. In any patient with bradycardia receiving digitalis and especially in patients with normo- or hyperkalemia and sinus bradycardia, potassium infusions may worsen bradycardia and conduction block.

—Potassium infusions are most effective for the digitalis-toxic patient with tachyarrhythmias and hypokalemia.

—Other treatments for digitalis-related arrhythmias include phenytoin, lidocaine, procainamide, and propranolol.

—Digitalis toxicity may also cause hyperkalemia, probably a result of inhibition of the Na-K pump by digitalis. Hyperkalemia may be severe enough to cause AV block or asystole.

—Elimination of digitalis is mainly through urinary excretion. Patients with impaired renal function will have prolonged digitalis elimination times.

Dose

—Intravenous loading dose for digoxin:

—Adults: Average digitalizing dose is 0.5–1.0 mg with 50% given as the first dose and the remainder in two doses at 4- to 8-hour intervals.

—Children:

—Premature neonates	15–25 µg/kg
—Full-term neonates	20–30 µg/kg
—1–24 months	30–50 µg/kg
—2–5 years	25–35 µg/kg
—5–10 years	15–30 µg/kg
—Older than 10 years	8–12 µg/kg

—The loading dose should be divided into three doses: The initial dose is usually 50% of the total loading dose, followed in 4–8 hours by 25% of the loading dose for two doses.

Digitalis Interactions with Anesthesia Drugs

Digitalis and albuterol

—Acute administration of albuterol either intravenously or orally resulted in a 16% reduction of digoxin concentration within 30 minutes in a number of patients with stable digoxin levels.

—Additionally, serum potassium concentrations also declined approximately 15% within 10 minutes of the albuterol dose.

Digitalis and bretylium

—Digitalis-induced arrhythmias generally should not be treated with bretylium. This is because bretylium initially releases catecholamines, which may potentiate the arrhythmias seen with digitalis toxicity.

Digitalis and calcium chloride, calcium gluconate

—Intravenous calcium has been reported to precipitate severe arrhythmias in patients taking digitalis glycosides. If such arrhythmias should occur, lowering of calcium levels may be effective.

Digitalis and ketamine

—Ketamine may have a protective effect against digitalis-induced arrhythmias by decreasing phase IV automaticity.

Digitalis and succinylcholine

—Succinylcholine may precipitate cardiac arrhythmias in digitalized patients.

—Possible explanations of this interaction include the potential of succinylcholine to cause a shift of potassium from the intracellular to extracellular compartments in muscle tissue.

Digitalis and thiazide diuretics

—Thiazide diuretics and other diuretics that can produce hypokalemia can interact with the digitalis glycosides by precipitating arrhythmias. The basis of this interaction is hypokalemia and, in some cases, hypomagnesemia.

Digitalis Interactions with Diseases

Digitalis and alkalosis

—Alkalosis, because of the relationship with hypokalemia, can precipitate or worsen digitalis toxicity.

—This interaction is a result of the fact that digitalis glycosides exert their effect on the heart by binding to the Na-K ATPase enzyme in cardiac tissue and inhibit this enzyme.

—Studies have shown that binding of digitalis to the Na-K ATPase enzyme is increased in hypokalemia.

Digitalis and hypokalemia

—Digitalis toxicity is potentiated by hypokalemia.

—This interaction is a result of the fact that digitalis glycosides exert their effect on the heart by binding to the Na-K ATPase enzyme in cardiac tissue and inhibit this enzyme.

—Studies have shown that binding of digitalis to the Na-K ATPase enzyme is increased in hypokalemia.

—Potassium infusion to patients with digitalis toxicity who are hypokalemic results in decreased binding of digitalis and may decrease cardiotoxicity.

—Caution with potassium infusions must be used, since in patients who have high potassium and digitalis toxicity further increases in serum potassium may worsen heart block associated with toxicity to digitalis.

Digitalis and malignant hyperthermia

—Digitalis is considered safe for use in patients with susceptibility for malignant hyperthermia.

Digitalis and Wolf–Parkinson–White syndrome

—Verapamil, diltiazem, digitalis, beta blockers, and lidocaine should not be used to acutely treat wide complex tachyarrhythmias associated with the Wolf–Parkinson–White syndrome.

—In tachyarrhythmias with wide QRS complexes, antegrade conduction must be assumed to be taking place via accessory paths. Conduction through these paths can be accelerated by verapamil, diltiazem, digitalis, lidocaine, or propranolol. Intravenous procainamide is the treatment of choice.

—If the QRS complex is narrow, indicating antegrade conduction via normal conduction paths, treatment can be with agents that slow conduction through the AV node: verapamil, propranolol, digitalis, procainamide, or diltiazem.

Digitalis Interactions with Patient Drugs

Digitalis and amphotericin B

—Treatment with amphotericin B may produce hypokalemia and therefore predispose to digitalis toxicity.

Digitalis and thiazide diuretics (chlorthalidone, indapamide, metolazone, quinethazone)

—Thiazide diuretics and other diuretics that can produce hypokalemia can interact with the digitalis glycosides by precipitating arrhythmias. The basis of this interaction is hypokalemia and, in some cases, hypomagnesemia.

DILTIAZEM (Cardizem)

Classification and indications

—Diltiazem is a calcium channel blocker.

—It is indicated for the treatment of angina, hypertension, and short-term treatment of some tachyarrhythmias.

Pharmacology

—Depolarization of cardiac and smooth muscle cells is associated with ion movement (sodium, calcium, potassium, chloride) through ion channels. These channels are voltage-gated, meaning that they are opened and closed according to changes in transmembrane potentials.

—With depolarization, there is rapid movement of sodium through "fast" channels, whereas calcium moves much more slowly through "slow" channels. It is by interfering with calcium movement through these slow calcium channels that calcium channel blockers mainly exert their effects.

—Some of the calcium channel blockers have more pronounced effects on cardiac conduction (verapamil, diltiazem), whereas others have greater effects on vascular smooth muscle, resulting in lower blood pressure and coronary vasodilation (nifedipine, nicardipine).

—Calcium channel blockers slow conduction through the AV node (verapamil, diltiazem) and increase nodal refractoriness. As a result, these agents can slow ventricular rate in patients with atrial fibrillation or flutter and in patients with paroxysmal supraventricular tachycardia.

—A negative inotropic effect (decreased myocardial contractility) is associated mainly with verapamil but can also be seen with diltiazem and nicardipine.

—Elimination of diltiazem depends on hepatic metabolism and urinary excretion. Patients with impaired hepatic or renal function may experience more pronounced effects at usual doses. Reduced dosage is recommended in such patients.

Dose

—Intravenous dose:

—Initial dose: 0.25 mg/kg (20 mg for average adult). This may be repeated in 15 minutes if necessary at a higher dose of 0.35 mg/kg (25 mg for average adult).

—Continuous infusion: 5–15 mg/hr (usual dose is 10 mg/hr). This infusion is not recommended for more than 24 hours until further experience with prolonged infusions is available.

Diltiazem Interactions with Anesthesia Drugs

Diltiazem and muscle relaxants (atracurium, doxacurium, gallamine, metocurine, mivacurium, pancuronium, pipercuronium, rocuronium, tubocurarine, vecuronium)

—Calcium channel blockers have been associated with prolongation of neuromuscular blockade from non-depolarizing agents.

—This interaction is probably related to the depletion of intracellular calcium associated with chronic therapy. This can result in a decrease in acetylcholine release at the neuromuscular junction.

Diltiazem and beta blockers (esmolol, labetalol, propranolol)

—Verapamil and diltiazem can significantly potentiate the effects of beta blockers on cardiac conduction and contractility, particularly when used intravenously.

—Severe bradycardia and hypotension can occur when these medications are used concomitantly, especially in patients with abnormalities of cardiac conduction (sick sinus syndrome) or ventricular function (congestive heart failure).

Diltiazem and calcium chloride, calcium gluconate

—Calcium may antagonize some effects of calcium channel blockers.

—In some patients, intravenous calcium has reduced the hypotensive effects of nifedipine but not its ability to prevent angina. In other cases, calcium has caused a return of an arrhythmia that had been controlled with a calcium channel blocker.

—Because the response to calcium may not be completely predictable in patients treated with calcium channel blockers, caution should be exercised when using intravenous calcium in such patients.

Diltiazem and nitroprusside

—The combination of diltiazem and nitroprusside may reduce significantly the dose of nitroprusside required to lower arterial pressure.

—In a study of 20 patients to assess the interaction of these two medications, intravenous infusions of diltiazem reduced by up to 50% the dose of nitroprusside required to achieve a certain level of arterial blood pressure.

Diltiazem and thiazide diuretics

—Thiazide diuretics work to treat hypertension by causing vasodilation, among other mechanisms. Other drugs that produce vasodilation, such as calcium channel blockers and angiotensin-converting enzyme (ACE) inhibitors, may potentiate this effect and may require a decrease in dosage.

Diltiazem Interactions with Diseases

Diltiazem and atrial fibrillation or flutter

—Patients who have atrial fibrillation or flutter associated with Wolf–Parkinson–White syndrome should not be treated with verapamil or diltiazem.

—These medications may cause a worsening tachycardia that is thought to be due to reflex increases in sympathetic activity.

Diltiazem and autonomic dysfunction, Shy–Drager syndrome

—Patients whose autonomic nervous system responses are impaired by disease (Shy–Drager) or medication (beta blockers) may be unable to adequately compensate for vasodilation or negative inotropic and chronotropic effects of calcium channel blockers.

—In these patients, exaggerated hypotension or bradycardia may be seen with calcium channel blockers.

—Diltiazem would more likely be associated with hypotension and bradycardia rather than myocardial depression, which is more often seen with verapamil.

Diltiazem and cerebral edema, intracranial hypertension

—Most systemic vasodilators (nitroglycerin, nitroprusside, hydralazine, calcium channel blockers, and adenosine) can produce cerebrovascular vasodilation as well. As a result, cerebral blood volume is either maintained or increased even though systemic blood pressure is decreased.

—Trimethaphan, a ganglionic blocker, usually will not increase cerebral blood volume because ganglionic blockade normally does not cause vasodilation of the cerebral circulation.

Diltiazem and cirrhosis, liver disease

—Elimination of diltiazem depends on hepatic metabolism and urinary excretion. Patients with impaired hepatic or renal function may experience more pronounced effects at usual doses. Reduced dosage is recommended.

Diltiazem and congestive heart failure

—Some calcium channel blockers have negative inotropic activity (decreased myocardial contractility) and can worsen or precipitate congestive heart failure.

—Verapamil should be avoided in patients with impaired ventricular function. Although diltiazem and nicardipine have less potent negative inotropic effect than verapamil, they should be used cautiously in patients with decreased ventricular function.

—Nifedipine appears to have only slight negative inotropic actions.

Diltiazem and heart block (second, third degree)
—Patients with second degree, Mobitz II AV block or sick sinus syndrome may experience worsening conduction blockade from verapamil or diltiazem.
—Verapamil and diltiazem have both cardiac conduction and vascular actions. The other calcium channel blockers have primarily vascular actions (smooth muscle relaxation causing decreased blood pressure).
—The cardiac effects of verapamil and diltiazem include decreased sinus node automaticity, prolongation of AV nodal conduction time, an increase in the refractory time of the AV node, and depressed myocardial contractility.

Diltiazem and PIH (pregnancy-induced hypertension), preeclampsia/eclampsia, toxemia
—Patients with hypertensive disorders of pregnancy may require treatment with antihypertensives such as trimethaphan or magnesium sulfate (for preeclampsia/eclampsia). These medications can have significant interactions with anesthetic agents such as succinylcholine, non-depolarizing neuromuscular blocking agents, and calcium channel blockers.
—Magnesium potentiates the effect of calcium channel blockers and the combination may result in profound hypotension. This interaction is probably more likely to occur with calcium channel blockers that have more potent hypotensive effects (nifedipine, nicardipine, verapamil) than diltiazem.

Diltiazem and renal dysfunction
—Elimination of diltiazem depends on hepatic metabolism and urinary excretion. Patients with impaired hepatic or renal function may experience more pronounced effects at usual doses. Reduced dosage is recommended.

Diltiazem and sick sinus syndrome
—Diltiazem, verapamil, and beta blockers should be avoided or used with extreme caution in patients with sick sinus syndrome (SSS).
—Use of these drugs, which depress sinus node automaticity, may cause severe bradycardia even in patients with SSS who are experiencing supraventricular tachycardia.
—Digitalis may be effective in controlling supraventricular tachycardias.

Diltiazem and Wolf–Parkinson–White syndrome
—Verapamil, diltiazem, digitalis, beta blockers, and lidocaine should not be used to acutely treat wide complex tach-

yarrhythmias associated with the Wolf–Parkinson–White syndrome.

—In tachyarrhythmias with wide QRS complexes, antegrade conduction must be assumed to be taking place via accessory paths. Conduction through these paths can be accelerated by verapamil, diltiazem, digitalis, lidocaine, or propranolol. Intravenous procainamide is the treatment of choice.

—If the QRS complex is narrow, indicating antegrade conduction via normal conduction paths, treatment can be with agents that slow conduction through the AV node: verapamil, propranolol, digitalis, procainamide, or diltiazem.

Diltiazem Interactions with Patient Drugs

Diltiazem and beta blockers (acebutolol, atenolol, betaxolol, carteolol, labetalol, levobunolol, metoprolol, nadolol, penbutolol, pindolol, propranolol, timolol)

—Verapamil and diltiazem, particularly when used intravenously, can significantly potentiate the effects of beta blockers on cardiac conduction and contractility.

—Severe bradycardia and hypotension can occur when these medications are used concomitantly, especially in patients with abnormalities of cardiac conduction (sick sinus syndrome) or ventricular function (congestive heart failure).

Diltiazem and amiodarone

—Amiodarone increases refractoriness and slows conduction in most cardiac tissue. A number of medications, including class I antiarrhythmics like lidocaine, calcium channel blockers, and beta blockers, which have similar effects, can precipitate severe bradycardia when given to a patient taking amiodarone.

—A case was reported of a patient with sick sinus syndrome on amiodarone who developed profound sinus bradycardia after local anesthesia with lidocaine.

Diltiazem and flecainide

—Flecainide can cause decreased myocardial contractility, particularly at the onset of intravenous therapy. Patients most significantly affected are those with compromised left ventricular function (ejection fraction <30%).

—Beta blockers and some calcium channel blockers may have added negative inotropic effects with flecainide.

—Verapamil has more negative inotropic effect than diltiazem, nicardipine, or nifedipine.

Diltiazem and mefloquine

—Mefloquine is a derivative of quinine and has rarely been associated with bradycardia and prolonged QT interval. Beta blockers and calcium channel blockers should be used with caution in patients on this medication.

Diltiazem and nitroglycerin, isosorbide dinitrate, erythrityl tetranitrate

—Pronounced hypotension may be seen when patients receiving nitroglycerin are given diltiazem.

Diltiazem and rifampin

—Patients taking rifampin require significantly higher doses of calcium channel blockers. This interaction has been documented with verapamil, diltiazem, and nifedipine.

—The studies done demonstrated the increased requirement for both oral and intravenous forms of the calcium channel blockers, but requirements were higher for patients taking oral medications.

—The mechanisms of this interaction include an increased metabolism and reduced protein binding of the calcium channel blockers by rifampin.

DIPHENYLHYDANTOIN, PHENYTOIN (Dilantin)

Classification and indications

—Diphenylhydantoin is an anticonvulsant that also has antiarrhythmic properties.

—It is indicated for the management of seizures and atrial and ventricular tachycardias. It is considered a class IB antiarrhythmic (affecting only phase IV depolarization).

Pharmacology

—The anticonvulsant property of diphenylhydantoin results mainly from its ability to limit propagation of seizure activity (other agents may work by elevating seizure threshold).

—The antiarrhythmic properties involve a decrease in automaticity as well as a decrease in excitability of Purkinje fibers. Because of this effect, phenytoin is contraindicated in patients with sinus bradycardia, sinoatrial block, as well as patients with second and third degree heart block or with Stokes–Adams syndrome.

—Diphenylhydantoin is particularly effective for the treatment of ventricular arrhythmias caused by digitalis intoxication, but is not very useful for atrial arrhythmias.

—Toxicity associated with phenytoin administration includes hypotension, CNS depression, and cardiovascular collapse.

—Therapeutic concentrations for phenytoin are between 7.5 and 20 μg/mL. Intramuscular administration is not recommended due to erratic absorption.

—Following IV administration of 1–1.5 g, therapeutic concentrations are achieved in 1–2 hours.

—The average half-life is about 10–15 hours after intravenous administration and elimination is a result of hepatic metabolism.

Dose

—For cardiac arrhythmias: 100-mg boluses (no faster than 50 mg/min) every 5 minutes until arrhythmia is abolished or total of 1 g has been administered.

—For seizures:

—Adults: A loading dose of 10–15 mg/kg IV (no faster than 50 mg/min).

—Children: A loading dose of 15–20 mg/kg IV (no faster than 1–3 mg/kg/min).

Diphenylhydantoin Interactions with Anesthesia Drugs

Diphenylhydantoin and muscle relaxants (atracurium, doxacurium, gallamine, metocurine, mivacurium, pancuronium, pipercuronium, rocuronium, tubocurarine, vecuronium)

—Patients on chronic phenytoin therapy may be resistant to non-depolarizing muscle blockade. The studies involved metocurine and vecuronium, but may involve other non-depolarizing agents.

—The mechanism of this interaction is not known.

—Acute infusions of phenytoin may prolong non-depolarizing blockade. This was studied prospectively in a small number of patients who received a 10 mg/kg loading dose of phenytoin during steady-state muscle blockade with vecuronium. They had significant potentiation of their neuromuscular block compared to control patients.

Diphenylhydantoin and dopamine

—Several patients developed profound hypotension after receiving intravenous diphenylhydantoin while on dopamine infusions.

—The mechanism of this interaction is not known, and not all patients will experience this interaction.

Diphenylhydantoin Interactions with Diseases

Diphenylhydantoin and heart block (second, third degree), Stokes–Adams syndrome

—The antiarrhythmic properties of diphenylhydantoin involve a decrease in automaticity as well as a decrease in excitability of Purkinje fibers. Because of this effect, phenytoin is contraindicated in patients with sinus bradycardia, sinoatrial block, as well as patients with second and third degree heart block, or with Stokes–Adams syndrome.

Diphenylhydantoin Interactions with Patient Drugs

Diphenylhydantoin and dopamine

—Several patients have developed profound hypotension after receiving intravenous diphenylhydantoin while on dopamine infusions.

—The mechanism of this interaction is not known, and not all patients will experience this interaction.

DOBUTAMINE (Dobutrex)

Classification and indications

—Dobutamine is a sympathomimetic agent related to dopamine.

—It is used to increase cardiac output in patients with decreased myocardial contractility from myocardial infarction or cardiac surgery, for example.

Pharmacology

—Dobutamine increases myocardial contractility primarily by stimulation of beta 1 adrenergic receptors, although there is some stimulation of beta 2 and alpha receptors.

—Unlike dopamine, dobutamine does not release endogenous norepinephrine, nor does it cause renal or mesenteric vasodilation through stimulation of dopaminergic receptors.

—Though dobutamine is less commonly associated with tachycardia or cardiac arrhythmias than dopamine, heart rate increases of 30 beats per minute may occur. Hyper or hypotension may also be seen.

—Dobutamine increases conduction through the AV node and may result in higher ventricular rates in patients with atrial fibrillation or flutter. In such cases, use of an agent which can slow AV conduction, such as digitalis, may be necessary.

—The plasma half-life of dobutamine is short (2 minutes) and elimination is from metabolism in the liver followed by renal excretion.

Dose

—Usual intravenous dose: 2.5–15 µg/kg/min. Occasionally, much higher doses (up to 40 µg/kg/min) have been used.

Dobutamine Interactions with Patient Drugs

Dobutamine and guanadrel, guanethidine

—Patients receiving guanethidine and guanadrel can have an exaggerated hypertensive response to norepinephrine and other direct-acting catecholamines such as phenylephrine, dobutamine, and epinephrine.

—Indirect-acting catecholamines, such as ephedrine, metaraminol, mephentermine, and dopamine, may have fewer pressor effects than expected.

—Guanethidine and guanadrel deplete intraneuronal norepinephrine in postganglionic sympathetic neurons and in this way may diminish the response of indirect acting catecholamines, while sensitizing adrenergic receptors to direct-acting amines.

Dobutamine and monoamine oxidase inhibitors (isocarboxazid, phenelzine, selegilene tranylcypromine)

—Indirect-acting vasopressors (ephedrine, mephentermine, and metaraminol) act by releasing intraneuronal monoamines such as dopamine and norepinephrine. This is the explanation of the hypertensive crises seen when patients receiving monamine oxidase inhibitors are given these vasopressors.

—Direct-acting vasopressors such as phenylephrine, epinephrine, norepinephrine, and dobutamine may be potentiated by MAO inhibitors and should be used in smaller amounts than normally used.

—Dopamine has both direct and indirect actions and must be used with caution (perhaps one-tenth the normal dose).

DOPAMINE (Intropin)

Classification and indications

—Dopamine is an endogenous catecholamine. It is the immediate precursor of norepinephrine.

—It is indicated for the management of low cardiac output resulting from myocardial infarction, or cardiac surgery, for example.

Pharmacology

—Dopamine stimulates beta 1, alpha, and dopaminergic receptors. Also, unlike dobutamine, it causes release of endogenous norepinephrine from storage sites.

—Stimulation of the receptors is partly related to dose. At a dose of 0.5–2 μg/kg/min, there is primarily stimulation of dopaminergic receptors, producing vasodilation of coronary, renal, mesenteric, and cerebral vasculature.

—At doses of 2–10 μg/kg/min, there is also stimulation of beta 1 receptors resulting in increased myocardial contractility and some vasodilation. At doses above 10 μg/kg/min, alpha adrenergic receptor stimulation causes peripheral vasoconstriction.

—In summary, low or moderate doses cause increased urinary blood flow and variable levels of myocardial stimulation, while higher doses increase peripheral resistance by vasoconstriction. The vasoconstriction may affect the renal and mesenteric vasculature, depending on the dose.

—Dopamine may cause tachycardia, ectopy, and hypertension in some patients. Also, patients with depletion of catecholamines (such as chronic congestive heart failure) may not respond as well to dopamine, since release of endogenous catecholamines is an important mechanism of its action. In such cases, dobutamine may be more effective.

Dose

—Depending on the clinical situation, dopamine may be initiated at 1 to 5 μg/kg/min for less critical patients.

—For more critically ill patients, recommended infusion rates are 5 to 10 μg/kg/min up to as much as 50 μg/kg/min.

Dopamine Interactions with Anesthesia Drugs

Dopamine and beta blockers (esmolol, labetalol, propranolol)

—Use of beta blockers for treatment of supraventricular tachycardia may have undesirable effects in some patients; specifically, in patients requiring cardiovascular support with agents that are both inotropic and vasoconstrictive (dopamine, epinephrine, norepinephrine), blockade of beta receptors may result in decreased cardiac contractility in the face of systemic vasoconstriction, resulting in cardiac failure.

Dopamine and diphenylhydantoin, phenytoin

—Several patients have developed profound hypotension after receiving intravenous diphenylhydantoin while on dopamine infusions.

—The mechanism of this interaction is not known, and not all patients will experience this interaction.

Dopamine Interactions with Patient Drugs
Dopamine and ergot alkaloids (dihydroergotamine, ergonovine, ergotamine tartrate, methylergonovine)

—A case report of gangrene of the extremities was reported in a patient who received infusions intravenously of both dopamine and ergonovine.

—The proposed mechanism of this interaction is that the vasoconstrictive properties of these medications can be additive.

—Although the other ergot alkaloids have not specifically been identified as interacting in such a way with dopamine, it is reasonable to use caution with this combination.

Dopamine and guanadrel, guanethidine

—Patients receiving guanethidine and guanadrel can have an exaggerated hypertensive response to norepinephrine and other direct-acting catecholamines such as phenylephrine, dobutamine, and epinephrine.

—Indirect-acting catecholamines, such as ephedrine, metaraminol, mephentermine, and dopamine, may have fewer pressor effects than expected.

—Guanethidine and guanadrel deplete intraneuronal norepinephrine in postganglionic sympathetic neurons and in this way may diminish the response of indirect-acting catecholamines, while sensitizing adrenergic receptors to direct-acting amines.

Dopamine and monoamine oxidase inhibitors (isocarboxazid, phenelzine, selegilene tranylcypromine)

—Indirect-acting vasopressors (ephedrine, mephentermine, and metaraminol) act by releasing intraneuronal monoamines such as dopamine and norepinephrine. This is the explanation of the hypertensive crises seen when patients receiving monamine oxidase inhibitors are given these vasopressors.

—Direct-acting vasopressors such as phenylephrine, epinephrine, norepinephrine, and dobutamine may be potentiated by MAO inhibitors and should be used in smaller amounts than normally used.

—Dopamine has both direct and indirect actions and must be used with caution (perhaps one-tenth the normal dose).

DOXACURIUM (Nuromax)

Classification and indications

—Doxacurium is a non-depolarizing neuromuscular blocking agent.

—It is indicated for use as part of a general anesthetic for skeletal muscle relaxation during surgery. It can also be used for intubation.

Pharmacology

—Doxacurium antagonizes acetylcholine at the neuromuscular junction by competitively binding to acetylcholine receptors.

—Onset of action is slower than some other agents. After a dose of 0.05 mg/kg, intubating conditions are achieved after about 5 minutes. This dose has a clinical duration of about 90 minutes (25% recovery of control twitch height).

—There is no significant release of histamine and no effect on mean arterial blood pressure or heart rate.

—Elimination of doxacurium is dependent on renal excretion. Patients with impaired renal function will show prolonged effects from doxacurium.

—Prolonged neuromuscular blockade in patients with liver disease can be seen with doxacurium mivacurium, vecuronium, pancuronium, rocuronium, and tubocurarine.

—This interaction is complex, and may be due to decreased clearance, decreased hepatic uptake of the agent, or decreased synthesis of enzymes important for degradation of the neuromuscular blocker. An example of the latter is prolongation of mivacurium's duration of action as a result of decreased plasma cholinesterase from severe liver disease.

—Because of the increased volume of distribution of many drugs seen in patients with liver disease, initial doses of some muscle relaxants may need to be larger than in healthy patients. Once neuromuscular blockade is achieved, recovery may be prolonged.

Dose

—For induction: 0.05 mg/kg will result in intubating conditions in about 5 minutes and have a duration of about 90 minutes (25% recovery of control twitch height). Repeat doses should be about one third of initial dose.

—Following induction with succinylcholine: 0.025 mg/kg. Prior administration of succinylcholine has no significant effect on doxacurium.

Doxacurium Interactions with Anesthesia Drugs

Doxacurium and calcium channel blockers (diltiazem, nicardipine, nifedipine, verapamil)

—Calcium channel blockers have been associated with prolongation of neuromuscular blockade from non-depolarizing agents.

—This interaction is probably related to the depletion of intracellular calcium associated with chronic therapy. This can result in a decrease in acetylcholine release at the neuromuscular junction.

Doxacurium and inhalational anesthetics (desflurane, enflurane, halothane, isoflurane, sevoflurane)

—Desflurane, enflurane, halothane, isoflurane, and sevoflurane can significantly potentiate neuromuscular blockade, depending on the neuromuscular blocker used. Nitrous oxide has minimal effects.

—Tubocurarine and pancuronium are potentiated the most by inhalational agents, while atracurium and vecuronium are intensified significantly less.

—Potentiation by inhalational agents occurs through depression of spinal cord reflexes as well as effects at or distal to the neuromuscular junction.

Doxacurium and diphenylhydantoin, phenytoin

—Patients on chronic phenytoin therapy may be resistant to non-depolarizing muscle blockade. The studies involved metocurine and vecuronium but may involve other non-depolarizing agents.

—The mechanism of this interaction is not known.

—Acute infusions of phenytoin may prolong non-depolarizing blockade. This was studied prospectively in a small number of patients who received a 10 mg/kg loading dose of phenytoin during steady-state muscle blockade with vecuronium. They had significant potentiation of their neuromuscular block compared to control patients.

Doxacurium and furosemide

—Furosemide may potentiate neuromuscular blockade from tubocurarine and succinylcholine. This is based on a case report of several patients given furosemide and tubocurarine during surgery and on animal studies.

—The implication for this interaction for other neuromuscular blocking drugs is uncertain and the mechanism is not known.

Doxacurium and lidocaine
—Most local anesthetics can block neuromuscular transmission from non-depolarizing agents as well as depolarizing muscle relaxants. Of clinical significance to the anesthesiologist, lidocaine, given as a 50- to 100-mg bolus or even by infusion, can significantly increase a non-depolarizer block or a phase II block from succinylcholine.

Doxacurium and procainamide
—Procainamide can potentiate muscle relaxation from non-depolarizing agents. This is probably a result of decreased acetylcholine release at the neuromuscular junction caused by procainamide.

Doxacurium and quinidine
—Quinidine, procainamide, propranolol, and most local anesthetics have been shown to enhance the neuromuscular blockade from depolarizing and non-depolarizing agents.
—A number of well-documented cases have illustrated the ability of these agents, when given in the immediate postoperative period, to convert subclinical muscle weakness from neuromuscular blocking drugs into significant muscle weakness requiring reintubation.

Doxacurium and succinylcholine
—Prior administration of succinylcholine has been shown to potentiate neuromuscular blockade of some non-depolarizing agents.
—Although this interaction has been documented with pancuronium, it was not seen with doxacurium and may not be a consistent finding with non-depolarizing agents.

Doxacurium Interactions with Diseases
Doxacurium and advanced age
—Prolonged duration of neuromuscular blockade can be seen in older patients with several different non-depolarizing agents including doxacurium, mivacurium, and rocuronium. In some cases, delayed onset of muscle relaxation also occurs. This has been attributed to decreased perfusion of the neuromuscular junction as a result of advanced age.

Doxacurium and burns
—Patients with burn injuries are susceptible to a life threatening hyperkalemic response to succinylcholine and can have marked resistance to non-depolarizing muscle relaxants.
—Both of these altered responses to neuromuscular blocking agents have been attributed to proliferation of extrajunc-

tional acetylcholine receptors, similar to the patient with a denervation injury.

—Resistance to non-depolarizing agents appears to increase with larger area burns and, in fact, may not be significant in patients with less than 30% body surface area burns. In addition to proliferation of extrajunctional acetylcholine receptors, this abnormal response is probably also related to the increased metabolic rate and hepatic and renal clearance seen in burn patients. Doses of non-depolarizing agents may need to be increased by as much as 300%.

—Duration of this resistance usually is 2 months following the injury but has been reported in a patient 463 days after the burn.

Doxacurium and cirrhosis, liver disease

—Prolonged neuromuscular blockade in patients with liver disease can be seen with doxacurium, mivacurium, vecuronium, pancuronium, rocuronium, and tubocurarine.

—This interaction is complex and may be due to decreased clearance, decreased hepatic uptake of the agent, or decreased synthesis of enzymes important for degradation of the neuromuscular blocker. An example of the latter is prolongation of mivacurium's duration of action as a result of decreased plasma cholinesterase from severe liver disease.

—Because of the increased volume of distribution of many drugs seen in patients with liver disease, initial doses of muscle relaxants may need to be larger than in healthy patients. Once neuromuscular blockade is achieved, recovery may be prolonged.

Doxacurium and Eaton–Lambert syndrome

—Patients with Eaton–Lambert syndrome are very sensitive to both depolarizing and non-depolarizing neuromuscular blockade.

—This disorder is similar to myasthenia gravis and patients complain of skeletal muscle weakness, but it is usually associated with carcinoma (especially small cell tumors of the lung).

—If the diagnosis is known or suspected prior to surgery, reduced doses of muscle relaxants should be used. However, sometimes the diagnosis is first made when a patient has surgery for a lung tumor and has an unexpected, prolonged neuromuscular block.

—Anticholinesterases are unreliable in reversing muscle weakness.

Doxacurium and hyperthyroidism, thyrotoxicosis

—Muscle weakness is commonly seen with hyperthyroidism and affects proximal muscles, usually sparing respiratory function. In some cases, myopathy is the dominant feature of thyroid hormone excess and can resemble myasthenia. Lower doses of muscle relaxants may be indicated.

Doxacurium and hypokalemia

—Hypokalemia appears to potentiate the effects of neuromuscular blockade from non-depolarizing agents.

—The interaction is probably due to hyperpolarization of the muscle endplate and, therefore, resistance to depolarization. Hyperpolarization would more likely occur with more acute changes in potassium concentration since the potassium losses would be from the extracellular compartment rather than from intracellular sites.

—Chronic hypokalemia is more likely to be associated with potassium depletion from both extra and intracellular compartments with no significant change in transmembrane potential. As a result, significant effects on neuromuscular blockade would be less likely.

Doxacurium and hypothermia

—Non-depolarizing muscle blockade is prolonged by hypothermia. This interaction is a result of an effect on the neuromuscular blocking agents themselves rather than on the anticholinesterases used to reverse the neuromuscular blocking agents.

—Hypothermia appears to prolong the effect of the non-depolarizing agents by several mechanisms, including delayed metabolism into inactive metabolites as well as delayed excretion via the urinary and biliary routes.

Doxacurium and malignant hyperthermia

—Anesthetic agents considered safe for use in patients with known or suspected susceptibility for developing malignant hyperthermia (MH) include propofol, barbiturates, etomidate, ketamine, non-depolarizing neuromuscular blocking agents, narcotics, benzodiazepines, droperidol, epinephrine, norepinephrine, and anticholinesterases.

—Nitrous oxide is probably safe in the susceptible patient based on repeated use in MH-susceptible humans and swine.

—Local or regional anesthesia with either amide (such as lidocaine) or ester (such as procaine) anesthetics is now considered safe for MH- susceptible patients.

Doxacurium and myasthenia gravis

—Patients with myasthenia gravis are very sensitive to neuromuscular blockade from non-depolarizing agents.

—This is probably a result of decreased acetylcholine receptors from autoimmune destruction associated with myasthenia gravis.

—Although these patients are treated with the same or similar anticholinesterases used to antagonize muscle blockade, sensitivity (not resistance) to neuromuscular blockade is seen clinically.

Doxacurium and neuromuscular disease (amyotrophic lateral sclerosis, multiple sclerosis, syringomyelia)

—Patients with a wide variety of neuromuscular disorders may be more resistant than normal patients to the effects of non-depolarizing neuromuscular blockers.

—This includes patients with disuse atrophy of the muscles (such as bedridden patients with chronic disease) as well as patients with upper or lower motor neuron disease such as amyotrophic lateral sclerosis, multiple sclerosis, or syringomyelia.

—Disuse or denervation of muscle results in production of extrajunctional acetylcholine receptors on the muscle membrane. These receptors are less easily blocked by non-depolarizing agents but are activated by lower concentrations of depolarizing drugs (succinylcholine).

—When these receptors, which can be scattered over a large surface of the muscle, are depolarized by succinylcholine, ion flow takes place through the receptor channel. Large amounts of potassium may exit the muscle cell causing hyperkalemia.

—Despite initial resistance to blockade, such patients may demonstrate prolonged neuromuscular weakness as a result of decreased muscle strength and mass.

Doxacurium and PIH (pregnancy-induced hypertension), preeclampsia/eclampsia, toxemia

—Patients with hypertensive disorders of pregnancy may require treatment with antihypertensives such as trimethaphan or magnesium sulfate (for preeclampsia/eclampsia). These medications can have significant interactions with anesthetic agents such as succinylcholine, non-depolarizing neuromuscular blocking agents, or calcium channel blockers.

—Neuromuscular blockade produced by both depolarizing and non-depolarizing agents can be potentiated in patients receiving magnesium sulfate. The mechanisms involved include a decreased amount of acetylcholine released by the nerve impulse at the motor nerve terminal and a decrease in the depolarizing action of acetylcholine on the muscle.

Doxacurium Interactions with Patient Drugs

Doxacurium and antibiotics

—A number of antibiotics have significant interactions with neuromuscular blocking agents.

—These include the aminoglycosides (amikacin, gentamicin, kanamycin, neomycin, paromomycin, netilmicin, neomycin, streptomycin, tobramycin), as well as polymyxin B, colistin, amphotericin B, clindamycin, bacitracin, and lincomycin.

—All of the above antibiotics may potentiate non-depolarizing agents, but some (aminoglycosides, amphotericin B, clindamycin, colistin) can also potentiate succinylcholine blockade.

—These antibiotics potentiate neuromuscular blockade by different mechanisms, making management of these problems difficult. Although treatment with anticholinesterases or calcium has been recommended, results are inconsistent.

Doxacurium and amphotericin B

—Prolonged neuromuscular blockade can occur with depolarizing and non-depolarizing agents in patients receiving amphotericin B.

—The mechanism for this interaction is thought to be associated with the hypokalemia that can be caused by amphotericin B therapy.

Doxacurium and beta blockers, propranolol

—Beta blockers may potentiate non-depolarizing neuromuscular blocking agents. This interaction has been reported between propranolol and tubocurarine.

—Other beta blockers are also capable of causing weakness in patients with myasthenia gravis, but the mechanism or significance of these interactions is unclear.

Doxacurium and calcium channel blockers (amlodipine, bepridil, diltiazem, felodipine, isradipine, lidoflazine, nicardipine, nimodipine, nisoldipine, nitrendipine, verapamil)

—Calcium channel blockers have been associated with prolongation of neuromuscular blockade from non-depolarizing agents.

—This interaction is probably related to the depletion of intracellular calcium associated with chronic therapy. This can result in a decrease in acetylcholine release at the neuromuscular junction.

Doxacurium and diphenylhydantoin, phenytoin

—Patients on chronic phenytoin therapy may be resistant to non-depolarizing muscle blockade. The studies involved metocurine and vecuronium but may involve other non-depolarizing agents.

—The mechanism of this interaction is not known.

—Acute infusions of phenytoin may prolong non-depolarizing blockade. This was studied prospectively in a small number of patients who received a 10 mg/kg loading dose of phenytoin during steady-state muscle blockade with vecuronium. They had significant potentiation of their neuromuscular block compared to control patients.

Doxacurium and lidocaine

—Most local anesthetics can block neuromuscular transmission from non-depolarizing agents as well as depolarizing muscle relaxants. Of clinical significance to the anesthesiologist, lidocaine, given as a 50- to 100-mg bolus or even by infusion, can significantly increase a non-depolarizer block or a phase II block from succinylcholine.

Doxacurium and lithium

—Lithium has been reported to increase the duration of both non-depolarizing and depolarizing neuromuscular blocking drugs.

—The mechanism of this interaction is unknown and the clinical significance of this interaction is uncertain.

Doxacurium and magnesium sulfate

—Neuromuscular blockade produced by both depolarizing and non-depolarizing agents can be potentiated in patients receiving magnesium sulfate. The mechanisms involved include a decreased amount of acetylcholine released by the nerve impulse at the motor nerve terminal and a decrease in the depolarizing action of acetylcholine on the muscle.

Doxacurium and mexilitene

—Mexilitene, like lidocaine and most local anesthetics, can potentiate neuromuscular blockade from depolarizing and non-depolarizing agents.

Doxacurium and procainamide

—Procainamide can potentiate muscle relaxation from non-depolarizing agents. This is probably a result of decreased acetylcholine release at the neuromuscular junction caused by procainamide.

Doxacurium and quinidine

—Quinidine and quinine can potentiate muscle relaxation from both depolarizing and nondepolarizing agents.

—The mechanism of this interaction is a curare-like action at the myoneural junction. Also, plasma pseudocholinesterase is inhibited by quinidine (and quinine), resulting in possible prolongation of muscle relaxation from succinylcholine.

Doxacurium and tocainide

—Tocainide, an orally active form of lidocaine, can potentiate both depolarizing and non-depolarizing neuromuscular blockade. This is a property of most local anesthetics as well as a number of other medications.

DOXAPRAM HCL (Dopram)

Classification and indications

—Doxapram is a CNS stimulant.

—It is indicated for treatment of respiratory depression resulting from CNS depressant drugs (anesthetics, barbiturates, narcotics). Reversal of narcotic-induced respiratory depression is not associated with reversal of analgesia.

Pharmacology

—Doxapram increases respiration by stimulation of the peripheral carotid chemoreceptors at low doses and by central stimulation at higher doses.

—Because of its stimulatory effect on the CNS, doxapram may result in increases in heart rate, cardiac output, and blood pressure.

—Patients who may respond adversely to the stimulation produced by doxapram include those with hypermetabolic disorders such as hyperthyroidism or pheochromocytoma, patients with increased intracranial pressure, or those with tachyarrhythmias.

—After intravenous administration, onset of respiratory stimulation occurs in 20–40 seconds and lasts for 5–12 minutes.

—Doxapram is rapidly metabolized and metabolites are excreted in urine and feces.

Dose

—Postanesthetic respiratory depression

—Bolus: 0.5–1.0 mg/kg IV, every 5 minutes up to 2.0 mg/kg.

—Infusion: 5 mg/min of a solution of doxapram 1 mg/mL. If there is improvement or adverse reactions, the rate should be reduced to 1–3 mg/min. The total dose administered should not exceed 4 mg/kg or 3 g.

Doxapram HCl Interactions with Anesthesia Drugs
Doxapram HCl and vasopressors (ephedrine, epinephrine, metaraminol, methoxamine, norepinephrine, phenylephrine)

—Because of its central stimulatory effect, there may additive pressor effects between doxapram and sympathomimetic agents.

Doxapram HCl Interactions with Diseases
Doxapram HCl and cerebral edema, intracranial hypertension, epilepsy, hypertension, pheochromocytoma, hyperthyroidism, thyrotoxicosis

—Because of its mechanism of action, doxapram is contraindicated in a number of conditions, such as hypertension, convulsive disorders, hyperthyroidism, cerebral edema, and pheochromocytoma.

—Analeptic agents, such as doxapram, are CNS stimulants. Because CNS stimulation can elevate arterial pressure, decrease seizure thresholds, and have additive stimulatory effects in conditions such as the above disorders, doxapram is contraindicated in patients with these underlying conditions.

—Analeptic agents improve ventilation through their effect on the brainstem and, in the case of doxapram, the carotid chemoreceptors.

Doxapram HCl Interactions with Patient Drugs
Doxapram HCl and monoamine oxidase inhibitors (isocarboxazid, phenelzine, selegilene tranylcypromine)

—Doxapram, a CNS stimulant, can also produce tachycardia and hypertension. When used in patients taking monoamine oxidase inhibitors, exaggerated hypertension and arrhythmias can occur.

DROPERIDOL (Inapsine)

Classification and indications
—Droperidol is a butyrophenone derivative, related to haloperidol.
—It is used for sedation (either alone or with narcotics–neuroleptanalgesia), as an anxiolytic, as part of a general anesthetic, or as an antiemetic.

Pharmacology
—Droperidol, which is related to phenothiazines, shares some of the properties of this class of drugs. Sedation is a prominent effect and, like the phenothiazines, droperidol may produce extrapyramidal reactions (oculogyric crises, neck extension, flexed arms).
—Both droperidol and phenothiazines antagonize the effects of dopamine in the basal ganglia. Patients with Parkinson's disease (who receive the dopamine precursor levodopa) may be affected adversely by administration of these drugs.
—Droperidol has alpha receptor blocking properties and may cause hypotension. Because of this alpha blockade, administration of epinephrine should be avoided (skeletal muscle vasodilation is caused by epinephrine).
—Following IV administration, onset of action is about 3 minutes, but may require 30 minutes for peak effects. The sedative effects persist for 4 hours or more.
—Elimination is partly dependent on liver metabolism, with some renal excretion as well.

Dose
—Adults: 0.22–0.275 mg/kg IV or IM. Lower doses are frequently used (0.5 mg) by anesthesiologists and nurse anesthetists because other anesthetic agents are also administered.
—Children: 0.075–0.165 mg/kg IV or IM, with the same considerations as above.

Droperidol Interactions with Diseases
Droperidol and cerebral edema, intracranial hypertension
—Most intravenous anesthetic agents (except ketamine) can be safely used in patients with elevated intracranial pressure.
—Droperidol appears to have little effect on cerebral blood flow and cerebral metabolic rate.

Droperidol and malignant hyperthermia

—Anesthetic agents considered safe for use in patients with known or suspected susceptibility for developing malignant hyperthermia (MH) include propofol, barbiturates, etomidate, ketamine, non-depolarizing neuromuscular blocking agents, narcotics, benzodiazepines, droperidol, epinephrine, norepinephrine, and anticholinesterases.

—Nitrous oxide is probably safe in the susceptible patient based on repeated use in MH-susceptible humans and swine.

—Local or regional anesthesia with either amide (such as lidocaine) or ester (such as procaine) anesthetics is now considered safe for MH- susceptible patients.

Droperidol and Parkinson's disease

—Droperidol antagonizes the effects of dopamine in the basal ganglia and can worsen the condition of patients with Parkinson's disease.

Droperidol Interactions with Patient Drugs

Droperidol and carbidopa, levodopa

—Carbidopa and levodopa are used to increase dopamine concentrations in the brain. Butyrophenones (droperidol) block the dopaminergic effects of dopamine in the basal ganglia and can antagonize levodopa and carbidopa.

EDROPHONIUM (Enlon, Reversol, Tensilon)

Classification and indications

—Edrophonium is a synthetic parasympathomimetic agent.

—It is indicated for use as a reversal agent for non-depolarizing neuromuscular blocking agents (competitive inhibitors of acetylcholine). It is also used for testing for myasthenia gravis and has been used in the treatment of supraventricular tachycardias.

Pharmacology

—Edrophonium inhibits the destruction of acetylcholine by binding reversibly to acetylcholinesterase. As a result, acetylcholine accumulates at cholinergic synapses (such as the neuromuscular junction and the sinus node).

—Speed of reversal of the anticholinesterases depends on several factors, including depth of muscle blockade, neuromuscular blocker used, and dose and type of anticholinesterase.

—In general, onset of action is fastest with edrophonium, followed by neostigmine and pyridostigmine.

—At moderate levels of neuromuscular blockade (<90% twitch depression), neostigmine, edrophonium, and pyridostigmine are about equivalent in ability to induce reversal. When muscle blockade is profound (>90% twitch depression), edrophonium is not as effective as neostigmine.

—Pyridostigmine has the longest duration of action. Although edrophonium was thought to have a very short duration of action, studies with edrophonium doses of 0.5–1.0 mg/kg demonstrate a similar duration between edrophonium and neostigmine.

—Cardiac effects of parasympathomimetic agents, such as the anticholinesterases, result in bradycardia. To antagonize these responses, reversal agents are usually administered with either atropine or glycopyrrolate.

—Because of the rapid onset of edrophonium, atropine is usually recommended for coadministration, whereas glycopyrrolate (which is also slower in onset) is used for the slower onset of neostigmine and pyridostigmine.

Dose

—For reversal of neuromuscular blockade: edrophonium, 0.5–1.0 mg/kg with atropine, 7–10 μg/kg IV.

Edrophonium Interactions with Anesthesia Drugs

Edrophonium and quinidine

—Patients receiving anticholinesterase drugs for myasthenia gravis can have exacerbation of muscle weakness if given procainamide or quinidine.

—This is related to the ability of these drugs to enhance neuromuscular blockade from depolarizing and non-depolarizing agents.

—Lidocaine and propranolol would also be expected to have this interaction but appear to be safe for use in myasthenics.

Edrophonium and succinylcholine

—Neostigmine, edrophonium, pyridostigmine, and any other anticholinesterase can significantly prolong the duration of neuromuscular blockade from succinylcholine.

—Because these medications are nonspecific anticholinesterases, they also inhibit plasma pseudocholinesterase and therefore delay metabolism of succinylcholine.

—The exact time necessary to prevent this interaction after administering an anticholinesterase is not known. Since the duration of action of neostigmine is 50–90 minutes, this may be a minimum interval to avoid this interaction.

Edrophonium Interactions with Diseases

Edrophonium and acidosis (respiratory or metabolic)

—Alterations of the normal acid–base status may result in difficulty reversing non-depolarizing neuromuscular blockade.

—Respiratory acidosis ($pCO_2 > 50$) and metabolic alkalosis have been shown to prevent adequate reversal of pancuronium neuromuscular block. This interaction appears to be complex and is incompletely understood, but is probably related to changes in electrolytes and intracellular pH rather than simple changes in acid–base measurements.

Edrophonium and Eaton–Lambert syndrome

—Anticholinesterases are unreliable in reversing the muscle relaxation of non-depolarizing agents in patients with Eaton–Lambert syndrome.

—Patients with this syndrome may experience prolonged neuromuscular blockade with both non-depolarizing and depolarizing agents.

Edrophonium and hypocalcemia

—Reversal of neuromuscular blockade can be impaired in the presence of hypocalcemia.

—Stimulation of a motor nerve causes a nerve action potential which allows entry of calcium into the nerve ending. The calcium appears to cause release of acetylcholine from vesicles in the nerve ending into the neuromuscular junction, resulting in endplate depolarization.

—In the presence of inadequate ionized calcium, less acetylcholine is released, impairing the ability of acetylcholinesterase inhibitors to overcome the competitive blockade of acetylcholine receptors by neuromuscular blocking agents.

Edrophonium and hypokalemia

—Reversal of neuromuscular blockade in patients with hypokalemia may be more difficult. Although this has been demonstrated in animal studies, there is some controversy about the clinical importance of hypokalemia in reversal of muscle blockade in humans.

—Hypokalemia, particularly acute hypokalemia, can potentiate non-depolarizing neuromuscular blockers.

Edrophonium and hypothermia

—Non-depolarizing muscle blockade is prolonged by hypothermia. This interaction is a result of an effect on the neuromuscular blocking agents themselves rather than on the anticholinesterases used to reverse the neuromuscular blocking agents.

—Hypothermia appears to prolong the effect of the non-depolarizing agents by several mechanisms, including delayed metabolism into inactive metabolites as well as delayed excretion via the urinary and biliary routes.

Edrophonium and malignant hyperthermia

—Anesthetic agents considered safe for use in patients with known or suspected susceptibility for developing malignant hyperthermia (MH) include propofol, barbiturates, etomidate, ketamine, non-depolarizing neuromuscular blocking agents, narcotics, benzodiazepines, droperidol, epinephrine, norepinephrine, and anticholinesterases.

—Nitrous oxide is probably safe in the susceptible patient based on repeated use in MH-susceptible humans and swine.

—Local or regional anesthesia with either amide (such as lidocaine) or ester (such as procaine) anesthetics is now considered safe for MH- susceptible patients.

Edrophonium and myasthenia gravis

—Reversal of a non-depolarizing blockade in patients with myasthenia gravis is controversial.

—Because patients are treated chronically with anticholinesterases, anticholinesterase inhibition is already nearly maximized.

—Conservative recommendations are to not use anticholinesterases for reversal of muscle blockade but rather to allow spontaneous recovery.

ENALAPRIL (ENALAPRILAT) (Vasotec)

Classification and indications

—Enalapril is an angiotensin-converting enzyme (ACE) inhibitor.

—It is indicated for the management of hypertension, either alone or in combination with other antihypertensive agents. It is also used in the management of congestive heart failure.

Pharmacology

—Enalaprilat is formed from hydrolysis of enalapril. Its mechanism of action appears to be competitive inhibition of the enzyme (angiotensin-converting enzyme, ACE) that converts angiotensin I to angiotensin II, which is a vasoconstrictor.

—Arterial pressure is reduced as a result of arteriolar dilation as well as possible venous dilation.

—Additionally, enalaprilat probably has some other antihypertensive action because, even in patients with low-renin hypertension, there is a hypotensive effect.

—Cardiac effects are indirect, mainly the result of changes in peripheral resistance and venous tone. There is usually no change or an increase in cardiac output and stroke volume.

—Onset of hypotensive effect can be seen after intravenous administration in 5–15 minutes, with maximum effects after 1–4 hours.

—Elimination of enalaprilat depends on hepatic metabolism and renal excretion. Patients with liver or renal disease may have prolonged effects from the drug.

Dose

—For hypertension: 1.25 mg IV slowly over a 5-minute period, every 6 hours, if needed. Higher doses (up to 5 mg every 6 hours) have been well tolerated.

Enalapril (enalaprilat) Interactions with Diseases
Enalapril (enalaprilat) and pregnancy

—ACE inhibitors are not considered safe for use in pregnant women.

—Especially in the second and third trimesters, fetal abnormalities have been linked to ACE therapy.

Enalapril (enalaprilat) Interactions with Patient Drugs
Enalapril (enalaprilat) and bumetanide, ethacrynic acid, furosemide

—ACE inhibitors used to treat hypertension in a patient who is being diuresed with the loop diuretics may produce a profound drop in blood pressure.

—This response has been seen as early as 2–3 hours after initiation of ACE inhibitors.

—The mechanisms of this interaction may include hypovolemia from diuretic therapy or, in some patients, high levels of renin and angiotensin.

—The setting in which this interaction may be significant for anesthesiologists might be a hypertensive patient who presents for urgent surgery while receiving intensive diuretic treatment for cardiac decompensation. Use of ACE inhibitor therapy in the perioperative setting may precipitate the interaction described.

ENFLURANE (Ethrane)

Classification and indications
—Enflurane is a nonflammable, halogenated ether.
—It is indicated for use as an inhalational anesthetic.

Pharmacology
—The minimal alveolar concentration (MAC) of enflurane is 1.7%.
—It has a blood/gas partition coefficient of 1.9, making it similar to isoflurane (1.4) but about four times more soluble than nitrous oxide or desflurane. This results in slower induction and emergence from anesthesia than less soluble agents.
—Higher solubility in blood results in slower induction and emergence from anesthesia.
—Approximately 2–10% of enflurane is metabolized in the liver, releasing fluoride ion. The renal threshold for toxicity from fluoride ion is thought to be >40 µmol, which is above levels normally encountered during enflurane anesthesia.
—Like other halogenated ethers, enflurane causes a reversible decrease in myocardial contractility.
—Decreased arterial blood pressure is a result of peripheral vasodilation.
—Enflurane has been associated with electroencephalographic changes during deep anesthesia.
—At high concentrations of enflurane (2.5%) and/or low pCO_2 (<25 torr), the likelihood of seizure activity is highest. Facial twitching as well as limb muscle contraction has been associated with electroencephalographic changes in both normal and epileptic patients.
—Characteristic changes in the EEG consist of high frequency and voltage pattern progressing to spike and dome complexes. Electrical seizure activity has been documented, however, not only at high concentrations but at concentrations as low as 1% in normal children.
—Although there is considerable controversy about the ability of enflurane to elicit clinically significant seizures, most recommendations are to avoid enflurane in patients with such disorders.

Dose
—Induction: Enflurane, isoflurane, and desflurane are irritating to the airways and are generally not recommended for inhalational induction.

—Maintenance: Use of other anesthetic agents (opioids, benzo-diazepines, barbiturates, propofol, etc.) can reduce the MAC of inhalational anesthetics. As a result, depending on the anesthetic technique used, the type of operation, and vari-ability of patient response, maintenance requirements for inhalational agents are highly variable.

Enflurane Interactions with Anesthesia Drugs

Enflurane and muscle relaxants (atracurium, doxacurium, gallamine, metocurine, mivacurium, pancuronium, pipercuronium, rocuronium, tubocurarine, vecuronium)

—Halothane, isoflurane, and ethrane can significantly poten-tiate neuromuscular blockade, depending on the neuro-muscular blocker used. Nitrous oxide has minimal effects.

—Tubocurarine and pancuronium are potentiated the most by inhalational agents, while atracurium and vecuronium are intensified significantly less.

—Potentiation by inhalational agents occurs through depres-sion of spinal cord reflexes as well as effects at or distal to the neuromuscular junction.

Enflurane and clonidine

—Clonidine has been shown to reduce the MAC of inhaled and opioid anesthetics.

—This effect may be related to clonidine's inhibition of the sympathetic outflow from the vasomotor center in the medulla (clonidine is a central alpha 2 receptor agonist, which results in inhibition of CNS sympathetic centers).

Enflurane and epinephrine, norepinephrine

—Halothane and, to a lesser extent, isoflurane and ethrane reduce the threshold for arrhythmias from epinephrine and norepinephrine. The mechanism of this "sensitization" of the myodium to these sympathomimetic amines includes an increase in automaticity and changes in depolarization.

—Although exact numbers are not agreed on, a general guide-line for safe administration of epinephrine based on some clinical studies is to use no more than 10 mL of 1:100,000 (1 µg/mL) epinephrine solution every 10 minutes with a limit of 30 mL/hr. with isoflurane or ethrane, a slightly larger amount can probably be used.

Enflurane and succinylcholine

—Succinylcholine neuromuscular blockade may be potenti-ated by desflurane and isoflurane.

—Halothane and enflurane probably have clinically insignificant interactions with succinylcholine.

Enflurane Interactions with Diseases

Enflurane and alcohol—acute intoxication

—Patients with acute alcohol intoxication (including chronic abusers of alcohol) have a lower minimal alveolar concentration (MAC) for inhalational anesthetics.

—The mechanism of this interaction appears to be additive CNS depressant effects between alcohol and inhalational agents.

Enflurane and alcohol—chronic abuse

—Chronic abuse of alcohol has complex and incompletely understood effects on a patient's response to anesthetic agents. In general, these patients tend to be more tolerant (in a nonintoxicated state) to barbiturates, benzodiazepines, narcotics, and inhalational agents.

—Exceptions to this generalization include the alcoholic patient with a cardiomyopathy who may demonstrate increased sensitivity to myocardial depression from inhalational agents.

—Also, the patient with severe liver disease may have impaired ability to metabolize succinylcholine due to decreased levels of plasma pseudocholinesterase.

Enflurane and cerebral edema, intracranial hypertension

—All commonly used inhalational volatile anesthetics (halothane > enflurane > isoflurane) cause an increased cerebral blood flow (CBF). Less is known about sevoflurane and desflurane, but they are believed to have effects similar to those of isoflurane. Nitrous oxide has minimal effects on CBF.

—The volatile anesthetics, although they depress cerebral metabolic rate, cause cerebrovascular dilation that results in increased CBF. Hyperventilation to a $PaCO_2$ between 25 and 35 mm Hg will effectively prevent increased CBF from isoflurane but not the other volatile anesthetics.

Enflurane and epilepsy

—Although there is considerable controversy about the ability of enflurane to elicit clinically significant seizures, most recommendations are to avoid enflurane in patients with such disorders.

—At high concentrations of enflurane (2.5%) and/or low pCO_2 (<25 torr), the likelihood of seizure activity is highest. Facial twitching as well as limb muscle contraction has been associated with electroencephalographic changes in both normal and epileptic patients.

—Characteristic changes in the EEG consist of high frequency and voltage pattern progressing to spike and dome complexes. Electrical seizure activity has been documented, however, not only at high concentrations but at concentrations as low as 1% in normal children.

Enflurane and hepatitis

—All forms of anesthesia, including general, regional, and nitrous-narcotic, are associated with postoperative liver function test abnormalities. The exact mechanism of this reaction is not known but is likely related to reduced liver blood flow from anesthesia and surgery.

—The presence of hepatitis or any liver disease has been shown to increase the morbidity and mortality in patients receiving anesthesia. The mechanism of this increase in morbidity and mortality is not clear but is most likely related to changes in hepatic blood flow as a result of anesthesia and surgery.

—Since there is no known method of avoiding exacerbation of preexisting liver disease by anesthesia, most recommendations are to postpone surgery in patients suspected of having acute hepatitis.

—There is no evidence that enflurane, isoflurane, desflurane, or sevoflurane is hepatotoxic.

—Halothane, however, can occasionally cause fulminant hepatic necrosis in both adults and children. A milder form of hepatotoxicity is also seen with halothane anesthesia.

Enflurane and malignant hyperthermia

—Halothane, isoflurane, enflurane, desflurane, sevoflurane, as well as other, older inhalational agents all are potent triggering agents of malignant hyperthermia (MH) in the susceptible patient.

—Succinylcholine, decamethonium, and possibly tubocurarine are also triggering agents.

—Anesthetic agents considered safe for use in patients with known or suspected susceptibility for developing malignant hyperthermia include propofol, barbiturates, etomidate, ketamine, non-depolarizing neuromuscular blocking agents, narcotics, benzodiazepines, droperidol, epinephrine, norepinephrine, and anticholinesterases.

—Nitrous oxide is probably safe in the susceptible patient based on repeated use in MH-susceptible humans and swine.

—Local or regional anesthesia with either amide (such as lidocaine) or ester (such as procaine) anesthetics is now considered safe for MH- susceptible patients.

Enflurane and myotonia

—Inhalational anesthetics may cause exaggerated cardiac depression in patients with myotonia dystrophica.

—Patients with myotonia dystrophica, but not the other myotonic syndromes, are likely to have some degree of cardiomyopathy even in the absence of clinical symptoms. As a result, these patients may be very sensitive to any myocardial depressant.

Enflurane and porphyria

—Inhalational agents are considered to be safe for use in patients with porphyria, as are narcotics, depolarizing and non-depolarizing muscle relaxants, etomidate, anticholinesterases, and propofol.

—Barbiturates are contraindicated in three of the four hepatic porphyrias (acute intermittent porphyria, variegate porphyria, and hereditary coproporphyria). Porphyria cutanea tarda and the erythropoietic porphyrias are not exacerbated by barbiturates.

—It is theorized that barbiturates can provoke an attack of porphyria by inducing the enzyme aminolevulinic acid synthetase, which results in synthesis of more porphyrin compounds and their precursors.

Enflurane and pregnancy

—Pregnancy is associated with significant reductions in minimal alveolar concentrations (MAC) for inhalational agents.

—In animal studies and some human studies, decreases in MAC of up to 40% have been documented.

—The suggested mechanism for this decreased MAC includes increases in progesterone and endorphin levels associated with pregnancy.

Enflurane and renal dysfunction

—Enflurane, isoflurane, halothane, and desflurane are considered safe for administration to patients with renal dysfunction.

—Although enflurane undergoes biotransformation with the formation of inorganic fluoride to a greater extent than other agents (with the exception of methoxyflurane, which is very nephrotoxic), even 4 hours of anesthesia with enflurane produce nontoxic fluoride levels. There is some question, however, of renal toxicity after prolonged (9 hours) anesthesia with enflurane.

—Sevoflurane is also biotransformed to inorganic fluoride, but at potentially nephrotoxic levels (50 μmol/L), according to some studies.

—All inhaled anesthetic agents can cause a transient, reversible decrease in renal function as reflected in lowered glomerular filtration rate (GFR), urine output, and urinary sodium excretion.

—The mechanism for this action may include alterations in antidiuretic hormone, vasopressin, or renin, as well as decreases in renal blood flow.

Enflurane Interactions with Patient Drugs

Enflurane and amiodarone

—Amiodarone, an antiarrhythmic that increases refractoriness and slows conduction in most cardiac tissue, has been associated with severe cardiac complications including arrhythmias, low cardiac output, and decreased systemic vascular resistance in patients having general anesthesia with inhalational agents.

—The mechanism of these interactions is not known.

Enflurane and clonidine

—Clonidine has been shown to reduce the MAC of inhaled and opioid anesthetics.

—This effect may be related to clonidine's inhibition of the sympathetic outflow from the vasomotor center in the medulla (clonidine is a central alpha 2 receptor agonist, which results in inhibition of CNS sympathetic centers).

Enflurane and disulfiram

—Profound hypotension may occur when patients taking disulfiram are exposed to halogenated anesthetics (enflurane, isoflurane, and halothane).

Enflurane and isoniazid

—Normally, fluoride levels with enflurane use remain well below nephrotoxic levels. In patients taking isoniazid, however, fluoride levels may reach nephrotoxic levels.

EPHEDRINE

Classification and indications

—Ephedrine is a sympathomimetic found naturally in a genus of plants *(Ephedra)*.

—It is indicated for the management of hypotension and/or bradycardia when patient positioning or fluid therapy is impractical, ineffective, or contraindicated.

Pharmacology

—Ephedrine directly stimulates beta and alpha receptors and also causes release of stored norepinephrine.

—Stimulation of beta 2 receptors causes bronchial smooth muscle relaxation and dilation of skeletal muscle arterioles, whereas beta 1 stimulation produces increased myocardial contractility and tachycardia. Arrhythmias may be seen.

—Blood pressure responses may be unpredictable because ephedrine causes dilation of skeletal muscle arterioles (beta 2 effect) and vasoconstriction of skin and viscera (alpha receptor stimulation). Usually blood pressure increases because of combined cardiac stimulation and vasoconstriction.

—Coronary arteries may be dilated as a result of cardiac stimulation and coronary blood flow may be increased due to increased blood pressure. However, decreased coronary blood flow has occurred.

—Repeated or prolonged use of ephedrine may result in depletion of norepinephrine stores and decreased pressor responses.

Dose

—Adult: 10–25 mg IM, SC, or IV slowly.

—Pediatric: 0.5–1 mg/kg/dose IM, SC, or IV slowly. Maximum 3 mg/kg/day.

Ephedrine Interactions with Anesthesia Drugs

Ephedrine and cocaine

—Cocaine may potentiate the vasopressor responses to sympathomimetic agents.

—The mechanism of this interaction involves the inhibition of reuptake of catecholamines by cocaine. This property probably accounts for the vasoconstriction caused by cocaine use.

—Cardiovascular symptoms of hypertension, arrhythmias, and tachycardia from cocaine use are related to both central and sympathetic nervous system effects of cocaine.

Ephedrine and oxytocin, ergot alkaloids (methylergonovine)

—Severe hypertension has been associated with administration of oxytocin to patients who had received a prophylactic vasoconstrictor up to 4 hours previously for a caudal block.

—This interaction is more likely to be seen in patients with underlying mild hypertension and in those receiving an ergot alkaloid (such as methylergonovine).

—The safest method of administering an oxytocic is a dilute intravenous infusion of oxytocin.

Ephedrine and phentolamine

—Blockade of alpha 1 receptors can result in unresponsiveness to vasopressors, depending on the vasopressor being used.

—Ephedrine and mephentermine have significant beta 2 stimulation along with beta 1 and alpha adrenergic activity. As a result, it is possible that hypotension could worsen in patients on alpha blockers given ephedrine due to the unopposed vasodilation resulting from beta 2 stimulation.

—Although good documentation of this interaction is scarce, this is similar to the response that can be seen with epinephrine.

—Because norepinephrine has beta 1 activity, it is more likely to be effective in treating hypotension in patients on alpha blockers.

Ephedrine Interactions with Diseases
Ephedrine and hyperthyroidism, thyrotoxicosis

—Agents that stimulate the sympathetic nervous system (catecholamines, ephedrine, phenylephrine, dopram, ketamine) may have exaggerated effects in patients with hyperthyroidism. Although most evident in untreated patients, even patients receiving treatment for excess thyroid hormone may demonstrate this response.

—Excess thyroid hormone causes stimulation of metabolism of most body tissues. As a result, cardiac output increases by 50% or more to remove the extra metabolic byproducts. Also, direct stimulatory effects on the myocardium at even slightly elevated thyroid hormone levels causes tachycardia and increased contractility.

—At higher thyroid hormone levels, myocardial depression may occur as a result of excess demands or a direct myocardial depression.

Ephedrine and pheochromocytoma

—Blockade of alpha 1 receptors can result in unresponsiveness to vasopressors, depending on the vasopressor being used.

—Ephedrine and mephentermine have significant beta 2 stimulation along with beta 1 and alpha adrenergic activity. As a result, it is possible that hypotension could worsen in patients on alpha blockers given ephedrine due to the unopposed vasodilation resulting from beta 2 stimulation.

—Although good documentation of this interaction is scarce, it is similar to the response that can be seen with epinephrine.

—Because norepinephrine has beta 1 activity, it is more likely to be effective in treating hypotension in patients on alpha blockers.

Ephedrine and pregnancy

—Ephedrine, mephentermine, and metaraminol are the preferred agents for treatment of hypotension in pregnancy.

—The above agents have both alpha and beta agonist activity and are not associated with reduced placental blood flow.

—Phenylephrine, norepinephrine, angiotensin, and methoxamine are predominantly alpha adrenergic agents that act peripherally and can cause uterine artery vasoconstriction and placental hypoperfusion.

Ephedrine Interactions with Patient Drugs

Ephedrine and alpha adrenergic blockers (doxazasin, phenoxybenzamine, phentolamine, prazosin, terazosin)

—Blockade of alpha 1 receptors can result in unresponsiveness to vasopressors, depending on the vasopressor being used.

—Ephedrine and mephentermine have significant beta 2 stimulation along with beta 1 and alpha adrenergic activity. As a result, it is possible that hypotension could worsen in patients on alpha blockers given ephedrine due to the unopposed vasodilation resulting from beta 2 stimulation.

—Although good documentation of this interaction is scarce, it is similar to the response that can be seen with epinephrine.

—Because norepinephrine has beta 1 activity, it is more likely to be effective in treating hypotension in patients on alpha blockers.

Ephedrine and ergot alkaloids (dihydroergonovine, ergonovine, ergotamine tartrate, methylergonovine)

—Severe hypertension has been associated with administration of oxytocin to patients who had received a prophylactic vasoconstrictor up to 4 hours previously for a caudal block.

—This interaction is more likely to be seen in patients with underlying mild hypertension and in those receiving an ergot alkaloid (such as methylergonovine).

—The safest method of administering an oxytocic is a dilute intravenous infusion of oxytocin.

Ephedrine and guanadrel, guanethidine

—Patients receiving guanethidine and guanadrel can have an exaggerated hypertensive response to norepinephrine and other direct-acting catecholamines such as phenylephrine, dobutamine, and epinephrine.

—Indirect-acting catecholamines, such as ephedrine, metaraminol, mephentermine, and dopamine may have fewer pressor effects than expected.

—Guanethidine and guanadrel deplete intraneuronal norepinephrine in postganglionic sympathetic neurons and in this way may diminish the response of indirect acting catecholamines, while sensitizing adrenergic receptors to direct-acting amines.

Ephedrine and monoamine oxidase inhibitors (isocarboxazid, phenelzine, selegilene tranylcypromine)

—Indirect-acting vasopressors (ephedrine, mephentermine, and metaraminol) act by releasing intraneuronal monoamines such as dopamine and norepinephrine. This is the explanation of the hypertensive crises seen when patients receiving monamine oxidase inhibitors are given these vasopressors.

—Direct acting vasopressors such as phenylephrine, epinephrine, norepinephrine, and dobutamine may be potentiated by MAO inhibitors and should be used in smaller amounts than normally used.

—Dopamine has both direct and indirect actions and must be used with caution (perhaps one tenth the normal dose).

Ephedrine and oxytocin

—Oxytocin administration has been associated with severe hypertension in patients who had received a prophylactic vasoconstrictor up to 4 hours previously for a caudal block.

—Severe hypertension is more likely to occur in patients with existing mild hypertension and in those patients who receive an ergot alkaloid (such as methylergonovine) rather than a dilute solution of oxytocin.

Ephedrine and ritodrine

—Ritodrine and terbutaline, beta 2 agonists, may potentiate other sympathomimetic agents.

—The mechanism of this interaction is probably related to the beta 1 adrenergic stimulation that can be seen with either ritodrine or terbutaline administration, particularly when these agents are used at higher dosage.

EPINEPHRINE

Classification and indications

—Epinephrine is an endogenous catecholamine secreted by the adrenal gland.

—It is indicated for the management of hypotension, anaphylaxis, bronchospasm, and cardiac arrest. It is also used with local anesthetics to decrease systemic absorption and prolong the duration of action.

Pharmacology

—Epinephrine directly stimulates alpha and beta adrenergic receptors.

—At usual therapeutic parenteral doses, the major effects of alpha and beta stimulation by epinephrine are:

—Bronchial smooth muscle relaxation (beta 2 stimulation).

—Cardiac stimulation results in increased heart rate and contractility (beta 1 stimulation).

—Skeletal muscle arteriolar dilation causes decreased peripheral resistance (beta 2 stimulation).

—Although alpha receptor stimulation causes vasoconstriction of skin, mucous membranes, and viscera, the arteriolar dilation of skeletal muscle usually results in a decrease in peripheral resistance. At higher doses, however, vasoconstriction of skeletal vasculature can occur.

—Because of the increased heart rate and cardiac output, the usual effect of epinephrine is to increase blood pressure, although diastolic pressure may decrease somewhat.

—Constriction of renal blood vessels may reduce glomerular filtration rate and urine output, unless the increase in cardiac output and blood pressure overcome this effect.

—Parenterally administered epinephrine is metabolized in the liver and other tissues by enzymes.

—Onset of action is very rapid after intravenous administration and within 5–10 minutes of subcutaneous injection. Following oral administration, bronchodilation begins within one minute and effects are mainly confined to the respiratory tract, unless larger doses are used (such as 1 mg for cardiac resuscitation).

Dose

—*Bronchospasm and anaphylaxis:*

—Adults:

　—Subcutaneously or IM: 0.1–0.5 mg every 20 minutes for 3 doses.

　—Intravenously: 0.1–0.25 mg as necessary or by intravenous infusion of 1–4 μg/min.

—Children:

　—Subcutaneously: 0.01 mg/kg, but not greater than 0.5 mg/dose. This dose may be repeated at 20-minute intervals for 3 or 4 doses.

　—Intravenously: a 1:10,000 dilution (0.1 mg/mL) may be administered at a dose of 0.1 mL/kg/dose. A continuous infusion may be administered at a rate of 0.1 μg/kg/min.

　—Inhalation: Using a 1% solution (10 mg/mL), 0.03 mL (0.3 mg) in 3 mL of saline may be administered by inhalation.

—*Cardiac arrest:*

—Adults: 0.5–1.0 mg every 5 minutes IV or by continuous infusion of 1 to 4 μg/min. (5–10 mL of a 1:10,000 solution).

—Children: 0.01 mg/kg every 5 minutes.

—Administration via the endotracheal tube should be at the same doses as for intravenous route.

Epinephrine Interactions with Anesthesia Drugs

Epinephrine and beta blockers (esmolol, labetalol, propranolol)

—Epinephrine, used in local anesthesia or intravenously, can cause unexpected severe hypertension in patients on chronic beta blocker therapy. The mechanism for this interaction is the unrestricted alpha stimulation from epinephrine in patients who are beta-blocked.

Epinephrine and chlorpromazine

—Neuroleptic drugs, particularly chlorpromazine, thioridazine, and clozapine, may produce an unexpected hypotensive response with epinephrine.

—The mechanism for this interaction involves the alpha receptor blockade associated with neuroleptic drugs, leaving the vasodilating beta receptors unopposed.

—Hypotension is possibly better treated with more selective alpha adrenergic agents such as phenylephrine.

—This interaction is not likely to be seen with neuroleptic agents other than the three listed above.

Epinephrine and cocaine

—Cocaine may potentiate the vasopressor responses to sympathomimetic agents.

—The mechanism of this interaction involves the inhibition of reuptake of catecholamines by cocaine. This property probably accounts for the vasoconstriction caused by cocaine use.

—Cardiovascular symptoms of hypertension, arrhythmias, and tachycardia from cocaine use are related to both central and sympathetic nervous system effects of cocaine.

Epinephrine and doxapram HCl

—There may additive pressor effects between doxapram and sympathomimetic agents.

Epinephrine and enflurane, halothane, Isoflurane

—Halothane and, to a lesser extent, isoflurane and ethrane reduce the threshold for arrhythmias from epinephrine and norepinephrine. The mechanism of this "sensitization" of the myodium to these sympathomimetic amines includes an increase in automaticity and changes in depolarization.

—Although exact numbers are not agreed on, a general guideline for safe administration of epinephrine based on some clinical studies is to use no more than 10 mL of 1:100,000 (1 μg/mL) epinephrine solution every 10 minutes with a limit of 30 mL/hr. with isoflurane or ethrane, a slightly larger amount can probably be used.

Epinephrine and methylergonovine

—Oxytocics (oxytocin, ergonovine, methylergonovine) may interact with vasopressors to produce hypertension, which is more likely to be severe in patients with a predisposition to hypertension.

—The use of an intramuscular or intravenous ergot alkaloid (such as IM methylergonovine) either preceded or followed by a vasopressor may result in severe hypertension. The safest method of administering an oxytocic is a dilute intravenous infusion of oxytocin.

Epinephrine and oxytocin

—Severe hypertension has been associated with administration of oxytocin to patients who had received a prophylactic vasoconstrictor up to 4 hours previously for a caudal block.

—This interaction is more likely to be seen in patients with underlying mild hypertension and in those receiving an ergot alkaloid (such as methylergonovine) rather than a dilute solution of oxytocin.

Epinephrine and phentolamine

—Blockade of alpha 1 receptors can result in unresponsiveness to vasopressors, depending on the vasopressor being used.

—Epinephrine has significant beta 2 stimulation along with beta 1 and alpha adrenergic activity. As a result, it is possible that hypotension could worsen in patients on alpha blockers given epinephrine due to the unopposed vasodilation resulting from beta 2 stimulation.

—Because norepinephrine has beta 1 activity, it is more likely to be effective in treating hypotension in patients on alpha blockers.

Epinephrine Interactions with Diseases

Epinephrine and hyperthyroidism, thyrotoxicosis

—Agents that stimulate the sympathetic nervous system (catecholamines, ephedrine, phenylephrine, dopram, ketamine) may have exaggerated effects in patients with hyperthyroidism. Although most evident in untreated patients, even patients receiving treatment for excess thyroid hormone may demonstrate this response.

—Excess thyroid hormone causes stimulation of metabolism of most body tissues. As a result, cardiac output increases by 50% or more to remove the extra metabolic byproducts. Also, direct stimulatory effects on the myocardium at even slightly elevated thyroid hormone levels causes tachycardia and increased contractility.

—At higher thyroid hormone levels, myocardial depression may occur as a result of excess demands or a direct myocardial depression.

Epinephrine and malignant hyperthermia

—Anesthetic agents considered safe for use in patients with known or suspected susceptibility for developing malignant hyperthermia include propofol, barbiturates, etomidate, ketamine, non-depolarizing neuromuscular blocking

agents, narcotics, benzodiazepines, droperidol, epinephrine, norepinephrine, and anticholinesterases.
—Nitrous oxide is probably safe in the susceptible patient based on repeated use in MH-susceptible humans and swine.
—Local or regional anesthesia with either amide (such as lidocaine) or ester (such as procaine) anesthetics is now considered safe for MH-susceptible patients.

Epinephrine and pheochromocytoma
—Blockade of alpha 1 receptors can result in unresponsiveness to vasopressors, depending on the vasopressor being used.
—Epinephrine has significant beta 2 stimulation along with beta 1 and alpha adrenergic activity. As a result, it is possible that hypotension could worsen in patients on alpha blockers given epinephrine due to the unopposed vasodilation resulting from beta 2 stimulation.
—Because norepinephrine has beta 1 activity, it is more likely to be effective in treating hypotension in patients on alpha blockers.

Epinephrine and pregnancy
—Ephedrine, mephentermine, and metaraminol are the preferred agents for treatment of hypotension in pregnancy.
—The above agents have both alpha and beta agonist activity and are not associated with reduced placental blood flow.
—Epinephrine has both alpha and beta effects, depending on the dose. At higher doses, alpha effects predominate and can result in decreased uterine blood flow.
—Phenylephrine, norepinephrine, angiotensin, and methoxamine are predominantly alpha adrenergic agents that act peripherally and can cause uterine artery vasoconstriction and placental hypoperfusion.

Epinephrine Interactions with Patient Drugs
Epinephrine and alpha adrenergic blockers (doxazosin, phenoxybenzamine, phentolamine, prazosin, terazosin)
—Blockade of alpha 1 receptors can result in unresponsiveness to vasopressors, depending on the vasopressor being used.
—Epinephrine has significant beta 2 stimulation along with beta 1 and alpha adrenergic activity. As a result, it is possible that hypotension could worsen in patients on alpha blockers given epinephrine due to the unopposed vasodilation resulting from beta 2 stimulation.

—Because norepinephrine has beta 1 activity, it is more likely to be effective in treating hypotension in patients on alpha blockers.

Epinephrine and beta blockers (acebutolol, atenolol, betaxolol, carteolol, labetalol, levobunolol, metoprolol, nadolol, penbutolol, pindolol, propranolol, timolol)

—Epinephrine, used in local anesthesia or intravenously, can cause unexpected severe hypertension in patients on chronic beta blocker therapy. The mechanism for this interaction is the unrestricted alpha stimulation from epinephrine in patients who are beta-blocked.

Epinephrine and ergot alkaloids (dihydroergotamine, ergonovine, ergotamine tartrate, methylergonovine)

—Ergot alkaloids may interact with vasopressors to produce hypertension, which is more likely to be severe in patients with a predisposition to hypertension.

—Because of possibly additive vasoconstrictive effects, the administration of vasopressors to patients receiving ergot alkaloids may produce unexpected degrees of hypertension.

Epinephrine and guanadrel, guanethidine

—Patients receiving guanethidine and guanadrel can have an exaggerated hypertensive response to norepinephrine and other direct-acting catecholamines such as phenylephrine, dobutamine, and epinephrine.

—Indirect-acting catecholamines, such as ephedrine, metaraminol, mephentermine, and dopamine, may have fewer pressor effects than expected.

—Guanethidine and guanadrel deplete intraneuronal norepinephrine in postganglionic sympathetic neurons and in this way may diminish the response of indirect-acting catecholamines while sensitizing adrenergic receptors to direct-acting amines.

Epinephrine and monoamine oxidase inhibitors (isocarboxazid, phenelzine, selegilene, tranylcypromine)

—Indirect-acting vasopressors (ephedrine, mephentermine, and metaraminol) act by releasing intraneuronal monoamines such as dopamine and norepinephrine. This is the explanation of the hypertensive crises seen when patients receiving monamine oxidase inhibitors are given these vasopressors.

—Direct-acting vasopressors such as phenylephrine, epinephrine, norepinephrine, and dobutamine may be potentiated by MAO inhibitors and should be used in smaller amounts than normally used.

—Dopamine has both direct and indirect actions and must be used with caution (perhaps one tenth the normal dose).

Epinephrine and oxytocin

—Oxytocin administration has been associated with severe hypertension in patients who had received a prophylactic vasoconstrictor up to 4 hours previously for a caudal block.

—Severe hypertension is more likely to occur in patients with existing mild hypertension and in patients who receive an ergot alkaloid (such as methylergonovine) rather than a dilute solution of oxytocin.

Epinephrine and phenothiazines (chlorpromazine, methdilazine, prochlorperazine, promazine, promethazine)

—Phenothiazines, particularly chlorpromazine, thioridazine, and clozapine, may produce an unexpected hypotensive response with epinephrine.

—The mechanism for this interaction involves the alpha receptor blockade associated with neuroleptic drugs, leaving the vasodilating beta receptors unopposed.

—Hypotension is possibly better treated with more selective alpha adrenergic agents such as phenylephrine.

—This interaction is not likely to be seen with phenothiazines other than the three listed above, although vasopressors other than epinephrine are recommended in patients taking these medications.

Epinephrine and ritodrine, terbutaline

—Ritodrine and terbutaline, beta 2 agonists, may potentiate other sympathomimetic agents.

—The mechanism of this interaction is probably related to the beta 1 adrenergic stimulation that can be seen with ritodrine or terbutaline administration, particularly when these drugs are used at higher dosages.

Epinephrine and tricyclic antidepressants (amitriptyline, amoxapine, clomipramine, desipramine, doxepin, imipramine, maprotilene, nortriptyline, protriptyline, trimipramine)

—Patients taking tricyclic antidepressant drugs (TCAs) develop an exaggerated pressor response, consisting of hypertension and cardiac arrhythmias, when given epinephrine intravenously. The mechanism of this interaction is unclear but is probably related to blockade of norepinephrine reuptake that is caused by TCA medications.

—Although patient studies have documented the above interaction for intravenous epinephrine, it is possible that intramuscular, infiltration (for local anesthesia), or inhalational (for respiratory therapy) epinephrine could have the same results.

ESMOLOL (Brevibloc)

Classification and indications

—Esmolol is a short-acting, beta 1–selective blocking agent.

—It is indicated for the management of supraventricular tachyarrhythmias and for hypertension. Because of the short-acting nature of esmolol, it is particularly useful in the perioperative setting, where short-term control of hypertension and/or tachycardia may be necessary (associated with tracheal intubation, for example).

Pharmacology

—Esmolol competitively inhibits beta 1 receptors, with little effect on beta 2 receptors (bronchial and vascular smooth muscle). At high doses (>300 μg/kg/min), this selectivity is decreased.

—Beta 1 blockade results in a decrease in contractility and heart rate. Myocardial oxygen consumption decreases, which may be beneficial in cases of ischemia.

—Esmolol also decreases systolic and diastolic blood pressure. The exact mechanism of this action is not clear but may involve a direct vasodilating effect.

—The antiarrhythmic effect is a result of a prolongation of the recovery time of the sinus node, slowing of conduction through the atrioventricular node, and other effects.

—Following intravenous administration, depending on the dose, effects on heart rate, blood pressure, and PR interval can be seen in about 1–5 minutes. Ninety percent recovery from these effects occurs in about 8–15 minutes.

—Elimination of esmolol depends on plasma esterases (but not pseudocholinesterase), with little hepatic or renal metabolism. Pharmacodynamics are not affected even in patients undergoing dialysis.

—Esmolol has some interactions with potential significance for patients receiving anesthesia.

—Muscle blockade from succinylcholine is prolonged in some patients for 5–8 minutes when these patients are given esmolol.

—In patients receiving morphine and esmolol, an increase (up to 46%) in steady-state concentrations of esmolol has been documented.

Dose

—For supraventricular tachycardias:
  —Loading dose: 0.5 mg/kg
  —Maintenance dose: Initial infusion rate of 50 μg/kg/min of a solution of 10 mg/mL. Infusion rate may be increased up to 200 μg/kg/min, with additional loading doses of 0.5 mg/kg for every increase of 50 μg/kg/min.
—For hypertension:
  —Loading dose: 0.5 to 1 mg/kg.
  —Maintenance dose: 50 to 150 μg/kg/minute, titrated up or down as needed.

Esmolol Interactions with Anesthesia Drugs

Esmolol and cocaine

—Beta blockers have been demonstrated to potentiate coronary vasoconstriction caused by cocaine.
—This interaction was documented in the cardiac catheterization lab using intranasal cocaine followed by administration of propranolol.
—Although the significance of this interaction to clinical practice is not clear, patients who develop hypertension, tachycardia, and angina from cocaine may be best treated by an agent such as labetalol, which has alpha blocking properties.

Esmolol and diazoxide

—The hypotensive response to diazoxide may be accentuated in patients taking beta blockers.
—This may be due to blunting of the normal sympathetic response that would otherwise occur.

Esmolol and diltiazem, verapamil

—Verapamil and diltiazem, particularly when used intravenously, can significantly potentiate the effects of beta blockers on cardiac conduction and contractility.
—Severe bradycardia and hypotension can occur when these medications are used concomitantly, especially in patients with abnormalities of cardiac conduction (sick sinus syndrome) or ventricular function (congestive heart failure).

Esmolol and dopamine

—Use of esmolol for treatment of supraventricular tachycardia may have undesirable effects in some patients; specifically, in patients requiring cardiovascular support with agents that are both inotropic and vasoconstrictive (dopamine, epinephrine, norepinephrine), blockade of beta receptors may result in decreased cardiac contractility in the face of systemic vasoconstriction, resulting in cardiac failure.

Esmolol and epinephrine, norepinephrine

—Use of esmolol for treatment of supraventricular tachycardia may have undesirable effects in some patients; specifically, in patients requiring cardiovascular support with agents that are both inotropic and vasoconstrictive (dopamine, epinephrine, norepinephrine), blockade of beta receptors may result in decreased cardiac contractility in the face of systemic vasoconstriction, resulting in cardiac failure.

Esmolol and isoproterenol

—Patients who are receiving beta blockers may be more resistant to the bronchodilator effects of isoproterenol. The nonselective beta blockers, such as propranolol, are more likely to have an interaction of greater magnitude than selective blockers, such as metoprolol.

Esmolol and ketamine

—Ketamine may produce myocardial depression if there is interference with the normal sympathetic response, as seen in patients on beta blockers.

Esmolol and morphine

—Coadministration of esmolol and morphine has resulted in significant increases (up to almost 50%) in steady-state levels of esmolol, but not morphine.

Esmolol and phenylephrine

—Phenylephrine produces mostly alpha stimulation. In patients who are receiving beta blockers, it has been associated with exaggerated hypertensive response. This is due to the unopposed vasoconstriction from beta blockade. A similar response is seen with epinephrine.

—This interaction is more likely to occur with nonselective beta blockers such as propranolol, nadolol, timolol, and pindolol.

Esmolol and succinylcholine

—Coadministration of esmolol and succinylcholine may result in a slight (5–8 minute) prolongation of the neuromuscular blockade in some patients.

—The onset of the neuromuscular blockade is not affected.

Esmolol Interactions with Diseases
Esmolol and asthma
—Use of beta blockers in patients with reactive airway disease (asthma, coronary obstructive pulmonary disease) can result in significant increases in airway resistance.

—Although noncardioselective beta blockers (labetalol, propranolol) are most likely to precipitate bronchospasm in these patients, even selective beta 1 blockers (esmolol) have enough beta 2 blocking properties to require caution.

Esmolol and congestive heart failure
—Beta blockers can precipitate congestive heart failure in patients with compromised cardiac function. In patients in congestive heart failure, there may be deterioration in cardiac status.

—The exception to these consequences might be the situation in which tachyarrhythmias may be precipitating acute cardiac decompensation by increasing the myocardial oxygen demand.

—Beta 1 adrenergic blockade reduces heart rate, myocardial contractility, and, therefore, cardiac ouput. Also, atrioventricular node conduction time is prolonged and sinus node automaticity are decreased.

Esmolol and heart block (second, third degree)
—Use of beta blockers in patients with second or third degree heart block can cause dangerous decreases in heart rate.

—Beta 1 adrenergic blockade results in a decrease in sinus node automaticity as well as a prolongation of atrioventricular conduction time.

—If beta blockers are used in patients with heart block, cardiac pacing may be necessary.

Esmolol and Raynaud's phenomenon
—Beta blockers must be used with extreme caution in patients with Raynaud's phenomenon because of the capacity of these drugs to worsen or precipitate digital vasospasm.

—Arteriovenous shunts exist in the fingertips and dilate with beta adrenergic stimulation. Beta 1 blockade can result in vasoconstriction. Labetalol, because of its ability to block alpha receptors, would be less likely to cause this problem.

Esmolol and sick sinus syndrome
—Diltiazem, verapamil, and beta blockers should be avoided or used with extreme caution in patients with sick sinus syndrome.

—Use of these drugs, which depress sinus node automaticity, may cause severe bradycardia even in patients with SSS who are experiencing supraventricular tachycardia.

—Digitalis may be effective in controlling supraventricular tachycardias.

Esmolol and Wolf–Parkinson–White syndrome

—Verapamil, diltiazem, digitalis, beta blockers, and lidocaine should not be used to acutely treat wide complex tachyarrhythmias associated with the Wolf–Parkinson–White syndrome.

—In tachyarrhythmias with wide QRS complexes, antegrade conduction must be assumed to take place via accessory paths. Conduction through these paths can be accelerated by verapamil, diltiazem, digitalis, lidocaine, or propranolol. Intravenous procainamide is the treatment of choice.

—If the QRS complex is narrow, indicating antegrade conduction via normal conduction paths, treatment can be with agents that slow conduction through the AV node: verapamil, propranolol, digitalis, procainamide, or diltiazem.

Esmolol Interactions with Patient Drugs
Esmolol and amiodarone

—Metoprolol and propranolol have both been associated with life-threatening arrhythmias (severe bradycardia, cardiac arrest, or ventricular fibrillation) in patients taking amiodarone. In all cases, these arrhythmias developed within 1 hour to several hours after initiation of these beta blockers and after only one or two doses.

—Although these cases involved oral beta blockers, intravenous esmolol or propranolol could have similar results.

—Other beta blockers have not been associated with this interaction.

Esmolol and dopamine

—Use of beta blockers for treatment of supraventricular tachycardia may have undesirable effects in some patients; specifically, in patients requiring cardiovascular support with agents that are both inotropic and vasoconstrictive (dopamine, epinephrine, norepinephrine), blockade of beta receptors may result in decreased cardiac contractility in the face of systemic vasoconstriction, resulting in cardiac failure.

Esmolol and flecainide

—Flecainide can cause decreased myocardial contractility, particularly at the onset of intravenous therapy. Patients most significantly affected are those with compromised left ventricular function (ejection fraction less than 30%).

—Beta blockers and some calcium channel blockers may have added negative inotropic effects with flecainide.

Esmolol and mefloquine

—Mefloquine is a derivative of quinine and has rarely been associated with bradycardia and prolonged QT interval. Beta blockers and calcium channel blockers should be used with caution in patients on this medication.

Esmolol and methyldopa

—Patients taking methyldopa for hypertension may experience a hypertensive response when given beta blockers. This has been reported in a patient on methyldopa who was given a slow intravenous injection of propranolol.

—The mechanism for this response is thought to be related to the accumulation of methylnorepinephrine, which is a result of methyldopa therapy. This substance has both vasoconstricting and vasodilating properties. The latter, when blocked by beta blockers, could leave unopposed vasoconstriction resulting in hypertension.

Esmolol and morphine

—Coadministration of esmolol and morphine has resulted in significant increases (up to almost 50%) in steady-state levels of esmolol, but not morphine.

Esmolol and ritodrine, terbutaline

—Beta blockers may inhibit the effects of ritodrine and terbutaline, which are beta 2 selective blockers used for uterine relaxation.

ETOMIDATE (Amidate)

Classification and indications

—Etomidate is a hypnotic, nonanalgesic agent.

—It is indicated for the induction of general anesthesia and for supplementation of brief anesthetics using nitrous oxide/oxygen (such as for dilatation and curettage).

Pharmacology

—Etomidate rapidly produces hypnosis, possibly through effects on neurotransmitters (GABA).

—Cerebral blood flow and cerebral metabolic rate are decreased without decreasing mean arterial pressure.

—At normal induction doses (0.3 mg/kg), cardiovascular effects are minimal. Even at higher doses, cardiac index, heart rate, pulmonary artery pressure, stroke volume, and systemic vascular resistance are minimally affected.

—Etomidate does not cause histamine release, even in patients with reactive airway disease.

—A reversible, dose-dependent inhibition of adrenocortical function has been demonstrated following induction doses or infusions of etomidate. Temporary (6 hours postoperatively) adrenocortical suppression resulted from induction and infusion of etomidate.

—The significance of this response is not clear. In patients in the intensive care unit who received etomidate infusions for 5 or more days, there was increased mortality. In anesthetized patients, even undergoing prolonged procedures, no increase in morbidity or mortality has been documented.

—Pain on injection, myoclonus, and postoperative nausea and vomiting may be associated with use of etomidate.

—Redistribution is the mechanism that results in termination of the effect of etomidate.

Dose

—Induction: 0.3 mg/kg (range 0.2–0.6 mg/kg) IV over 30–60 seconds.

Etomidate Interactions with Anesthesia Drugs

Etomidate and verapamil

—A case report of two patients who received verapamil, one on a chronic basis and one who had received a 10-mg intravenous dose prior to anesthesia, described prolonged anesthesia and respiratory depression following etomidate.

—The mechanism of this interaction or its significance is not known.

Etomidate Interactions with Diseases

Etomidate and advanced age

—A reduced induction dose is recommended for thiopental, etomidate, and propofol in most elderly patients.

—Reduction in the dose requirements for these drugs may be a result of a decreased volume of distribution, decreased elimination, or a combination of effects brought about by aging.

Etomidate and alcohol—acute intoxication

—Patients who are acutely intoxicated with alcohol (including chronic alcoholics) usually demonstrate increased sensitivity to general anesthesia.

—Although the precise mechanism of interactions are not agreed on, it appears that alcohol intoxication has additive CNS depression with barbiturates, benzodiazepines, and narcotics, as well as inhalational agents.

Etomidate and alcohol—chronic abuse

—Chronic abuse of alcohol has complex and incompletely understood effects on a patient's response to anesthetic agents. In general, these patients tend to be more tolerant (in a nonintoxicated state) to barbiturates, benzodiazepines, narcotics, and inhalational agents.

—Exceptions to this generalization include the alcoholic patient with a cardiomyopathy who may demonstrate increased sensitivity to myocardial depression from inhalational agents.

—Also, the patient with severe liver disease may have impaired ability to metabolize succinylcholine due to decreased levels of plasma pseudocholinesterase.

Etomidate and malignant hyperthermia

—Anesthetic agents considered safe for use in patients with known or suspected susceptibility for developing malignant hyperthermia (MH) include propofol, barbiturates, etomidate, ketamine, non-depolarizing neuromuscular blocking agents, narcotics, benzodiazepines, droperidol, epinephrine, norepinephrine, and anticholinesterases.

—Nitrous oxide is probably safe in the susceptible patient based on repeated use in MH-susceptible humans and swine.

—Local or regional anesthesia with either amide (such as lidocaine) or ester (such as procaine) anesthetics is now considered safe for MH-susceptible patients.

Etomidate and porphyria

—Anesthesia can be safely administered to these patients using narcotics, depolarizing and non-depolarizing muscle relaxants, etomidate, anticholinesterases, and inhalational agents.

—Use of propofol is considered probably safe.

—Barbiturates are contraindicated in 3 of the 4 hepatic porphyrias (acute intermittent porphyria, variegate porphyria, and hereditary coproporphyria). Porphyria cutanea tarda and the erythropoietic porphyrias are not exacerbated by barbiturates.

—It is theorized that barbiturates can provoke an attack of porphyria by inducing the enzyme aminolevulinic acid synthetase, which results in synthesis of more porphyrin compounds and their precursors.

Etomidate and renal dysfunction

—Renal dysfunction has not been demonstrated to cause significant changes in pharmacokinetics or pharmacodynamics of benzodiazepines, narcotics (with the possible exception of butorphanol), barbiturates, or propofol.
—In patients with renal dysfunction, the above drugs may appear to have an increase in duration or intensity. This has been explained as a response to the systemic effects of renal dysfunction rather than specific effects on the metabolism of theses drugs.
—Some muscle relaxants are significantly affected by renal failure.

FENTANYL (Sublimaze)

Classification and indications

—Fentanyl is an opioid analgesic.
—It is indicated for use in patients being anesthetized for surgery. It can be used as part of a technique for general anesthesia (such as nitrous/narcotic) or as part of a regimen for intravenous sedation (such as with propofol or midazolam). Fentanyl can also be administered in the epidural space as part of a regional anesthetic or for postoperative analgesia.

Pharmacology

—Fentanyl, like other narcotics, exerts its analgesic effects through opioid receptors in the CNS (brain and spinal cord).
—Although narcotics used in anesthesia are potent analgesics, there is controversy about the level of amnesia induced with even large doses of narcotics. To avoid awareness during anesthesia, use of other anesthetic agents (benzodiazepines, inhalation agents, etc.) is recommended.
—Somatosensory evoked potentials (SEPs) are not significantly affected by narcotics.
—Although there is some controversy about increases in intracranial pressure from opioids, in general, opioids cause slight decreases in cerebral blood flow, metabolic rate, and intracranial pressure.

—Cardiovascular effects of alfentanil, sufentanil, and fentanyl include variable degrees of bradycardia and hypotension. This is thought to be mostly from decreased central sympathetic outflow, although some direct effects have been suggested.

—Like other narcotics, fentanyl causes respiratory depression and reduced hypoxic ventilatory drive.

—Muscle rigidity, particularly of the chest wall, has been associated with rapid administration of narcotics. The mechanism of this action is not clear, but older patients seem more prone to this response. It has also been associated most frequently with alfentanil.

—Muscle rigidity can occur not only during induction but on emergence from anesthesia or, rarely, hours after the last opioid dose.

—Onset of analgesia is rapid, but not as rapid as with alfentanil. Peak analgesia after intravenous administration occurs within several minutes. After a dose of 50–100 μg, the duration of action is 30–60 minutes.

—For comparison, the elimination half-lives of fentanyl, sufentanil, and alfentanil are 219, 164, and 90 minutes, respectively.

—Elimination of alfentanil, sufentanil, and fentanyl is a result of hepatic metabolism.

—Fentanyl pharmacokinetics are not significantly affected by cirrhosis, unless liver disease is severe. Higher than normal doses of fentanyl may be required in patients who consume large amounts of alcohol chronically.

—Older patients are more sensitive to opioids and in general have prolonged elimination times.

Dose
—Adults:
 —*Intravenous*
 —Noncardiac surgery: 2 μg/kg on induction with thiopental or propofol. Depending on the anesthetic regimen used, initial doses of fentanyl up to 20 μg/kg can be used.
 —Cardiac surgery: 20 to 50 μg/kg on induction, with additional doses of 25 to 50 μg as needed.
 —*Epidural*
 —Bolus: 50–100 μg bolus in preservative—free saline.
 —Infusion: 50–100 μg/hr.

—Children: 1.5 to 3 µg/kg IV on induction with thiopental or propofol.

Fentanyl Interactions with Anesthesia Drugs

Fentanyl and clonidine

—Clonidine has been shown to potentiate narcotics and reduce the MAC of inhaled anesthetics.

—This effect may be related to clonidine's inhibition of the sympathetic outflow from the vasomotor center in the medulla (clonidine is a central alpha 2 receptor agonist, which results in inhibition of CNS sympathetic centers).

Fentanyl and naloxone

—Cases of pulmonary edema, hypertension, and ventricular arrhythmias have occurred in postoperative patients receiving naloxone for reversal of respiratory depression induced by narcotics. The precise etiology of these reactions is not known.

Fentanyl Interactions with Diseases

Fentanyl and advanced age

—Elderly patients may require lower doses of narcotics than younger adults.

—This may be a result of reduced metabolism of this class of drugs or represent an increased brains sensitivity to narcotics as a result of aging.

Fentanyl and alcohol—acute intoxication

—Patients who are acutely intoxicated with alcohol (including chronic alcoholics) usually demonstrate increased sensitivity to general anesthesia.

—Although the precise mechanism of interactions are not agreed on, it appears that alcohol intoxication has additive CNS depression with barbiturates, benzodiazepines, and narcotics, as well as inhalational agents.

Fentanyl and alcohol—chronic abuse

—chronic abuse of alcohol has complex and incompletely understood effects on a patient's response to anesthetic agents. In general, these patients tend to be more tolerant (in a nonintoxicated state) to barbiturates, benzodiazepines, narcotics, and inhalational agents.

—Exceptions to this generalization include the alcoholic patient with a cardiomyopathy who may demonstrate increased sensitivity to myocardial depression from inhalational agents.

—Also, the patient with severe liver disease may have impaired ability to metabolize succinylcholine due to decreased levels of plasma pseudocholinesterase.

Fentanyl and cerebral edema, intracranial hypertension
—Most intravenous anesthetics cause a reduction in cerebral blood flow (CBF) and intracranial pressure (ICP) or have no effect on ICP. Although this effect is primarily from depression of cerebral metabolic rate (CMR), in some cases a direct vasoconstriction occurs.
—The exception to the above is ketamine, which causes an increased CMR and CBF with an increase in ICP.
—All of the narcotics, as well as barbiturates, etomidate, benzodiazepines, and propofol, have been associated with a reduction or maintenance of ICP during anesthesia.

Fentanyl and malignant hyperthermia
—Anesthetic agents considered safe for use in patients with known or suspected susceptibility for developing malignant hyperthermia (MH) include propofol, barbiturates, etomidate, ketamine, non-depolarizing neuromuscular blocking agents, narcotics, benzodiazepines, droperidol, epinephrine, norepinephrine, and anticholinesterases.
—Nitrous oxide is probably safe in the susceptible patient based on repeated use in MH-susceptible humans and swine.
—Local or regional anesthesia with either amide (such as lidocaine) or ester (such as procaine) anesthetics is now considered safe for MH-susceptible patients.

Fentanyl and porphyria
—Narcotics are considered safe anesthetics for use in porphyrias.
—Not all of the porphyrias have significance for the anesthesiologist. Three of the four hepatic porphyrias (acute intermittent, variegate, hereditary coproporphyria) and none of the erythropoietic porphyrias are associated with neurologic symptoms that can be triggered by certain medications: barbiturates, etomidate, and corticosteroids.
—Benzodiazepines and etomidate are considered to be questionable triggering agents, whereas safe anesthetics are inhalational agents, narcotics, muscle relaxants, anticholinesterases, and propofol.

Fentanyl and renal dysfunction
—Renal dysfunction has not been demonstrated to cause significant changes in pharmacokinetics or pharmacodynamics of benzodiazepines, narcotics (with the possible exception of butorphanol), barbiturates, or propofol.
—In patients with renal dysfunction, the above drugs may appear to have an increase in duration or intensity. This has

been explained as a response to the systemic effects of renal dysfunction rather than specific effects on the metabolism of theses drugs.

—Some muscle relaxants are significantly affected by renal failure.

Fentanyl Interactions with Patient Drugs

Fentanyl and cimetidine

—Cimetidine may potentiate narcotics, causing greater respiratory depression and sedation than expected. This may be related to the alteration of hepatic metabolism of narcotics produced by cimetidine.

—This effect is seen less with morphine than other narcotics and is probably related to the fact that morphine undergoes a different metabolic process than some other narcotics such as fentanyl or meperidine.

—Ranitidine is not associated with this interaction.

Fentanyl and clonidine

—Clonidine has been shown to potentiate narcotics and reduce the minimal alveolar concentration (MAC) of inhaled anesthetics.

—This effect may be related to clonidine's inhibition of the sympathetic outflow from the vasomotor center in the medulla (clonidine is a central alpha 2 receptor agonist, which results in inhibition of CNS sympathetic centers).

FUROSEMIDE (Lasix)

Classification and indications

—Furosemide is a loop diuretic.

—It is indicated for the management of congestive heart failure (even in patients with significant renal dysfunction) and for hypertension.

Pharmacology

—Furosemide and ethacrynic acid are loop diuretics that function by blocking reabsorption of sodium and chloride ions in the ascending limb of the loop of Henle. This results in an osmotic diuresis from the increased solute load (unabsorbed ions). Also, by decreasing ion reabsorption, the concentration of medullary interstitial fluid decreases and, therefore, promotes diuresis.

—The result of interference with ion reabsorption is loss of sodium, potassium, chloride, and hydrogen ions (as well as others). Patients on chronic therapy or who are receiving very large doses usually require some replacement of these ions.

—Furosemide decreases both renal and peripheral vascular resistance as well as increasing venous capacitance. This results in increased renal blood flow, decreased venous return to the heart, and decreased blood pressure.

—In patients with chronic renal insufficiency, large doses may increase glomerular filtration rate temporarily.

—Following intravenous administration, onset of diuresis occurs within 5 minutes, peaks at about 20–60 minutes, and lasts for 2 hours.

—Tinnitus and permanent or reversible hearing loss have been associated with rapid IV or IM administration of furosemide, usually with doses much greater than 20–40 mg. Also, coadministration of furosemide and aminoglycoside antibiotics may increase ototoxicity.

Dose

—Acute pulmonary edema:

—Adults: 40 mg IV slowly. After 1 hour, dose may be increased to 80 mg if necessary.

—Children: 1 mg/kg IV slowly. Dose may be increased to 2 mg/kg in 2 hours if necessary.

Furosemide Interactions with Anesthesia Drugs

Furosemide and muscle relaxants (atracurium, doxacurium, gallamine, metocurine, mivacurium, pancuronium, pipercuronium, rocuronium, succinylcholine, tubocurarine, vecuronium)

—Furosemide may potentiate neuromuscular blockade from tubocurarine and succinylcholine.

—This is based on a case report of several patients given furosemide and tubocurarine during surgery and on animal studies.

—The implication for this interaction for other neuromuscular blocking drugs is uncertain and the mechanism is not known.

Furosemide Interactions with Patient Drugs

Furosemide and aminoglycoside antibiotics (amikacin, gentamicin, kanamycin, netilmicin, streptomycin, tobramycin)

—Some sources suggest that furosemide may increase the potential for ototoxicity or nephrotoxicity of aminoglycoside antibiotics. In fact, there is little persuasive evidence of this interaction.

GALLAMINE (Flaxedil)

Classification and indications
—Gallamine is a non-depolarizing neuromuscular blocker.
—It is used for skeletal muscle relaxation during intubation and for maintenance of muscle relaxation during general anesthesia and surgery.

Pharmacology
—Gallamine competes with acetylcholine at the neuromuscular junction of skeletal muscle by binding to acetylcholine receptors.
—It has strong vagolytic properties that result in tachycardia. This effect is seen at doses well below those necessary for complete muscle relaxation and probably contributes to the hypertensive effect sometimes associated with use of gallamine.
—After doses of 4–6 mg/kg, conditions for intubation are achieved within minutes. The clinical duration of muscle relaxation after this dose is about 90–120 minutes.
—Elimination of gallamine is entirely dependent on renal excretion. The drug undergoes no metabolism and is excreted unchanged in the urine.

Dose
—Intubation: 4–6 mg/kg.
—Maintenance: 0.3–0.5 mg/kg will have a duration of about 30–40 minutes.

Gallamine Interactions with Anesthesia Drugs

Gallamine and calcium channel blockers (diltiazem, nicardipine, nifedipine, verapamil)
—Calcium channel blockers have been associated with prolongation of neuromuscular blockade from non-depolarizing agents.
—This interaction is probably related to the depletion of intracellular calcium associated with chronic therapy. This can result in a decrease in acetylcholine release at the neuromuscular junction.

Gallamine and inhalational anesthetics (desflurane, enflurane, halothane, isoflurane, sevoflurane)
—Desflurane, enflurane, halothane, isoflurane, and sevoflurane can significantly potentiate neuromuscular blockade,

depending on the neuromuscular blocker used. Nitrous oxide has minimal effects.

—Tubocurarine and pancuronium are potentiated the most by inhalational agents, whereas atracurium and vecuronium are intensified significantly less.

—Potentiation by inhalational agents occurs through depression of spinal cord reflexes as well as effects at or distal to the neuromuscular junction.

Gallamine and diphenylhydantoin, phenytoin

—Patients on chronic phenytoin therapy may be resistant to non-depolarizing muscle blockade. The studies involved metocurine and vecuronium but may involve other non-depolarizing agents.

—The mechanism of this interaction is not known.

—Acute infusions of phenytoin may prolong non-depolarizing blockade. This was studied prospectively in a small number of patients who received a 10 mg/kg loading dose of phenytoin during steady-state muscle blockade with vecuronium. They had significant potentiation of their neuromuscular block compared to control patients.

Gallamine and furosemide

—Furosemide may potentiate neuromuscular blockade from tubocurarine and succinylcholine.

—This is based on a case report of several patients given furosemide and tubocurarine during surgery and on animal studies.

—The implication for this interaction for other neuromuscular blocking drugs is uncertain and the mechanism is not known.

Gallamine and lidocaine

—Most local anesthetics can block neuromuscular transmission from non-depolarizing agents as well as depolarizing muscle relaxants. Of clinical significance to the anesthesiologist, lidocaine, given as a 50- to 100-mg bolus or even by infusion, can significantly increase a non-depolarizer block or a phase II block from succinylcholine.

Gallamine and procainamide

—Procainamide can potentiate muscle relaxation from non-depolarizing agents. This is probably a result of decreased acetylcholine release at the neuromuscular junction caused by procainamide.

Gallamine and quinidine

—Quinidine, procainamide, propranolol, and most local anesthetics have been shown to enhance the neuromuscular blockade from depolarizing and non-depolarizing agents.

—A number of well-documented cases have illustrated the ability of these agents, when given in the immediate postoperative period, to convert subclinical muscle weakness from neuromuscular blocking drugs into significant muscle weakness requiring reintubation.

Gallamine and succinylcholine

—Prior administration of succinylcholine has been shown to potentiate neuromuscular blockade of some non-depolarizing agents.

—Although this interaction has been documented with pancuronium, it was not seen with doxacurium and may not be a consistent finding with non-depolarizing agents.

Gallamine Interactions with Diseases

Gallamine and advanced age

—Prolonged duration of neuromuscular blockade can be seen in older patients with several different non-depolarizing agents including doxacurium, mivacurium, and rocuronium.

—In some cases, delayed onset of muscle relaxation also occurs. This has been attributed to decreased perfusion of the neuromuscular junction as a result of advanced age.

Gallamine and burns

—Patients with burn injuries are susceptible to a life-threatening hyperkalemic response to succinylcholine and can have marked resistance to non-depolarizing muscle relaxants.

—Both of these altered responses to neuromuscular blocking agents have been attributed to proliferation of extrajunctional acetylcholine receptors, similar to the patient with a denervation injury.

—Resistance to non-depolarizing agents appears to increase with larger area burns and, in fact may not be significant in patients with <30% body surface area burns. In addition to proliferation of extrajunctional acetylcholine receptors, this abnormal response is probably also related to the increased metabolic rate and hepatic and renal clearance seen in burn patients. Doses of non-depolarizing agents may need to be increased by as much as 300%.

—Duration of this resistance usually is 2 months following the injury, but has been reported in a patient 463 days after the burn.

Gallamine and cirrhosis, liver disease

—Prolonged neuromuscular blockade in patients with liver disease can be seen with doxacurium, mivacurium, vecuronium, pancuronium, rocuronium, and tubocurarine.

—This interaction is complex and may be due to decreased clearance, decreased hepatic uptake of the agent, or decreased synthesis of enzymes important for degradation of the neuromuscular blocker. An example of the latter is prolongation of mivacurium's duration of action as a result of decreased plasma cholinesterase from severe liver disease.

—Because of the increased volume of distribution of many drugs seen in patients with liver disease, initial doses of muscle relaxants may need to be larger than in healthy patients. Once neuromuscular blockade is achieved, recovery may be prolonged.

Gallamine and Eaton–Lambert syndrome

—Patients with Eaton–Lambert syndrome are very sensitive to both depolarizing and non-depolarizing neuromuscular blockade.

—This disorder is similar to myasthenia gravis and patients complain of skeletal muscle weakness, but it is usually associated with carcinoma (especially small cell tumors of the lung).

—If the diagnosis is known or suspected prior to surgery, reduced doses of muscle relaxants should be used, but sometimes the diagnosis is first made when a patient has surgery for a lung tumor and has an unexpected, prolonged neuromuscular block.

—Anticholinesterases are unreliable in reversing muscle weakness.

Gallamine and hyperthyroidism, thyrotoxicosis

—Muscle weakness is commonly seen with hyperthyroidism and affects proximal muscles, usually sparing respiratory function. In some cases, myopathy is the dominant feature of thyroid hormone excess and can resemble myasthenia. Lower doses of muscle relaxants may be indicated.

Gallamine and hypokalemia

—Hypokalemia appears to potentiate the effects of neuromuscular blockade from non-depolarizing agents.

—The interaction is probably due to hyperpolarization of the muscle endplate and, therefore, resistance to depolarization. Hyperpolarization would more likely occur with more acute changes in potassium concentration since the potassium losses would be from the extracellular compartment rather than from intracellular sites.

—Chronic hypokalemia is more likely to be associated with potassium depletion from both extra- and intracellular compartments with no significant change in transmembrane potential. As a result, significant effects on neuromuscular blockade would be less likely.

Gallamine and hypothermia

—Non-depolarizing muscle blockade is prolonged by hypothermia. This interaction is a result of an effect on the neuromuscular blocking agents themselves rather than on the anticholinesterases used to reverse the neuromuscular blocking agents.

—Hypothermia appears to prolong the effect of the non-depolarizing agents by several mechanisms, including delayed metabolism into inactive metabolites as well as delayed excretion via the urinary and biliary routes.

Gallamine and malignant hyperthermia

—Anesthetic agents considered safe for use in patients with known or suspected susceptibility for developing malignant hyperthermia (MH) include propofol, barbiturates, etomidate, ketamine, non-depolarizing neuromuscular blocking agents, narcotics, benzodiazepines, droperidol, epinephrine, norepinephrine, and anticholinesterases.

—Nitrous oxide is probably safe in the susceptible patient based on repeated use in MH-susceptible humans and swine.

—Local or regional anesthesia with either amide (such as lidocaine) or ester (such as procaine) anesthetics is now considered safe for MH-susceptible patients.

Gallamine and myasthenia gravis

—Patients with myasthenia gravis are very sensitive to neuromuscular blockade from non-depolarizing agents.

—This is probably a result of decreased acetylcholine receptors from autoimmune destruction associated with myasthenia gravis.

—Although these patients are treated with the same or similar anticholinesterases used to antagonize muscle blockade, sensitivity (not resistance) to neuromuscular blockade is seen clinically.

Gallamine and neuromuscular disease (amyotrophic lateral sclerosis, multiple sclerosis, syringomyelia)

—Patients with a wide variety of neuromuscular disorders may be more resistant than normal patients to the effects of non-depolarizing neuromuscular blockers.

—This includes patients with disuse atrophy of the muscles (such as bedridden patients with chronic disease) as well as patients with upper or lower motor neuron disease such as amyotrophic lateral sclerosis, multiple sclerosis, or syringomyelia.

—Disuse or denervation of muscle results in production of extrajunctional acetylcholine receptors on the muscle membrane. These receptors are less easily blocked by non-depolarizing agents but are activated by lower concentrations of depolarizing drugs (succinylcholine).

—When these receptors, which can be scattered over a large surface of the muscle, are depolarized by succinylcholine, ion flow takes place through the receptor channel. Large amounts of potassium may exit the muscle cell causing hyperkalemia.

—Despite initial resistance to blockade, such patients may demonstrate prolonged neuromuscular weakness as a result of decreased muscle strength and mass.

Gallamine and PIH (pregnancy-induced hypertension), preeclampsia/eclampsia, toxemia

—Patients with hypertensive disorders of pregnancy may require treatment with antihypertensives such as trimethaphan or magnesium sulfate (for preeclampsia/eclampsia). These medications can have significant interactions with anesthetic agents such as succinylcholine, non-depolarizing neuromuscular blocking agents, or calcium channel blockers.

—Neuromuscular blockade produced by both depolarizing and non-depolarizing agents can be potentiated in patients receiving magnesium sulfate. The mechanisms involved include a decreased amount of acetylcholine released by the nerve impulse at the motor nerve terminal and a decrease in the depolarizing action of acetylcholine on the muscle.

Gallamine Interactions with Patient Drugs
Gallamine and antibiotics

—A number of antibiotics have significant interactions with neuromuscular blocking agents.

—These include the aminoglycosides (amikacin, gentamicin, kanamycin, neomycin, paromomycin, netilmicin, neomycin, streptomycin, tobramycin), as well as polymyxin B, colistin, amphotericin B, clindamycin, bacitracin, and lincomycin.

—All of the above antibiotics may potentiate non-depolarizing agents, but some (aminoglycosides, amphotericin B, clindamycin, colistin) can also potentiate succinylcholine blockade.

—These antibiotics potentiate neuromuscular blockade by different mechanisms, making management of these problems difficult. Although treatment with anticholinesterases or calcium has been recommended, results are inconsistent.

Gallamine and amphotericin B

—Prolonged neuromuscular blockade can occur with depolarizing and non-depolarizing agents in patients receiving amphotericin B.

—The mechanism for this interaction is thought to be associated with the hypokalemia that can be caused by amphotericin B therapy.

Gallamine and beta blockers, propranolol

—Beta blockers may potentiate non-depolarizing neuromuscular blocking agents. This interaction has been reported between propranolol and tubocurarine.

—Other beta blockers are also capable of causing weakness in patients with myasthenia gravis, but the mechanism or significance of these interactions is unclear.

Gallamine and calcium channel blockers (amlodipine, bepridil, diltiazem, felodipine, isradipine, lidoflazine, nicardipine, nimodipine, nisoldipine, nitrendipine, verapamil)

—Calcium channel blockers have been associated with prolongation of neuromuscular blockade from non-depolarizing agents.

—This interaction is probably related to the depletion of intracellular calcium associated with chronic therapy. This can result in a decrease in acetylcholine release at the neuromuscular junction.

Gallamine and diphenylhydantoin, phenytoin

—Patients on chronic phenytoin therapy may be resistant to non-depolarizing muscle blockade. The studies involved metocurine and vecuronium but may involve other non-depolarizing agents.

—The mechanism of this interaction is not known.

—Acute infusions of phenytoin may prolong non-depolarizing blockade. This was studied prospectively in a small number of patients who received a 10 mg/kg loading dose of phenytoin during steady-state muscle blockade with vecuronium. They had significant potentiation of their neuromuscular block compared to control patients.

Gallamine and lidocaine

—Most local anesthetics can block neuromuscular transmission from non-depolarizing agents as well as depolarizing muscle relaxants. Of clinical significance to the anesthesiologist, lidocaine, given as a 50- to 100-mg bolus or even by infusion, can significantly increase a non-depolarizer block or a phase II block from succinylcholine.

Gallamine and lithium

—Lithium has been reported to increase the duration of both non-depolarizing and depolarizing neuromuscular blocking drugs.

—The mechanism of this interaction is unknown and the clinical significance of this interaction is uncertain.

Gallamine and magnesium sulfate

—Neuromuscular blockade produced by both depolarizing and non-depolarizing agents can be potentiated in patients receiving magnesium sulfate. The mechanisms involved include a decreased amount of acetylcholine released by the nerve impulse at the motor nerve terminal and a decrease in the depolarizing action of acetylcholine on the muscle.

Gallamine and mexilitene

—Mexilitene, like lidocaine and most local anesthetics, can potentiate neuromuscular blockade from depolarizing and non-depolarizing agents.

Gallamine and procainamide

—Procainamide can potentiate muscle relaxation from non-depolarizing agents. This is probably a result of decreased acetylcholine release at the neuromuscular junction caused by procainamide.

Gallamine and quinidine

—Quinidine and quinine can potentiate muscle relaxation from both depolarizing and non-depolarizing agents.

—The mechanism of this interaction is a curare-like action at the myoneural junction. Also, plasma pseudocholinesterase is inhibited by quinidine (and quinine), resulting in possible prolongation of muscle relaxation from succinylcholine.

Gallamine and tocainide
—Tocainide, an orally active form of lidocaine, can potentiate both depolarizing and non-depolarizing neuromuscular blockade. This is a property of most local anesthetics as well as a number of other medications.

HALOTHANE (Fluothane)

Classification and indications
—Halothane is a nonflammable, halogenated ether.
—It is indicated for induction and maintenance of general anesthesia in adults and children.

Pharmacology
—The minimal alveolar concentration (MAC) of halothane is 0.75%.
—It has a blood/gas partition coefficient of 2.4, which makes it significantly more soluble than all of the other commonly used inhalational agents.
—Higher solubility in blood results in slower induction and emergence from anesthesia.
—Although halothane is extensively metabolized, release of fluoride ion under normal clinical situations is not enough to produce renal toxicity.
—Halothane anesthesia has been associated with two distinct forms of post-anesthetic hepatic toxicity. The more common form is a non-specific hepatitis characterized by mild elevation of aminotransferases.
—The fulminant hepatic necrosis associated with halothane occurs between 1 in 22,000–35,000 administrations, according to the National Halothane Study, a retrospective study of 850,000 surgical patients.
—Fulminant hepatic necrosis following halothane administration is believed to be an immunologic reaction. Antibodies to hepatocytes are formed from an interaction between halothane metabolites (trifluoroacetyl halide) and liver microsomal proteins.
—All the volatile inhalational anesthetics produce a reduction in both myocardial contractility and thus stroke volume in a

dose-dependent manner. However, systemic vascular resistance, heart rate, and cardiac output (stroke volume ↔ heart rate) are affected differently by the different agents.

—Isoflurane and desflurane appear to maintain cardiac output by increasing heart rate while significantly decreasing systemic vascular resistance. Enflurane and halothane decrease cardiac output more than isoflurane and desflurane because of no associated increase in heart rate.

—Cerebral blood flow is increased by all the inhalational anesthetics. This is a result of cerebrovascular dilation and is partly opposed by a reduction in cerebral metabolic rate. The greatest increase in cerebral blood flow is associated with use of halothane, followed by enflurane and isoflurane. Sevoflurane and desflurane are similar to isoflurane.

Dose

—Induction:

—Halothane and nitrous oxide can be used for induction through inhalation since they are minimally irritating to the airways. Sevoflurane may also be suitable for inhalational induction.

—Isoflurane, enflurane, and desflurane are irritating to the airways and are generally not recommended for inhalational induction.

—Maintenance: Use of other anesthetic agents (opioids, benzodiazepines, barbiturates, propofol, etc.) can reduce the MAC of inhalational anesthetics. As a result, depending on the anesthetic technique used, the type of operation, and variability of patient response, maintenance requirements for inhalational agents are highly variable.

Halothane Interactions with Anesthesia Drugs

Halothane and clonidine

—Clonidine has been shown to reduce the MAC of inhaled and opioid anesthetics.

—This effect may be related to clonidine's inhibition of the sympathetic outflow from the vasomotor center in the medulla (clonidine is a central alpha 2 receptor agonist, which results in inhibition of CNS sympathetic centers).

Halothane and epinephrine, norepinephrine

—Halothane and, to a lesser extent, isoflurane and ethrane reduce the threshold for arrhythmias from epinephrine and norepinephrine. The mechanism of this "sensitization" of the myodium to these sympathomimetic amines

includes an increase in automaticity and changes in depolarization.

—Although exact numbers are not agreed on, a general guideline for safe administration of epinephrine based on some
clinical studies is to use no more than 10 mL of 1:100,000
(1 μg/mL) epinephrine solution every 10 minutes with a
limit of 30 ml/hr. with isoflurane or ethrane, a slightly
larger amount can probably be used.

Halothane and muscle relaxants (atracurium, doxacurium, gallamine, metocurine, mivacurium, pancuronium, pipercuronium, rocuronium, tubocurarine, vecuronium)

—Halothane, isoflurane, and ethrane can significantly potentiate neuromuscular blockade, depending on the neuromuscular blocker used. Nitrous oxide has minimal effects.

—Tubocurarine and pancuronium are potentiated the most
by inhalational agents, whereas atracurium and vecuronium
are intensified significantly less.

—Potentiation by inhalational agents occurs through depression of spinal cord reflexes as well as effects at or distal to
the neuromuscular junction.

Halothane Interactions with Diseases

Halothane and alcohol—acute intoxication

—Patients with acute alcohol intoxication (including chronic
abusers of alcohol) have a lower minimal alveolar concentration (MAC) for inhalational anesthetics.

—The mechanism of this interaction appears to be additive
CNS depressant effects between alcohol and inhalational
agents.

Halothane and alcohol—chronic abuse

—Chronic abuse of alcohol has complex and incompletely
understood effects on a patient's response to anesthetic
agents. In general, these patients tend to be more tolerant
(in a nonintoxicated state) to barbiturates, benzodiazepines,
narcotics, and inhalational agents.

—Exceptions to this generalization include the alcoholic
patient with a cardiomyopathy who may demonstrate
increased sensitivity to myocardial depression from inhalational agents.

—Also, the patient with severe liver disease may have impaired
ability to metabolize succinylcholine due to decreased levels
of plasma pseudocholinesterase.

Halothane and cerebral edema, intracranial hypertension

—All commonly used inhalational volatile anesthetics (halothane > enflurane > isoflurane) cause an increased cerebral blood flow (CBF). Less is known about sevoflurane and desflurane, but they are believed to have effects similar to isflurane. Nitrous oxide has minimal effects on CBF.

—The volatile anesthetics, although they depress cerebral metabolic rate, cause cerebrovascular dilation which results in increased CBF. Hyperventilation to a $PaCO_2$ between 25 and 35 mm Hg will effectively prevent increased CBF from isoflurane but not the other volatile anesthetics.

Halothane and halothane hepatitis

—Mild elevation of liver enzymes may occur in up to 20% of patients that have multiple exposures to halothane and perhaps other anesthetic agents. One patient in 35,000–40,000 exposed to halothane may develop a fulminant and fatal hepatic necrosis.

—Fatal hepatitis associated with halothane may begin 1 day to 2 weeks following halothane administration. The syndrome consists of fever, anorexia, nausea, and, sometimes, rash.

—Marked eosinophilia, elevated liver enzymes, and hyperbilirubinemia accompany severe hepatic necrosis.

—The National Halothane Study was unable to identify a clear-cut histologic lesion associated with hepatitis from halothane and the precise mechanism for this disorder is unknown.

—Use of halothane in pediatric patients, even repeat use after short intervals, has not been associated with the liver dysfunctions described above.

Halothane and hepatitis

—The presence of hepatitis or any liver disease has been shown to increase the morbidity and mortality in patients receiving anesthesia. The mechanism of this increase in morbidity and mortality is not clear but is most likely related to changes in hepatic blood flow as a result of anesthesia and surgery.

—All forms of anesthesia, including general, regional, and nitrous–narcotic can cause postoperative changes in liver function tests, though in most cases the changes are transient. Since there is no known method of avoiding exacerbation of preexisting liver disease by anesthesia, most recommendations are to postpone surgery in patients suspected of having acute hepatitis.

—(See also halothane hepatitis.)

Halothane and malignant hyperthermia

—Halothane, isoflurane, enflurane, desflurane, sevoflurane, as well as other, older inhalational agents all are potent triggering agents of malignant hyperthermia (MH) in the susceptible patient.

—Succinylcholine, decamethonium, and possibly tubocurarine are also triggering agents.

—Anesthetic agents considered safe for use in patients with known or suspected susceptibility for developing MH include propofol, barbiturates, etomidate, ketamine, nondepolarizing neuromuscular blocking agents, narcotics, benzodiazepines, droperidol, epinephrine, norepinephrine, and anticholinesterases.

—Nitrous oxide is probably safe in the susceptible patient based on repeated use in MH-susceptible humans and swine.

—Local or regional anesthesia with either amide (such as lidocaine) or ester (such as procaine) anesthetics is now considered safe for MH-susceptible patients.

Halothane and myotonia

—Inhalational anesthetics may cause exaggerated cardiac depression in patients with myotonia dystrophica.

—Patients with myotonia dystrophica, but not the other myotonic syndromes, are likely to have some degree of cardiomyopathy even in the absence of clinical symptoms. As a result, these patients may be very sensitive to any myocardial depressant.

Halothane and porphyria

—Inhalational agents are considered to be safe for use in patients with porphyria, as are narcotics, depolarizing and non-depolarizing muscle relaxants, etomidate, anticholinesterases, and propofol.

—Barbiturates are contraindicated in three of the four hepatic porphyrias (acute intermittent porphyria, variegate porphyria, and hereditary coproporphyria). Porphyria cutanea tarda and the erythropoietic porphyrias are not exacerbated by barbiturates.

—It is theorized that barbiturates can provoke an attack of porphyria by inducing the enzyme aminolevulinic acid synthetase, which results in synthesis of more porphyrin compounds and their precursors.

Halothane and pregnancy

—Pregnancy is associated with significant reductions in minimal alveolar concentrations (MACs) for inhalational agents.

—In animal studies and some human studies, decreases in MAC of up to 40% have been documented.

—The suggested mechanism for this decreased MAC includes increases in progesterone and endorphin levels associated with pregnancy.

Halothane and renal dysfunction

—Enflurane, isoflurane, halothane, and desflurane are considered safe for administration to patients with renal dysfunction.

—Although enflurane undergoes biotransformation with the formation of inorganic fluoride to a greater extent than other agents (with the exception of methoxyflurane which is very nephrotoxic), even 4 hours of anesthesia with enflurane produces nontoxic fluoride levels. There is some question, however, of renal toxicity after prolonged (9 hours) anesthesia with enflurane.

—Sevoflurane is also biotransformed to inorganic fluoride, but at potentially nephrotoxic levels (50 µmol/L), according to some studies.

—All inhaled anesthetic agents can cause a transient, reversible decrease in renal function as reflected in lowered glomerular filtration rate (GFR), urine output, and urinary sodium excretion.

—The mechanism for this action may include alterations in antidiuretic hormone, vasopressin, or renin, as well as decreases in renal blood flow.

Halothane Interactions with Patient Drugs

Halothane and amiodarone

—Amiodarone, an antiarrhythmic that increases refractoriness and slows conduction in most cardiac tissue, has been associated with severe cardiac complications including arrhythmias, low cardiac output, and decreased systemic vascular resistance in patients having general anesthesia with inhalational agents.

—The mechanism of these interactions is not known.

Halothane and clonidine

—Clonidine has been shown to reduce the MAC of inhaled and opioid anesthetics.

—This effect may be related to clonidine's inhibition of the sympathetic outflow from the vasomotor center in the medulla (clonidine is a central alpha 2 receptor agonist, which results in inhibition of CNS sympathetic centers).

Halothane and disulfiram

—Profound hypotension may occur when patients taking disulfiram are exposed to halogenated anesthetics (enflurane, isoflurane, and halothane).

HEPARIN

Classification and indications

—Heparin is a glycosaminoglycan that is naturally present in mast cells. Commercially available heparin is prepared from porcine intestine or bovine lung.

—It is used for treatment and prophylaxis of venous thrombosis, arterial thrombosis or embolism, consumptive coagulopathies (disseminated intravascular coagulation), and as an anticoagulant for extracorporeal circuits (dialysis, cardiopulmonary bypass).

Pharmacology

—Normally, antithrombin III slowly neutralizes thrombin and factor X. In the presence of heparin, this reaction is almost immediate and also affects factors IX, XI, XII, and plasmin, resulting in anticoagulation.

—Because it has no fibrinolytic activity, heparin cannot lyse existing thrombi but can prevent formation and extension of clots.

—At high doses, heparin can interfere with platelet aggregation and prolong the bleeding time, but this effect requires 2 or more days of therapy.

—Heparin resistance may be a result of low antithrombin III levels by inheritance or as a result of diseases (cirrhosis, nephrotic syndrome, disseminated intravascular coagulation). Normally, patients with hereditary deficiencies have levels 40–60% of normal and have a normal response to usual doses of heparin.

—Other potential causes of higher heparin requirements are patients with hypereosinophilia, advanced age, and use of oral contraceptives.

—Monitoring of anticoagulation includes measurement of activated partial thrombloplastin time (aPTT), heparin-protamine titration, and activated coagulation time (ACT).

—Following a dose of 4 mg/kg, the half-life of heparin in healthy adults is about 90 minutes. It is probably cleared mainly by the reticuloendothelial system.

—Reversal of the anticoagulant effect of heparin is accomplished with protamine, which binds to heparin and inactivates it.

Dose

—For cardiopulmonary bypass: 3–4 mg/kg (1 mg is approximately 100 units). At this dose, the ACT is usually prolonged from the normal of 70–110 seconds to about 400–600 seconds.

Heparin Interactions with Anesthesia Drugs
Heparin and diazepam

—The administration of heparin to patients given diazepam prior to cardiac bypass may cause a transient but very significant period of hypotension.

—The mechanism of this interaction may be related to a large increase in the concentration of unbound diazepam that has been documented after heparin administration.

Heparin and nitroglycerin

—Nitroglycerin infusions have been shown in several studies to increase requirements of heparin to maintain anticoagulation. However, this effect was demonstrated in long-term infusions over a 72-hour period or more. In studies of 1–2 hours, no interaction was found.

Heparin Interactions with Diseases
Heparin and Advanced age

—Older patients may demonstrate resistance to anticoagulation from heparin compared to younger patients.

—This interaction is believed to result from lower antithrombin III levels seen in some older patients.

HYDRALAZINE (Apresoline)

Classification and indications

—Hydralazine is an antihypertensive agent.

—It is indicated for the management of hypertension.

Pharmacology

—Hydralazine lowers blood pressure by vasodilation and reduction of peripheral vascular resistance. It has a direct vasodilatory effect which is greater on arterioles than veins.

—Cardiovascular effects include a reflex increase in heart rate, cardiac output, and stroke volume.

—Vasodilation also affects coronary arteries resulting in coronary vasodilation.

—Pulmonary artery pressures may increase in response to hydralazine, particularly in patients with mitral valve disease.

—Cerebral vascular dilation from hydralazine therapy may increase cerebral blood flow. This may result in increased intracranial pressure.

—After intravenous administration, onset of hypotensive effect begins in 5–20 minutes and lasts 2–6 hours, depending on the dose.

Dose

—Adults: 5–10 mg IV every 20 minutes as necessary to control blood pressure.

Hydralazine Interactions with Diseases

Hydralazine and cerebral edema, intracranial hypertension

—Most systemic vasodilators (nitroglycerin, nitroprusside, hydralazine, calcium channel blockers, and adenosine) can produce cerebrovascular vasodilation as well. As a result, cerebral blood volume is either maintained or increased even though systemic blood pressure is decreased.

—Trimethaphan, a ganglionic blocker, usually will not increase cerebral blood volume because ganglionic blockade normally does not cause vasodilation of the cerebral circulation.

ISOFLURANE (Forane)

Classification and indications

—Isoflurane is a nonflammable, halogenated ether.

—It is indicated for use as a general anesthetic.

Pharmacology

—The minimal alveolar concentration (MAC) of isoflurane is 1.15.

—It has a blood/gas partition coefficient of 1.4, which makes it similar to enflurane (1.9), but significantly more soluble than nitrous oxide, desflurane, or sevoflurane.

—Higher solubility in blood results in slower induction and emergence from anesthesia.

—A very small portion (0.2%) of inhaled isoflurane is metabolized, generating negligible amounts of fluoride ion or other metabolites. As a result, isoflurane has minimal toxicity for the liver or kidneys.

—All the volatile inhalational anesthetics produce a reduction in both myocardial contractility and thus stroke volume in a dose-dependent manner. However, systemic vascular resistance, heart rate, and cardiac output (stroke volume ↔ heart rate) are affected differently by the different agents.

—Isoflurane and desflurane appear to maintain cardiac output by increasing heart rate while significantly decreasing systemic vascular resistance. Enflurane and halothane decrease cardiac output more than isoflurane and desflurane because of no associated increase in heart rate.

—Cerebral blood flow is increased by all the inhalational anesthetics. This is a result of cerebral vascular dilation and is partly opposed by a reduction in cerebral metabolic rate. The greatest increase in cerebral blood flow is associated with use of halothane, followed by enflurane and isoflurane. Sevoflurane and desflurane are similar to isoflurane.

Dose
—Induction:
  —Halothane and nitrous oxide can be used for induction through inhalation because they are minimally irritating to the airways. Sevoflurane may also be suitable for inhalational induction.
  —Isoflurane, enflurane, and desflurane are irritating to the airways and are generally not recommended for inhalational induction.
—Maintenance: Use of other anesthetic agents (opioids, benzodiazepines, barbiturates, propofol, etc.) can reduce the MAC of inhalational anesthetics. As a result, depending on the anesthetic technique used, the type of operation, and variability of patient response, maintenance requirements for inhalational agents are highly variable.

Isoflurane Interactions with Anesthesia Drugs
Isoflurane and clonidine
—Clonidine has been shown to reduce the MAC of inhaled and opioid anesthetics.
—This effect may be related to clonidine's inhibition of the sympathetic outflow from the vasomotor center in the

medulla (clonidine is a central alpha 2 receptor agonist, which results in inhibition of CNS sympathetic centers).

Isoflurane and epinephrine, norepinephrine

—Halothane and, to a lesser extent, isoflurane and ethrane reduce the threshold for arrhythmias from epinephrine and norepinephrine. The mechanism of this "sensitization" of the myodium to these sympathomimetic amines includes an increase in automaticity and changes in depolarization.

—Although exact numbers are not agreed upon, a general guideline for safe administration of epinephrine based on some clinical studies is to use no more than 10 mL of 1:100,000 (1 μg/mL) epinephrine solution every 10 minutes with a limit of 30 mL/hr. with isoflurane or ethrane, a slightly larger amount can probably be used.

Isoflurane and muscle relaxants (atracurium, doxacurium, gallamine, metocurine, mivacurium, pancuronium, pipercuronium, rocuronium, tubocurarine, vecuronium)

—Halothane, isoflurane, and ethrane can significantly potentiate neuromuscular blockade, depending on the neuromuscular blocker used. Nitrous oxide has minimal effects.

—Tubocurarine and pancuronium are potentiated the most by inhalational agents, while atracurium and vecuronium are intensified significantly less.

—Potentiation by inhalational agents occurs through depression of spinal cord reflexes as well as effects at or distal to the neuromuscular junction.

Isoflurane and succinylcholine

—Succinylcholine neuromuscular blockade may be potentiated by desflurane and isoflurane.

—Halothane and enflurane probably have clinically insignificant interactions with succinylcholine.

Isoflurane Interactions with Diseases

Isoflurane and alcohol—acute intoxication

—Patients with acute alcohol intoxication (including chronic abusers of alcohol) have a lower minimal alveolar concentration (MAC) for inhalational anesthetics.

—The mechanism of this interaction appears to be additive CNS depressant effects between alcohol and inhalational agents.

Isoflurane and alcohol—chronic abuse

—Chronic abuse of alcohol has complex and incompletely understood effects on a patient's response to anesthetic agents. In general, these patients tend to be more tolerant (in a nonintoxicated state) to barbiturates, benzodiazepines, narcotics, and inhalational agents.

—Exceptions to this generalization include the alcoholic patient with a cardiomyopathy who may demonstrate increased sensitivity to myocardial depression from inhalational agents.

—Also, the patient with severe liver disease may have impaired ability to metabolize succinylcholine due to decreased levels of plasma pseudocholinesterase.

Isoflurane and cerebral edema, intracranial hypertension

—All commonly used inhalational volatile anesthetics (halothane > enflurane > isoflurane) cause an increased cerebral blood flow (CBF). Less is known about sevoflurane and desflurane, but they are believed to have effects similar to those of isoflurane. Nitrous oxide has minimal effects on CBF.

—The volatile anesthetics, although they depress cerebral metabolic rate, cause cerebrovascular dilation which results in increased CBF. Hyperventilation to a $PaCO_2$ between 25 and 35 mm Hg will effectively prevent increased CBF from isoflurane, but not the other volatile anesthetics.

Isoflurane and hepatitis

—All forms of anesthesia, including general, regional, and nitrous–narcotic, are associated with postoperative liver function test abnormalities. The exact mechanism of this reaction is not known but is likely related to reduced liver blood flow from anesthesia and surgery.

—The presence of hepatitis or any liver disease has been shown to increase the morbidity and mortality in patients receiving anesthesia. The mechanism of this increase in morbidity and mortality is not clear but is most likely related to changes in hepatic blood flow as a result of anesthesia and surgery.

—Because there is no known method of avoiding exacerbation of pre-existing liver disease by anesthesia, most recommendations are to postpone surgery in patients suspected of having acute hepatitis.

—There is no evidence that enflurane, isoflurane, desflurane, or sevoflurane is hepatotoxic. Halothane, however, can occasionally cause fulminant hepatic necrosis in both adults and children. A milder form of hepatotoxicity is also seen with halothane anesthesia.

Isoflurane and malignant hyperthermia

—Halothane, isoflurane, enflurane, desflurane, sevoflurane, as well as other, older inhalational agents all are potent triggering agents of malignant hyperthermia (MH) in the susceptible patient.

—Succinylcholine, decamethonium, and possibly tubocurarine are also triggering agents.

—Anesthetic agents considered safe for use in patients with known or suspected susceptibility for developing malignant hyperthermia include propofol, barbiturates, etomidate, ketamine, non-depolarizing neuromuscular blocking agents, narcotics, benzodiazepines, droperidol, epinephrine, norepinephrine, and anticholinesterases.

—Nitrous oxide is probably safe in the susceptible patient based on repeated use in MH-susceptible humans and swine.

—Local or regional anesthesia with either amide (such as lidocaine) or ester (such as procaine) anesthetics is now considered safe for MH-susceptible patients.

Isoflurane and myotonia

—Inhalational anesthetics may cause exaggerated cardiac depression in patients with myotonia dystrophica.

—Patients with myotonia dystrophica, but not the other myotonic syndromes, are likely to have some degree of cardiomyopathy even in the absence of clinical symptoms. As a result, these patients may be very sensitive to any myocardial depressant.

Isoflurane and porphyria

—Inhalational agents are considered to be safe for use in patients with porphyria, as are narcotics, depolarizing and non-depolarizing muscle relaxants, etomidate, anticholinesterases, and propofol.

—Barbiturates are contraindicated in three of the four hepatic porphyrias (acute intermittent porphyria, variegate porphyria, and hereditary coproporphyria). Porphyria cutanea tarda and the erythropoietic porphyrias are not exacerbated by barbiturates.

—It is theorized that barbiturates can provoke an attack of porphyria by inducing the enzyme aminolevulinic acid synthetase, which results in synthesis of more porphyrin compounds and their precursors.

Isoflurane and pregnancy

—Pregnancy is associated with significant reductions in minimal alveolar concentrations (MAC) for inhalational agents.

—In animal studies and some human studies, decreases in MAC of up to 40% have been documented.

—The suggested mechanism for this decreased MAC includes increases in progesterone and endorphin levels associated with pregnancy.

Isoflurane and renal dysfunction

—Enflurane, isoflurane, halothane, and desflurane are considered safe for administration to patients with renal dysfunction.

—Although enflurane undergoes biotransformation with the formation of inorganic fluoride to a greater extent than other agents (with the exception of methoxyflurane which is very nephrotoxic), even 4 hours of anesthesia with enflurane produce nontoxic fluoride levels. There is some question, however, of renal toxicity after prolonged (9 hours) anesthesia with enflurane.

—Sevoflurane is also biotransformed to inorganic fluoride, but at potentially nephrotoxic levels (50 μmol/L), according to some studies.

—All inhaled anesthetic agents can cause a transient, reversible decrease in renal function as reflected in lowered glomerular filtration rate (GFR), urine output, and urinary sodium excretion.

—The mechanism for this action may include alterations in antidiuretic hormone, vasopressin, or renin, as well as decreases in renal blood flow.

Isoflurane Interactions with Patient Drugs

Isoflurane and amiodarone

—Amiodarone, an antiarrhythmic that increases refractoriness and slows conduction in most cardiac tissue, has been associated with severe cardiac complications including arrhythmias, low cardiac output, and decreased systemic vascular resistance in patients having general anesthesia with inhalational agents.

—The mechanism of these interactions is not known.

Isoflurane and clonidine

—Clonidine has been shown to reduce the MAC of inhaled and opioid anesthetics.

—This effect may be related to clonidine's inhibition of the sympathetic outflow from the vasomotor center in the medulla (clonidine is a central alpha 2 receptor agonist, which results in inhibition of CNS sympathetic centers).

Isoflurane and disulfiram

—Profound hypotension may occur when patients taking disulfiram are exposed to halogenated anesthetics (enflurane, isoflurane, and halothane).

ISOPROTERENOL (Isuprel)

Classification and indications

—Isoproterenol is a synthetic sympathomimetic agent that acts on beta adrenergic receptors.

—It is indicated for treatment of bronchospasm and for atropine-resistant bradycardia. It has also been used for some low cardiac output states (cardiogenic shock, septic shock).

Pharmacology

—Isoproterenol is an almost pure beta adrenergic agonist with little, if any, alpha agonist activity.

—It is a nonselective beta agonist and stimulates both beta 1 and beta 2 receptors.

—Beta 1 stimulation results in a positive chronotropic (increased heart rate) and inotropic (increased contractility) effect. Atrioventricular conduction is increased and the refractory period is shortened.

—Cardiac output and stroke volume are usually increased, as well as increased myocardial oxygen consumption.

—Increased coronary blood flow from isoproterenol may not match the increase in oxygen consumption.

—Beta 2 stimulation results in bronchial dilation. This effect occurs after parenteral as well as inhalational administration.

—Beta 2 stimulation also results in relaxation of skeletal muscle arterioles and a reduced peripheral vascular resistance. However, increased heart rate and cardiac output usually prevent any decrease in blood pressure.

—Onset of effects are almost immediate following either intravenous or inhalational therapy and persist for 1–2 hours.

—Tissue uptake is primarily responsible for termination of the effects of isoproterenol.

Dose
—Bronchospasm:
Adults:
    —Metered inhaler: 1–2 inhalations every 4–6 hours. For acute attacks, one or two inhalations may be given every 1–5 minutes, up to 6 times in 1 hour (but only for 1 hour per 24 hours).
    —Nebulization: 2.5 mL of a 1% solution.
    —Intravenous: 0.01–0.02 mg (of a diluted solution) IV. This may be repeated as necessary.
Children:
    —Metered inhaler: same as adults (the smaller ventilatory capacity of children results in less medication inhaled).
    —Nebulization: 0.01 mL/kg/dose of a 1% solution (10 mg/mL). Maximum dose is 0.05 mL/dose. This may be repeated every 4 hours.
    —Intravenous: 0.1–1.5 µg/kg/min.
—Bradycardia or shock
—Adults: 2 to 20 µg/min of a solution of isoproterenol 1 mg/250 mL NS (4 µg/mL).
—Children: 0.1–1.5 µg/kg/min.

Isoproterenol Interactions with Anesthesia Drugs
Isoproterenol and beta blockers (esmolol, labetalol, propranolol)
    —Patients who are receiving beta blockers may be more resistant to the bronchodilator effects of isoproterenol. The nonselective beta blockers, such as propranolol, are more likely to have an interaction of greater magnitude than selective blockers, such as metoprolol.

Isoproterenol Interactions with Patient Drugs
Isoproterenol and beta blockers (acebutolol, atenolol, betaxolol, carteolol, labetalol, levobunolol, metoprolol, nadolol, penbutolol, pindolol, propranolol, timolol)
    —Patients who are receiving beta blockers may be more resistant to the bronchodilator effects of isoproterenol. The nonselective beta blockers, such as propranolol, are more likely to have an interaction of greater magnitude than selective blockers, such as metoprolol.
Isoproterenol and ritodrine, terbutaline
    —Terbutaline and ritodrine, both beta adrenergic agonists, may potentiate the cardiovascular effects of sympathomimetic agents.

KETAMINE (Ketalar)

Classification and indications
—Ketamine is a phencyclidine derivative.
—It is indicated for induction and maintenance of anesthesia. It also can be used for sedation, particularly for preoperative sedation of children.

Pharmacology
—Ketamine has multiple effects in the CNS, including depression of certain parts of the cerebral cortex, stimulation of parts of the limbic system, and possibly some opioid receptor activity (explaining analgesic properties).
—CNS effects include an increase in cerebral metabolic rate, cerebral blood flow, and intracranial pressure. These responses can be blunted by thiopental, benzodiazepines, or hyperventilation.
—The cardiovascular system is stimulated by ketamine, resulting in increases in blood pressure, heart rate, and cardiac output. These responses are thought to be a result of central stimulation, which overcomes the direct myocardial depressant action of ketamine.
—The cardiac stimulation of ketamine can be blunted by administration of benzodiazepines or volatile anesthetics.
—The respiratory effects of ketamine include bronchial smooth muscle relaxation and increased secretions, especially in children.
—Apnea is rarely produced by ketamine unless very high doses are used. Also, premedication with other sedatives is more likely to result in respiratory depression. Children are most susceptible to respiratory depression from ketamine, particularly when it is administered by bolus dose.
—Onset of anesthetic action is rapid, usually within 30 seconds. Termination of effect is also rapid (10–15 minutes after a single dose of 2 mg/kg IV) and is the result of redistribution.
—Metabolism occurs in the liver and metabolic products are excreted in the urine.

Dose
General anesthesia:
　　—Intravenous induction: 0.5–2 mg/kg IV.
　　—Intramuscular induction: 4–6 mg/kg IM.
Maintenance:
　　—Infusion: 10–50 μg/kg/min with nitrous oxide and oxygen (higher doses required if no nitrous used).

—Bolus: 0.5–1.0 mg IV prn.

Sedation:

—Infusion: 10–20 µg/kg/min.

—Bolus: 0.2–8 mg/kg IV.

—Intramuscular: 2–4 mg/kg IM.

Ketamine Interactions with Anesthesia Drugs

Ketamine and beta blockers (esmolol, labetalol, propranolol)

—Ketamine may produce myocardial depression if there is interference with the normal sympathetic response, as seen in patients on beta blockers.

Ketamine and digitalis

—Ketamine may have a protective effect against digitalis-induced arrhythmias by decreasing phase IV automaticity.

Ketamine Interactions with Diseases

Ketamine and angina, coronary artery disease

—Ketamine has significant, mostly stimulatory, effects on the cardiovascular system. Cardiovascular stimulation in patients with coronary artery disease can cause an undesirable increase in myocardial oxygen demand.

—Other clinical situations in which ketamine would be contraindicated because of the cardiovascular stimulation are aortic or intracranial aneurysms, thyrotoxicosis, and inadequately controlled hypertension.

—Ketamine causes an increase in heart rate, cardiac output, and arterial pressure (as much as 25%) by stimulation of the CNS and inhibition of neuronal norepinephrine reuptake.

—In severely ill patients, such as those in septic shock or in chronic congestive heart failure, the cardiovascular system is resistant to indirect stimulation. In these cases, the direct myocardial depressant effects of ketamine may be manifested by hypotension.

Ketamine and cerebral edema, intracranial hypertension

—Ketamine is contraindicated for use in patients with elevated intracranial pressure or intracranial aneurysm.

—Ketamine stimulates the cardiovascular system indirectly via the CNS and inhibition of neuronal norepinephrine reuptake. The result of these actions is an increase in heart rate, cardiac output, and arterial pressure (up to 25% increase). Ketamine also causes an increase in cerebrospinal fluid pressure and intracranial blood flow.

—Some of the cardiovascular effects of ketamine can be blocked with benzodiazepines and/or labetalol.

Ketamine and congestive heart failure

—Ketamine has significant cardiovascular stimulatory effects that usually contraindicate its use in patients with congestive heart failure from ischemic heart disease.

—Cardiovascular stimulation by ketamine is a result of central nervous stimulation and inhibition of neuronal norepinephrine reuptake. The consequence of these actions is an increase in cardiac output, heart rate, and peripheral vasoconstriction. Additionally, ketamine can cause an increase in pulmonary vascular resistance, placing added strain on the right ventricle.

—Some patients are resistant to indirect cardiovascular stimulation, such as those with septic shock or chronic congestive heart failure. In these patients, the direct myocardial depressant effects of ketamine may be evident.

Ketamine and hypertension

—Ketamine should be used cautiously in patients with hypertension, especially those with inadequate control.

—Ketamine causes hypertension by indirect cardiovascular stimulation, by inhibition of neuronal reuptake of norepinephrine, and by peripheral vasoconstriction.

—Some of the cardiovascular effects can be blunted by administration of benzodiazepines and/or labetalol.

Ketamine and hyperthyroidism, thyrotoxicosis

—Anesthesia drugs that stimulate the sympathetic nervous system (catecholamines, ephedrine, phenylephrine, dopram, ketamine) may have exaggerated effects in patients with hyperthyroidism. Although most evident in untreated patients, even patients receiving treatment for excess thyroid hormone may demonstrate this response.

—Excess thyroid hormone causes stimulation of metabolism of most body tissues. As a result, cardiac output increases by 50% or more to remove the extra metabolic by-products. Also, direct stimulatory effects on the myocardium at even slightly elevated thyroid hormone levels causes tachycardia and increased contractility.

—At higher thyroid hormone levels, myocardial depression may occur as a result of excess demands or a direct myocardial depression.

Ketamine and malignant hyperthermia

—Anesthetic agents considered safe for use in patients with known or suspected susceptibility for developing malignant hyperthermia (MH) include propofol, barbiturates, etomidate, ketamine, non-depolarizing neuromuscular blocking agents, narcotics, benzodiazepines, droperidol, and anticholinesterases.

—Nitrous oxide is probably safe in the susceptible patient, based on repeated use in MH-susceptible humans and swine.

Ketamine and porphyria

—Ketamine is not known to precipitate attacks of porphyria; however, its ability to induce psychosis postoperatively can be confused with psychosis from the disease.

—Not all of the porphyrias have significance for the anesthesiologist. Three of the four hepatic porphyrias (acute intermittent, variegate, hereditary coproporphyria) and none of the erythropoietic porphyrias are associated with neurologic symptoms that can be triggered by certain medications: barbiturates, etomidate, and corticosteroids.

—Benzodiazepines and etomidate are considered to be questionable triggering agents, whereas safe anesthetics are inhalational agents, narcotics, muscle relaxants, anticholinesterases, and propofol.

Ketamine and pregnancy

—Ketamine appears to be safe for use in pregnancy or for anesthesia for caesarean section if the dose is <2 mg/kg. Doses above this appear to be associated with fetal depression.

Ketamine and pulmonary hypertension

—Ketamine can cause an increase in pulmonary vascular resistance and should be used cautiously in patients with pulmonary hypertension.

—Cardiovascular stimulation by ketamine is a result of central nervous stimulation and inhibition of neuronal norepinephrine reuptake. The consequence of these actions is an increase in cardiac output, heart rate, and peripheral vasoconstriction.

—Some patients are resistant to indirect cardiovascular stimulation, such as those with septic shock or chronic congestive heart failure. In these patients, the direct myocardial depressant effects of ketamine may be evident.

Ketamine and thyrotoxicosis

—Ketamine can produce significant stimulatory effects on the cardiovascular system. This stimulation could lead to severe hypertension in a patient with thyrotoxicosis, and its use in this clinical situation is contraindicated.

—Ketamine causes hypertension by stimulation of the CNS, inhibition of neuronal reuptake of norepinephrine, and peripheral vasoconstriction.

—Some of these effects can be blunted by administration of ketamine with benzodiazepines and/or labetalol.

Ketamine Interactions with Patient Drugs

Ketamine and beta blockers (acebutolol, atenolol, betaxolol, carteolol, labetalol, levobunolol, metoprolol, nadolol, penbutolol, pindolol, propranolol, timolol)

—Ketamine may produce myocardial depression if there is interference with the normal sympathetic response, as seen in patients on beta blockers.

Ketamine and digitalis

—Ketamine may have a protective effect against digitalis-induced arrhythmias by decreasing phase IV automaticity.

Ketamine and thyroxine

—Ketamine may produce unexpected hypertension and tachycardia in patients taking thyroid medication.

—This is based on a case report of two patients and the significance and mechanism of this interaction is unclear.

KETOROLAC (Toradol)

Classification and indications

—Ketorolac is a nonsteroidal antiinflammatory drug (NSAID).

—It is indicated for the short-term treatment of moderately severe pain.

Pharmacology

—Ketorolac is an inhibitor of prostaglandin synthesis, like aspirin and other NSAIDs.

—Inhibition of prostaglandin synthesis is the basis of the antiinflammatory and analgesic properties of this class of drugs. However, it is also the basis for some of the adverse effects.

—Gastric ulceration and bleeding can result from both a local irritant effect of orally administered aspirin or NSAIDs, but it is also a result of prostaglandin synthesis inhibition when these drugs are given parenterally.

—Some of the gastric prostaglandins (which are also inhibited by these drugs) cause reduced gastric acid production and promote secretion of protective mucus. Inhibition of the production of these prostaglandins may result in gastrointestinal ulceration.

—Inhibition of the formation by platelets of thromboxane A2 (which is a potent aggregating agent) results in decreased platelet adhesiveness. A prolonged bleeding time can result.

—Unlike aspirin, the effect of ketorolac on platelets disappears in 24–48 hours following discontinuation of the medication.

—Prostaglandins play a role in renal vascular dilation. In healthy patients, these prostaglandins may be insignificant. However, in patients with decreased renal perfusion from any cause (congestive heart failure, renal disease, hypovolemia), inhibition of these vasodilatory prostaglandins may significantly decrease renal function. The result may be worsened renal function or even acute renal failure.

—Ketorolac is contraindicated in labor and delivery because prostaglandin synthesis inhibition may impair uterine contractions and a prolonged bleeding time may increase postpartum bleeding.

—Use of ketorolac in nursing mothers is also contraindicated because blood levels of ketorolac have been detected in breast milk and are thought to be of potential risk to the neonate.

—Ketorolac is completely absorbed after oral, intramuscular, or intravenous administration.

—Onset of analgesia occurs in 30–60 minutes, with peak analgesia after about 1–2 hours and a duration of 4–6 hours.

—Elimination of ketorolac is mainly a result of renal excretion. Patients with decreased renal function are likely to have decreased clearance of ketorolac, as are elderly patients (over 65 years old).

Dose*

—Single dose:

—Patients <65 years old: 60 mg IV or IM.

—Patients >65 years old or with renal disease: 30 mg IV or IM.

—Multiple dose:

—Patients <65 years old: 30 mg IV or IM every 6 hours (maximum 120 mg/day).

---

*Intravenous dosing should not be given over <15 seconds.

—Patients >65 years old, renal disease, or < 50 kg: 15 mg IV or IM every 6 hours (maximum 60 mg/day).

Ketorolac Interactions with Diseases

Ketorolac and advanced age

—Older patients (>65 years old) should receive lower doses of ketorolac because age-related reductions in renal function place these patients at higher risk for renal damage from ketorolac.

—In these patients, whose renal function may be very dependent on renal vascular dilation from prostaglandins, inhibition of these prostaglandins by ketorolac may worsen kidney function.

Ketorolac and congestive heart failure

—Ketorolac (a prostaglandin synthesis inhibitor) can worsen renal function in patients whose compromised renal function is very dependent on the presence of vasodilatory prostaglandins.

—Patients at risk for this interaction are those with renal dysfunction as a result of renal disease or advanced age (>65 years old) or poor renal perfusion from congestive heart failure or hypovolemia.

Ketorolac and pregnancy

—Ketorolac is contraindicated in labor and delivery or for nursing mothers.

—Because it is a prostaglandin synthesis inhibitor, ketorolac can interfere with platelet function and prolong the bleeding time, resulting in bleeding. It may also inhibit uterine contractions.

—Small amounts of ketorolac have been detected in the breast milk of nursing mothers who have been given the drug for postpartum analgesia. Because bleeding complications can potentially occur in the neonate, ketorolac is contraindicated in nursing mothers.

Ketorolac and renal dysfunction

—Ketorolac (a prostaglandin synthesis inhibitor) can worsen renal function in patients whose compromised renal function is very dependent on the presence of vasodilatory prostaglandins.

—Patients at risk for this interaction are those with renal dysfunction as a result of renal disease or advanced age (>65 years old) or poor renal perfusion from congestive heart failure or hypovolemia.

—Nonsteroidal agents may also cause interstitial nephritis, glomerulonephritis, or renal papillary necrosis.

—In these patients, reduced doses of ketorolac should be used.

LABETALOL (Normodyne, Normozide, Trandate)

Classification and indications
—Labetalol is an alpha and beta adrenergic blocking agent.

—It is indicated for the treatment of hypertension.

Pharmacology
—Labetalol is a nonselective beta blocker (both beta 1 and beta 2) and a selective alpha 1 blocker. After intravenous administration, the ratio of alpha to beta blockade is about 1:7.

—Beta 1 blockade results in decreased heart rate and contractility. As a result, patients with heart block (more than first degree), severe bradycardia, or congestive heart failure should not receive this medication.

—Alpha 1 blockade is associated with peripheral vascular dilation, decreased vascular resistance, and decreased blood pressure.

—Beta 2 blockade potentially may cause bronchial constriction and increased airway resistance. Offsetting this effect, however, is some apparent beta 2 agonist activity. Clinical studies have demonstrated that labetalol's tendency to produce bronchoconstriction is more equivalent to that of beta 1 selective blockers (such as atenolol).

—Maximal effects on blood pressure occur within about 5 minutes and the half-life after IV administration is approximately 6 hours.

—Elimination depends on liver metabolism and excretion through the biliary and urinary systems. Only patients with severe renal dysfunction are likely to experience prolonged effects.

Dose
—Intravenous:

—Bolus: 5 mg doses intravenously approximately every 5 minutes, as necessary. In patients not receiving other antihypertensive or sedative-hypnotic agents, manufacturer recommendations are to initiate dosage at 0.25 mg/kg, with repeat doses of 40–80 mg to a total of 300 mg, if necessary.

—Infusion: 2 mg/min of a solution containing 1 mg/mL. Once blood pressure is controlled the infusion should be stopped (since the half-life is about 5 hours).

Labetalol Interactions with Anesthesia Drugs
Labetalol and calcium channel blockers (diltiazem, verapamil)
—Verapamil and diltiazem, particularly when used intravenously, can significantly potentiate the effects of beta blockers on cardiac conduction and contractility.

—Severe bradycardia and hypotension can occur when these medications are used concomitantly, especially in patients with abnormalities of cardiac conduction (sick sinus syndrome) or ventricular function (congestive heart failure).

Labetalol and cocaine
—Beta blockers have been demonstrated to potentiate coronary vasoconstriction caused by cocaine.

—This interaction was documented in the cardiac catheterization lab using intranasal cocaine followed by administration of propranolol.

—Although the significance of this interaction to clinical practice is not clear, patients who develop hypertension, tachycardia, and angina from cocaine may be best treated by an agent such as labetalol, which has alpha blocking properties.

Labetalol and diazoxide
—The hypotensive response to diazoxide may be accentuated in patients taking beta blockers.

—This may be due to blunting of the normal sympathetic response that otherwise occurs.

Labetalol and isoproterenol
—Patients who are receiving beta blockers may be more resistant to the bronchodilator effects of isoproterenol. The nonselective beta blockers, such as propranolol, are more likely to have an interaction of greater magnitude than selective blockers, such as metoprolol.

Labetalol and ketamine
—Ketamine may produce myocardial depression if there is interference with the normal sympathetic response, as seen in patients on beta blockers.

Labetalol Interactions with Diseases
Labetalol and asthma
—Use of beta blockers in patients with reactive airway disease (asthma, chronic obstructive pulmonary disease) can result in significant increases in airway resistance.

—Although noncardioselective beta blockers (labetalol, propranolol) are most likely to precipitate bronchospasm in these patients, even selective beta 1 blockers (esmolol) have enough beta 2 blocking properties to require caution.

Labetalol and congestive heart failure

—Beta blockers can precipitate congestive heart failure in patients with compromised cardiac function. In patients in congestive heart failure, there may be deterioration in cardiac status.

—The exception to these consequences might be the situation in which tachyarrhythmias may be precipitating acute cardiac decompensation by increasing the myocardial oxygen demand.

—Because labetalol blocks both beta and alpha adrenergic receptors and is associated with vasodilation, it may be less likely to precipitate cardiac decompensation than pure beta blockers.

—Beta 1 adrenergic blockade reduces heart rate, myocardial contractility, and, therefore, cardiac ouput. Also, atrioventricular node conduction time is prolonged and sinus node automaticity is decreased.

Labetalol and heart block (second, third degree)

—Use of beta blockers in patients with second or third degree heart block can cause dangerous decreases in heart rate.

—Beta 1 adrenergic blockade results in a decrease in sinus node automaticity as well as a prolongation of atrioventricular conduction time.

—If beta blockers are used in patients with heart block, cardiac pacing may be necessary.

Labetalol and Raynaud's phenomenon

—Beta blockers must be used with extreme caution in patients with Raynaud's phenomenon because of the ability of these drugs to worsen or precipitate digital vasospasm.

—Arteriovenous shunts exist in the fingertips and dilate with beta adrenergic stimulation. Beta 1 blockade can result in vasoconstriction. Labetalol, because of its ability to block alpha receptors, would be less likely to cause this problem.

Labetalol and sick sinus syndrome

—Diltiazem, verapamil, and beta blockers should be avoided or used with extreme caution in patients with sick sinus syndrome (SSS).

—Use of these drugs, which depress sinus node automaticity, may cause severe bradycardia even in patients with SSS who are experiencing supraventricular tachycardia.

Labetalol and Wolf–Parkinson–White syndrome

—Verapamil, diltiazem, digitalis, beta blockers, and lidocaine should not be used to acutely treat wide complex tachyarrhythmias associated with the Wolf–Parkinson–White syndrome.

—In tachyarrhythmias with wide QRS complexes, antegrade conduction must be assumed to be taking place via accessory paths. Conduction through these paths can be accelerated by verapamil, diltiazem, digitalis, lidocaine, or propranolol. Intravenous procainamide is the treatment of choice.

—If the QRS complex is narrow, indicating antegrade conduction via normal conduction paths, treatment can be with agents that slow conduction through the AV node: verapamil, propranolol, digitalis, procainamide, or diltiazem.

Labetalol Interactions with Patient Drugs

Labetalol and amiodarone

—Metoprolol and propranolol have both been associated with life-threatening arrhythmias (severe bradycardia, cardiac arrest, or ventricular fibrillation) in patients taking amiodarone. In all cases, these arrhythmias developed within 1 hour to several hours after initiation of these beta blockers and after only one or two doses.

—Although these cases involved oral beta blockers, intravenous propranolol could have similar results.

—Other beta blockers have not been associated with this interaction.

Labetalol and flecainide

—Flecainide can cause decreased myocardial contractility, particularly at the onset of intravenous therapy. Patients most significantly affected are those with compromised left ventricular function (ejection fraction <30%).

—Beta blockers and some calcium channel blockers may have added negative inotropic effects with flecainide.

Labetalol and mefloquine

—Mefloquine is a derivative of quinine and has rarely been associated with bradycardia and prolonged QT interval. Beta blockers and calcium channel blockers should be used with caution in patients on this medication.

Labetalol and methyldopa

—Patients taking methyldopa for hypertension may experience a hypertensive response when given beta blockers. This has been reported in a patient on methyldopa who was given a slow intravenous injection of propranolol.

—The mechanism for this response is thought to be related to the accumulation of methylnorepinephrine that is a result of methyldopa therapy. This substance has both vasoconstricting and vasodilating properties. The latter, when blocked by beta blockers, could leave unopposed vasoconstriction, resulting in hypertension.

Labetalol and ritodrine

—Beta blockers may inhibit the effects of ritodrine and terbutaline, which are beta 2 selective blockers used for uterine relaxation.

LIDOCAINE (LidoPen, Xylocaine)

Classification and indications

—Lidocaine is a local anesthetic and a class IB antiarrhythmic agent.

—It is indicated for use as a local anesthetic for infiltration, nerve block, spinal, epidural, and caudal anesthesia. It is also indicated for treatment of ventricular arrhythmias.

Pharmacology

—Like all local anesthetics, lidocaine prevents the generation and conduction of nerve impulses by blocking the normal increase in sodium permeability that accompanies depolarization of nerve axons.

—The antiarrhythmic activity of lidocaine is a result of interference with phase IV depolarization, like all class I B drugs (lidocaine, tocainide, phenytoin, mexilitene). Class I A drugs are local anesthetics that interfere with phase 0 and phase IV depolarization (quinidine, procainamide, disopyramide).

—Onset of activity after intravenous administration of 50–100 mg is in 45–90 seconds and has a duration of 10–20 minutes. Loading doses are required to achieve therapeutic levels rapidly.

—When used for spinal anesthesia, lidocaine 5% has a duration of about 100 minutes for motor blockade and slightly longer for sensory blockade. For epidural or caudal anesthesia, the duration of 1.5–2% solutions is about 75–130 minutes. Addition of epinephrine slows the onset and increases the duration of blockade.

—Single dosage limits for lidocaine are 4.5 mg/kg (300 mg in adults) or 7 mg/kg with epinephrine.

—Elimination of lidocaine depends on liver metabolism. Conditions that decrease liver blood flow (congestive heart failure) can result in prolonged elimination times. Renal disease has no effect on duration of action.

Dose

—Ventricular arrhythmias:

—Bolus: 1–1.5 mg/kg (50–100 mg for average adult).

—Infusion: 20–50 µg/kg/min (1–4 mg/min).

—Spinal anesthesia: 1–1.5 mL of a 5% solution (50–75 mg). Higher doses (100 mg) are sometimes necessary.

—Epidural anesthesia: 10–15 mL of a 2% solution (200–300 mg).

—Caudal anesthesia: 20–30 mL of a 1% solution (200–300 mg).

Lidocaine Interactions with Anesthesia Drugs

Lidocaine and cimetidine

—In patients receiving oral, but not intravenous cimetidine, acute intravenous infusion of lidocaine may result in early signs of toxicity. This is due to the decrease in hepatic clearance of lidocaine caused by cimetidine.

—This interaction has been documented after single oral doses of cimetidine and may decrease lidocaine clearance by up to 30%.

—This interaction is not seen with other H2 receptor antagonists.

Lidocaine and muscle relaxants (atracurium, doxacurium, gallamine, metocurine, mivacurium, pancuronium, pipercuronium, rocuronium, tubocurarine, vecuronium)

—Most local anesthetics can block neuromuscular transmission from non-depolarizing agents as well as depolarizing muscle relaxants. Of clinical significance to the anesthesiologist, lidocaine, given as a 50- to 100-mg bolus or even by infusion, can significantly increase a non-depolarizer block or a phase II block from succinylcholine.

Lidocaine and succinylcholine

—Most local anesthetics can block neuromuscular transmission from non-depolarizing agents as well as depolarizing muscle relaxants.

—Bolus doses of lidocaine may prolong neuromuscular blockade from succinylcholine, but large doses of lidocaine (>3
mg/kg) are required for clinically significant interaction.

—Phase II block from succinylcholine can be prolonged from
normal bolus doses of lidocaine.

Lidocaine Interactions with Diseases

Lidocaine and advanced age

—Patients with congestive heart failure or compromised cardiac function can experience delayed elimination of lidocaine. This is a result of decreased hepatic blood flow.

—This interaction is significant mainly for patients receiving
prolonged infusions (>24 hours). Normal loading doses and
short-term infusion doses are appropriate.

Lidocaine and congestive heart failure

Lidocaine and malignant hyperthermia

—Local or regional anesthesia with either amide (such as lidocaine) or ester (such as procaine) anesthetics is now considered safe for malignant hyperthermia (MH)–susceptible
patients.

—Anesthetic agents considered safe for use in patients with
known or suspected susceptibility for developing MH
include propofol, barbiturates, etomidate, ketamine, non-
depolarizing neuromuscular blocking agents, narcotics,
benzodiazepines, droperidol, epinephrine, norepinephrine,
and anticholinesterases.

—Nitrous oxide is probably safe in the susceptible patient based
on repeated use in MH-susceptible humans and swine.

Lidocaine and Wolf–Parkinson–White syndrome

—Verapamil, diltiazem, digitalis, beta blockers, and lidocaine
should not be used to acutely treat wide complex tachyarrhythmias associated with the Wolf–Parkinson–White
syndrome.

—In tachyarrhythmias with wide QRS complexes, antegrade
conduction must be assumed to be taking place via accessory paths. Conduction through these paths can be accelerated by verapamil, diltiazem, digitalis, lidocaine, or propranolol. Intravenous procainamide is the treatment of choice.

—If the QRS complex is narrow, indicating antegrade conduction via normal conduction paths, treatment can be
with agents that slow conduction through the AV node: verapamil, propranolol, digitalis, procainamide, or diltiazem.

Lidocaine Interactions with Patient Drugs

Lidocaine and amiodarone

—Amiodarone increases refractoriness and slows conduction in most cardiac tissue. A number of medications, including class I antiarrhythmics like lidocaine, calcium channel blockers, and beta blockers, which have similar effects, can precipitate severe bradycardia when given to a patient taking amiodarone.

—A case was reported of a patient with sick sinus syndrome on amiodarone who developed profound sinus bradycardia after local anesthesia with lidocaine.

Lidocaine and beta blockers (acebutolol, atenolol, betaxolol, carteolol, labetalol, levobunolol, metoprolol, nadolol, penbutolol, pindolol, propranolol, timolol)

—Lidocaine clearance is reduced in patients taking beta blockers, which may result in higher serum levels of lidocaine than anticipated. This is attributed to a decreased cardiac output and decreased hepatic blood flow seen in patients taking beta blockers.

—Lidocaine with epinephrine used as a local anesthetic in large amounts can cause extreme hypertension in patients on chronic beta blocker therapy. This occurs because of unrestricted alpha stimulation in patients on beta blockers.

—Cardioselective beta blockers like acebutolol, atenolol, and metoprolol are less likely to be associated with a severe hypertensive interaction with epinephrine.

Lidocaine and cimetidine

—In patients receiving oral but not intravenous cimetidine, acute intravenous infusion of lidocaine may result in early signs of toxicity. This is due to the decrease in hepatic clearance of lidocaine caused by cimetidine.

—This interaction has been documented after single oral doses of cimetidine and may decrease lidocaine clearance by up to 30%.

—This interaction is not seen with other H2 receptor antagonists.

LORAZEPAM (Ativan)

Classification and indications

—Lorazepam is a benzodiazepine.

—It is indicated for use as a preoperative sedative, for intraoperative use as part of a general anesthetic, or for conscious sedation.

Pharmacology

—Benzodiazepines apparently exert some of their effects through GABA (gamma aminobutyric acid), but the exact mechanism of action is not known.

—Absorption after intramuscular injection is reliable and rapid with lorazepam and midazolam, but not with other benzodiazepines.

—Onset of sedative, anxiolytic, and anticonvulsant action is from 1 to 5 minutes after intravenous administration. Duration varies from 15 minutes to 1 hour for chlordiazepoxide and diazepam, <2 hours for midazolam, and 12–24 hours after IV lorazepam.

—Since benzodiazepines are metabolized in the liver, patients with liver disease can experience prolonged effects from usual doses. Also, geriatric patients may have prolonged elimination times.

Dose

—Preoperative sedation:

—Intramuscular: 0.05 mg/kg (up to 4 mg) intramuscularly 2 hours before surgery.

—Intravenously: 0.04 mg/kg (up to 2 mg) intravenously 15 to 20 minutes before surgery.

Lorazepam Interactions with Diseases

Lorazepam and advanced age

—Elderly patients may have decreased requirements for benzodiazepines.

—The exact mechanism for this response is controversial but may be related to decreased metabolism of this class of drugs. Alternatively, some elderly patients may be more sensitive to the CNS effects of these medications.

Lorazepam and alcohol—acute intoxication

—Patients who are acutely intoxicated with alcohol (including chronic alcoholics) usually demonstrate increased sensitivity to general anesthesia.

—Although the precise mechanism of interactions is not agreed on, it appears that alcohol intoxication has additive CNS depression with barbiturates, benzodiazepines, and narcotics, as well as inhalational agents.

Lorazepam and alcohol—chronic abuse

—Chronic abuse of alcohol has complex and incompletely understood effects on a patient's response to anesthetic agents. In general, these patients tend to be more tolerant (in a nonintoxicated state) to barbiturates, benzodiazepines, narcotics, and inhalational agents.

—Exceptions to this generalization include the alcoholic patient with a cardiomyopathy who may demonstrate increased sensitivity to myocardial depression from inhalational agents.

—Also, the patient with severe liver disease may have impaired ability to metabolize succinylcholine due to decreased levels of plasma pseudocholinesterase.

Lorazepam and cerebral edema, intracranial hypertension

—Most intravenous anesthetics cause a reduction in cerebral blood flow (CBF) and intracranial pressure (ICP) or have no effect on ICP. Although this effect is primarily from depression of cerebral metabolic rate (CMR), in some cases a direct vasoconstriction occurs.

—The exception to the above is ketamine, which causes an increased CMR and CBF with an increase in ICP.

—All of the narcotics, as well as barbiturates, etomidate, benzodiazepines, and propofol, have been associated with a reduction or maintenance of ICP during anesthesia.

Lorazepam and cirrhosis

—The benzodiazepines are metabolized extensively in the liver and patients with cirrhosis will demonstrate more prolonged effects of this class of drugs.

Lorazepam and liver disease

—Elimination of benzodiazepines is dependent on hepatic metabolism. Patients with liver dysfunction may experience prolonged effects from usual doses.

Lorazepam and malignant hyperthermia

—Anesthetic agents considered safe for use in patients with known or suspected susceptibility for developing malignant hyperthermia (MH) include propofol, barbiturates, etomidate, ketamine, non-depolarizing neuromuscular blocking agents, narcotics, benzodiazepines, droperidol, epinephrine, norepinephrine, and anticholinesterases.

—Nitrous oxide is probably safe in the susceptible patient based on repeated use in MH-susceptible humans and swine.

—Local or regional anesthesia with either amide (such as lidocaine) or ester (such as procaine) anesthetics is now considered safe for MH-susceptible patients.

Lorazepam and porphyria

—Benzodiazepines are considered to be questionable triggering agents for porphyria. This is based on their ability to provoke attacks of porphyria in rat models, though use in humans has not been associated with this reaction.

—Not all of the porphyrias have significance for the anesthesiologist. Three of the four hepatic porphyrias (acute intermittent, variegate, hereditary coproporphyria) and none of the erythropoietic porphyrias are associated with neurologic symptoms that can be triggered by certain medications: barbiturates, etomidate, and corticosteroids.

—Benzodiazepines and etomidate are considered to be questionable triggering agents, whereas safe anesthetics are inhalational agents, narcotics, muscle relaxants, anticholinesterases, and propofol.

Lorazepam and pregnancy

—Benzodiazepines may cause damage to the fetus, especially during the first trimester of pregnancy.

—Retrospective studies of chlordiazepoxide and diazepam have shown an increased risk of congenital malformations when administered to pregnant patients in their first trimester of pregnancy.

—Administration of preoperative benzodiazepines for obstetric procedures (such as caesarean sections) may produce CNS depression in neonates.

Lorazepam and renal dysfunction

—Renal dysfunction has not been demonstrated to cause significant changes in pharmacokinetics or pharmacodynamics of benzodiazepines, narcotics (with the possible exception of butorphanol), barbiturates, or propofol.

—In patients with renal dysfunction, the above drugs may appear to have an increase in duration or intensity. This has been explained as a response to the systemic effects of renal dysfunction rather than specific effects on the metabolism of these drugs.

—Some muscle relaxants are significantly affected by renal failure.

Lorazepam Interactions with Patient Drugs
Lorazepam and diphenylhydantoin, phenytoin

—Benzodiazepines, when given to a patient on chronic diphenylhydantoin therapy, may cause an increased serum level of diphenylhydantoin. This may be due to a decrease in the metabolism of diphenylhydantoin caused by benzodiazepines.

—The half-life of benzodiazepines can be decreased in patients on chronic diphenylhydantoin therapy.

MEPERIDINE (Demerol)

Classification and indications

—Meperidine is a synthetic opiate (phenylpiperidine derivative).

—It is used in anesthesia for preoperative sedation, as part of a general anesthetic, and for postoperative analgesia or control of shivering.

Pharmacology

—Meperidine, like other narcotics, exerts its analgesic effects through opioid receptors in the CNS (brain and spinal cord).

—Although narcotics used in anesthesia are potent analgesics, there is controversy about the level of amnesia induced with even large doses of narcotics. To avoid awareness during anesthesia, use of other anesthetic agents (benzodiazepines, inhalation agents, etc.) are recommended.

—Somatosensory evoked potentials (SEPs) are not significantly affected by narcotics.

—Although there is some controversy about increases in intracranial pressure from opioids, in general, opioids cause slight decreases in cerebral blood flow, metabolic rate, and intracranial pressure.

—Cardiovascular effects of meperidine include hypotension with anesthetic doses (resulting from histamine release) and tachycardia (probably related to structural similarity to atropine).

—Like other narcotics, meperidine causes respiratory depression and reduced hypoxic ventilatory drive.

—Muscle rigidity, particularly of the chest wall, has been associated with rapid administration of narcotics. The mechanism of this action is not clear, but older patients seem more prone to this response. It has also been associated most frequently with alfentanil.

—Muscle rigidity can occur not only during induction, but also on emergence from anesthesia or, rarely, hours after the last opioid dose.

—Peak analgesia following parenteral meperidine occurs within 1 hour and lasts for 2–4 hours.

—Elimination depends mainly on hepatic metabolism with some renal excretion. Patients with hepatic dysfunction may have drug accumulation after repeated high doses of meperidine.

Dose
—Adults:
  —Intramuscular: 50–150 mg IM every 3–4 hours as necessary.
  —Intravenous: 10–25 mg IV as necessary for supplementation of anesthesia or for analgesia.
  —For shivering: 25 mg IV.
—Children:
  —Intramuscular: 1–2 mg/kg IM every 3–4 hours as necessary.

Meperidine Interactions with Anesthesia Drugs
Meperidine and clonidine
—Clonidine has been shown to potentiate narcotics and reduce the MAC of inhaled anesthetics.
—This effect may be related to clonidine's inhibition of the sympathetic outflow from the vasomotor center in the medulla (clonidine is a central alpha 2 receptor agonist, which results in inhibition of CNS sympathetic centers).

Meperidine and naloxone
—Cases of pulmonary edema, hypertension, and ventricular arrhythmias have occurred in postoperative patients receiving naloxone for reversal of respiratory depression induced by narcotics. The precise etiology of these reactions is not known.
—A patient who receives multiple doses of meperidine over a prolonged period will accumulate a metabolite called normeperidine, which is a CNS stimulant with little analgesic qualities. When naloxone is used in such patients, the result of reversing the primarily CNS depressant effect of meperidine may be seizure activity.

Meperidine Interactions with Diseases
Meperidine and advanced age
—Elderly patients may require lower doses of narcotics than younger adults.
—This might be a result of reduced metabolism of this class of drugs or it might represent an increased brains sensitivity to narcotics as a result of aging.

Meperidine and alcohol—acute intoxication
—Patients who are acutely intoxicated with alcohol (including chronic alcoholics) usually demonstrate increased sensitivity to general anesthesia.

—Although the precise mechanism of interactions is not agreed on, it appears that alcohol intoxication has additive CNS depression with barbiturates, benzodiazepines, and narcotics, as well as inhalational agents.

Meperidine and alcohol—chronic abuse

—Chronic abuse of alcohol has complex and incompletely understood effects on a patient's response to anesthetic agents. In general, these patients tend to be more tolerant (in a nonintoxicated state) to barbiturates, benzodiazepines, narcotics, and inhalational agents.

—Exceptions to this generalization include the alcoholic patient with a cardiomyopathy who may demonstrate increased sensitivity to myocardial depression from inhalational agents.

—Also, the patient with severe liver disease may have impaired ability to metabolize succinylcholine due to decreased levels of plasma pseudocholinesterase.

Meperidine and cirrhosis, liver disease

—Elimination of meperidine depends mainly on hepatic metabolism with some renal excretion. Patients with hepatic dysfunction may have drug accumulation after repeated, high doses of meperidine.

Meperidine and malignant hyperthermia

—Anesthetic agents considered safe for use in patients with known or suspected susceptibility for developing malignant hyperthermia (MH) include propofol, barbiturates, etomidate, ketamine, non-depolarizing neuromuscular blocking agents, narcotics, benzodiazepines, droperidol, epinephrine, norepinephrine, and anticholinesterases.

—Nitrous oxide is probably safe in the susceptible patient based on repeated use in MH-susceptible humans and swine.

—Local or regional anesthesia with either amide (such as lidocaine) or ester (such as procaine) anesthetics is now considered safe for MH-susceptible patients.

Meperidine and porphyria

—Narcotics are considered safe anesthetics for use in porphyrias.

—Not all of the porphyrias have significance for the anesthesiologist. Three of the four hepatic porphyrias (acute intermittent, variegate, hereditary coproporphyria) and none of the erythropoietic porphyrias are associated with neurologic symptoms that can be triggered by certain medications: barbiturates, etomidate, and corticosteroids.

—Benzodiazepines and etomidate are considered to be questionable triggering agents, whereas safe anesthetics are inhalational agents, narcotics, muscle relaxants, anticholinesterases, and propofol.

Meperidine and renal dysfunction

—Renal dysfunction has not been demonstrated to cause significant changes in pharmacokinetics or pharmacodynamics of benzodiazepines, narcotics (with the possible exception of butorphanol), barbiturates, or propofol.

—In patients with renal dysfunction, the above drugs may appear to have an increase in duration or intensity. This has been explained as a response to the systemic effects of renal dysfunction rather than specific effects on the metabolism of theses drugs.

—Some muscle relaxants are significantly affected by renal failure.

Meperidine Interactions with Patient Drugs

Meperidine and cimetidine

—Cimetidine may potentiate narcotics, causing greater respiratory depression and sedation than expected. This may be related to the alteration of hepatic metabolism of narcotics produced by cimetidine.

—This effect is seen less with morphine than other narcotics and is probably related to the fact that morphine undergoes a different metabolic process than some other narcotics such as fentanyl or meperidine.

—Ranitidine is not associated with this interaction.

Meperidine and clonidine

—Clonidine has been shown to potentiate narcotics and reduce the MAC of inhaled anesthetics.

—This effect may be related to clonidine's inhibition of the sympathetic outflow from the vasomotor center in the medulla (clonidine is a central alpha 2 receptor agonist, which results in inhibition of CNS sympathetic centers).

Meperidine and monoamine oxidase inhibitors (isocarboxazid, phenelzine, selegilene, tranylcypromine)

—A syndrome of CNS excitation, hyperpyrexia, and seizures may occur when meperidine is administered to a patient taking monoamine oxidase inhibitors. The mechanism of this interaction is not clearly understood. Meperidine should be avoided in any patient receiving. MAO inhibitors and morphine or other narcotics should be used instead.

—Alternatively, potentiation of the narcotic effect can occur resulting in respiratory depression or even coma.

MEPHENTERMINE (Wyamine)

Classification and indications

—Mephentermine is a synthetic sympathomimetic amine, similar to methamphetamine and ephedrine.

—It is indicated for the management of hypotension when fluid therapy, patient positioning, or other specific corrective action (such as using inotropes for cardiogenic shock) is ineffective or contraindicated.

Pharmacology

—Mephentermine has both direct and indirect activity on adrenergic receptors, probably by releasing endogenous norepinephrine stores (as ephedrine does). As a result, there is stimulation of both alpha and beta receptors.

—Cardiovascular effects include an increase in myocardial contractility and cardiac output. Heart rate may be increased, but bradycardia may occur if increased blood pressure stimulates vagal tone.

—Systolic and diastolic blood pressures are normally increased by mephentermine, although there is vasodilation of arterioles in muscle and the mesentery.

—Onset of activity is almost immediate after intravenous administration and in 5–15 minutes of IM administration.

Dose

—Adults:
  —Intravenous: A slow infusion of 20–60 mg of a dilute solution (30 mg in 250 D5W).
  —Intramuscular: 15–30 mg, up to 0.5 mg/kg.
—Children:
  —Intramuscular: 0.4 mg/kg.

Mephentermine Interactions with Anesthesia Drugs
Mephentermine and methylergonovine

—Oxytocics (oxytocin, ergonovine, methylergonovine) may interact with vasopressors to produce hypertension, which is more likely to be severe in patients with a predisposition to hypertension.

—The use of an intramuscular or intravenous ergot alkaloid (such as IM methylergonovine) either preceded or followed by a vasopressor may result in severe hypertension. The safest method of administering an oxytocic is a dilute intravenous infusion of oxytocin.

Mephentermine and oxytocin

—Severe hypertension has been associated with administration of oxytocin to patients who had received a prophylactic vasoconstrictor up to 4 hours previously for a caudal block.

—This interaction is more likely to be seen in patients with underlying mild hypertension and in those receiving an ergot alkaloid (such as methylergonovine) rather than a dilute solution of oxytocin.

Mephentermine and phentolamine

—Blockade of alpha 1 receptors can result in unresponsiveness to vasopressors, depending on the vasopressor being used.

—Ephedrine and mephentermine have significant beta 2 stimulation along with beta 1 and alpha adrenergic activity. As a result, it is possible that hypotension could worsen in patients on alpha blockers given ephedrine due to the unopposed vasodilation resulting from beta 2 stimulation.

—Although good documentation of this interaction is scarce, this is similar to the response that can be seen with epinephrine.

—Because norepinephrine has beta 1 activity, it is more likely to be effective in treating hypotension in patients on alpha blockers.

Mephentermine Interactions with Diseases

Mephentermine and hyperthyroidism, thyrotoxicosis

—Agents that stimulate the sympathetic nervous system (such as mephentermine) may have exaggerated effects in patients with hyperthyroidism. Although most evident in untreated patients, even patients receiving treatment for excess thyroid hormone may demonstrate this response.

—Excess thyroid hormone causes stimulation of metabolism of most body tissues. As a result, cardiac output increases by 50% or more to remove the extra metabolic byproducts.

Also, direct stimulatory effects on the myocardium at even slightly elevated thyroid hormone levels cause tachycardia and increased contractility.

—At higher thyroid hormone levels, myocardial depression may occur as a result of excess demands or a direct myocardial depression.

Mephentermine and pheochromocytoma

—Blockade of alpha 1 receptors can result in unresponsiveness to vasopressors, depending on the vasopressor being used.

—Ephedrine and mephentermine have significant beta 2 stimulation along with beta 1 and alpha adrenergic activity. As a result, it is possible that hypotension could worsen in patients on alpha blockers given ephedrine due to the unopposed vasodilation resulting from beta 2 stimulation.

—Although good documentation of this interaction is scarce, this is similar to the response that can be seen with epinephrine.

—Because norepinephrine has beta 1 activity, it is more likely to be effective in treating hypotension in patients on alpha blockers.

Mephentermine and pregnancy

—Ephedrine, mephentermine, and metaraminol are the preferred agents for treatment of hypotension in pregnancy.

—The above agents have both alpha and beta agonist activity and are not associated with reduced placental blood flow.

—Phenylephrine, norepinephrine, angiotensin, and methoxamine are predominantly alpha adrenergic agents that act peripherally and can cause uterine artery vasoconstriction and placental hypoperfusion.

Mephentermine Interactions with Patient Drugs

Mephentermine and alpha adrenergic blockers (doxazasin, phenoxybenzamine, phentolamine, prazosin, terazosin)

—Blockade of alpha 1 receptors can result in unresponsiveness to vasopressors, depending on the vasopressor being used.

—Ephedrine and mephentermine have significant beta 2 stimulation along with beta 1 and alpha adrenergic activity. As a result, it is possible that hypotension could worsen in patients on alpha blockers given ephedrine due to the unopposed vasodilation resulting from beta 2 stimulation.

—Although good documentation of this interaction is scarce, this is similar to the response that can be seen with epinephrine.

—Because norepinephrine has beta 1 activity, it is more likely to be effective in treating hypotension in patients on alpha blockers.

Mephentermine and ergot alkaloids (dihydroergotamine, ergotamine tartrate, methylergonovine)

—Ergot alkaloids may interact with vasopressors to produce hypertension which is more likely to be severe in patients with a predisposition to hypertension.

—Because of possibly additive vasoconstrictive effects, the administration of vasopressors to patients receiving ergot alkaloids may produce unexpected degrees of hypertension.

Mephentermine and guanadrel, guanethidine

—Patients receiving guanethidine and guanadrel can have an exaggerated hypertensive response to norepinephrine and other direct-acting catecholamines such as phenylephrine, dobutamine, and epinephrine.

—Indirect-acting catecholamines, such as ephedrine, metaraminol, mephentermine, and dopamine may have fewer pressor effects than expected.

—Guanethidine and guanadrel deplete intraneuronal norepinephrine in postganglionic sympathetic neurons and in this way may diminish the response of indirect-acting catecholamines, while sensitizing adrenergic receptors to direct-acting amines.

Mephentermine and monoamine oxidase inhibitors (isocarboxazid, phenelzine, selegilene, tranylcypromine)

—Indirect-acting vasopressors (ephedrine, mephentermine, and metaraminol) act by releasing intraneuronal monoamines such as dopamine and norepinephrine. This is the explanation of the hypertensive crises seen when patients receiving monamine oxidase inhibitors are given these vasopressors.

—Direct-acting vasopressors such as phenylephrine, epinephrine, norepinephrine, and dobutamine may be potentiated by MAO inhibitors and should be used in smaller amounts than normally used.

—Dopamine has both direct and indirect actions and must be used with caution (perhaps 1/10 the normal dose).

Mephentermine and oxytocin
—Oxytocin administration has been associated with severe hypertension in patients who had received a prophylactic vasoconstrictor up to 4 hours previously for a caudal block.
—Severe hypertension is more likely to occur in patients with existing mild hypertension and in those patients who receive an ergot alkaloid (such as methylergonovine), rather than a dilute solution of oxytocin.

Mephentermine and ritodrine, terbutaline
—Ritodrine and terbutaline, beta 2 agonists, may potentiate other sympathomimetic agents.
—The mechanism of this interaction is probably related to the beta 1 adrenergic stimulation that can be seen with administration of these drugs.

METARAMINOL (Aramine)

Classification and indications
—Metaraminol is a synthetic sympathomimetic amine.
—It is indicated for the management of hypotension when fluid therapy, patient positioning, or other specific corrective action (such as using inotropes for cardiogenic shock) is ineffective or contraindicated.

Pharmacology
—Metaraminol is mainly an alpha adrenergic receptor agonist, but also stimulates beta 1 receptors. It also causes release of norepinephrine from storage sites.
—Cardiovascular effects relate to stimulation of alpha and beta 1 receptors. Vasoconstriction and the increase in peripheral resistance cause an increase in systolic and diastolic pressure. The increase in blood pressure results in vagal stimulation, which offsets the chronotropic effect of beta 1 receptor stimulation.
—Increased myocardial contractility is seen as a result of the beta 1 stimulation.
—Coronary artery constriction occurs, but may be offset by increased blood pressure and the increase in cardiac metabolism, which stimulates coronary artery vasodilation.
—Onset of action is in 1–2 minutes after IV and 10 minutes after IM administration.
—Elimination is by unknown mechanisms.

Dose
—Adults:
  —Intravenous: 0.5–5 mg IV or by infusion (15 to 100 mg in 500 mL D5W).
  —Intramuscular: 2–10 mg IM.
—Children:
  —Intravenous: 0.01 mg/kg or by infusion (10 mg in 250 mL D5W).
  —Intramuscular: 0.1 mg/kg.

Metaraminol Interactions with Anesthesia Drugs

Metaraminol and methylergonovine
—Oxytocics (oxytocin, ergonovine, methylergonovine) may interact with vasopressors to produce hypertension, which is more likely to be severe in patients with a predisposition to hypertension.
—The use of an intramuscular or intravenous ergot alkaloid (such as IM methylergonovine) either preceded or followed by a vasopressor may result in severe hypertension. The safest method of administering an oxytocic is a dilute intravenous infusion of oxytocin.

Metaraminol and oxytocin
—Severe hypertension has been reported in patients given oxytocin who had received a prophylactic vasoconstrictor up to 4 hours previously for a caudal block.
—This interaction is more likely to occur in patients with existing mild hypertension and who receive an ergot alkaloid (such as methylergonovine) rather than a dilute solution of oxytocin.

Metaraminol and phentolamine
—The pressor effects of vasopressors can be blunted in patients receiving alpha blockers.
—Norepinephrine and metaraminol stimulate mainly beta 1 (cardiac stimulation) and alpha receptors. When norepinephrine is given to patients on alpha blockers, the beta 1 stimulation may produce some increase in blood pressure. Hypotension is unlikely because of minimal beta 2 agonism.

Metaraminol Interactions with Diseases

Metaraminol and hyperthyroidism, thyrotoxicosis
—Agents which stimulate the sympathetic nervous system (such as metaraminol) may have exaggerated effects in

patients with hyperthyroidism. Although most evident in untreated patients, even patients receiving treatment for excess thyroid hormone may demonstrate this response.

—Excess thyroid hormone causes stimulation of metabolism of most body tissues. As a result, cardiac output increases by 50% or more to remove the extra metabolic byproducts. Also, direct stimulatory effects on the myocardium at even slightly elevated thyroid hormone levels causes tachycardia and increased contractility.

—At higher thyroid hormone levels, myocardial depression may occur as a result of excess demands or a direct myocardial depression.

Metaraminol and pheochromocytoma

—The pressor effects of vasopressors can be blunted in patients receiving alpha blockers.

—Norepinephrine and metaraminol stimulate mainly beta 1 (cardiac stimulation) and alpha receptors. When norepinephrine is given to patients on alpha blockers, the beta 1 stimulation may produce some increase in blood pressure. Hypotension is unlikely because of minimal beta 2 agonism.

Metaraminol and pregnancy

—Ephedrine, mephentermine, and metaraminol are the preferred agents for treatment of hypotension in pregnancy.

—The above agents have both alpha and beta agonist activity and are not associated with reduced placental blood flow.

—Phenylephrine, norepinephrine, angiotensin, and methoxamine are predominantly alpha adrenergic agents that act peripherally and can cause uterine artery vasoconstriction and placental hypoperfusion.

Metaraminol Interactions with Patient Drugs

Metaraminol and alpha adrenergic blockers (doxazasin, phenoxybenzamine, phentolamine, prazosin, terazosin)

—The pressor effects of vasopressors can be blunted in patients receiving alpha blockers.

—Norepinephrine and metaraminol stimulate mainly beta 1 (cardiac stimulation) and alpha receptors.

—When norepinephrine is given to patients on alpha blockers, the beta 1 stimulation may produce some increase in blood pressure. Hypotension is unlikely because of minimal beta 2 agonism.

Metaraminol and ergot alkaloids (dihydroergotamine, ergonovine, ergotamine tartrate, methylergonovine)

—Ergot alkaloids may interact with vasopressors to produce hypertension, which is more likely to be severe in patients with a predisposition to hypertension.

—Because of possibly additive vasoconstrictive effects, the administration of vasopressors to patients receiving ergot alkaloids may produce unexpected degrees of hypertension.

Metaraminol and guanadrel, guanethidine

—Patients receiving guanethidine and guanadrel can have an exaggerated hypertensive response to norepinephrine and other direct-acting catecholamines such as phenylephrine, dobutamine, and epinephrine.

—Indirect-acting catecholamines, such as ephedrine, metaraminol, mephentermine, and dopamine, may have fewer pressor effects than expected.

—Guanethidine and guanadrel deplete intraneuronal norepinephrine in postganglionic sympathetic neurons and in this way may diminish the response of indirect-acting catecholamines while sensitizing adrenergic receptors to direct-acting amines.

Metaraminol and monoamine oxidase inhibitors (isocarboxazid, phenelzine, selegilene, tranylcypromine)

—Indirect-acting vasopressors (ephedrine, mephentermine, and metaraminol) act by releasing intraneuronal monoamines such as dopamine and norepinephrine. This is the explanation of the hypertensive crises seen when patients receiving monamine oxidase inhibitors are given these vasopressors.

—Direct-acting vasopressors such as phenylephrine, epinephrine, norepinephrine, and dobutamine may be potentiated by MAO inhibitors and should be used in smaller amounts than normally used.

—Dopamine has both direct and indirect actions and must be used with caution (perhaps one tenth the normal dose).

Metaraminol and oxytocin

—Oxytocin administration has been associated with severe hypertension in patients who had received a prophylactic vasoconstrictor up to 4 hours previously for a caudal block.

—Severe hypertension is more likely to occur in patients with existing mild hypertension and in those patients who receive an ergot alkaloid (such as methylergonovine) rather than a dilute solution of oxytocin.

Metaraminol and ritodrine, terbutaline

—Ritodrine and terbutaline, beta 2 agonists, may potentiate other sympathomimetic agents.

—The mechanism of this interaction is probably related to the beta 1 adrenergic stimulation that can be seen with administration of these drugs.

METHOHEXITAL (Brevital)

Classification and indications

—Methohexital, a short-acting barbiturate, is a nonanalgesic, intravenous anesthetic agent.

—It is indicated for intravenous induction of anesthesia. It is also an anticonvulsant and has been used as an infusion for maintenance of anesthesia.

Pharmacology

—The barbiturates are believed to exert their effects through the GABA receptor. Gamma aminobutyric acid (GABA) is the main inhibitory neurotransmitter in the CNS. Barbiturates augment the activity of GABA.

—CNS effects of barbiturates include depression of the EEG, a decrease in the cerebral blood flow and metabolic rate, and a decrease in intracranial pressure (ICP). Cerebral perfusion pressure is maintained in spite of a decrease in mean arterial pressure because of a greater decrease in ICP.

—Cardiac effects following administration of methohexital include an initial decrease in blood pressure, a drop in cardiac output and contractility, but an increased heart rate. Although peripheral vascular resistance does not decrease, venodilation occurs.

—In patients who are very dependent on cardiac preload for hemodynamic stability (hypovolemia, congestive heart failure, tamponade, etc.), venodilation may result in profound decreases in cardiac output and blood pressure.

—Unlike etomidate, barbiturates do not inhibit adrenocortical responses to surgical stress.

—Although methohexital causes a dose-related histamine release, the clinical significance is low and is still safe for use in asthmatic patients.

—Onset of effect after induction doses is within 1 minute with a duration of 5–15 minutes, depending on the dose and the individual. Termination of the effect is a result of redistribution.

—Contraindications to the use of barbiturates are patients with acute intermittent, variegate, or hereditary coproporphyria.

Dose

—Induction:

—Intravenous: 1.5–2.5 mg/kg IV.

—Rectal: 20–30 mg per rectum.

Methohexital Interactions with Diseases

Methohexital and alcohol—chronic abuse

—Chronic abuse of alcohol has complex and incompletely understood effects on a patient's response to anesthetic agents. In general, these patients tend to be more tolerant (in a nonintoxicated state) to barbiturates, benzodiazepines, narcotics, and inhalational agents.

—Exceptions to this generalization include the alcoholic patient with a cardiomyopathy who may demonstrate increased sensitivity to myocardial depression from inhalational agents.

—Also, the patient with severe liver disease may have impaired ability to metabolize succinylcholine due to decreased levels of plasma pseudocholinesterase.

Methohexital and porphyria

—Barbiturates are contraindicated in three of the four hepatic porphyrias (acute intermittent porphyria, variegate porphyria, and hereditary coproporphyria). Porphyria cutanea tarda and the erythropoietic porphyrias are not exacerbated by barbiturates.

—It is theorized that barbiturates can provoke an attack of porphyria by inducing the enzyme aminolevulinic acid synthetase, which results in synthesis of more porphyrin compounds and their precursors.

—Anesthesia can be safely administered to these patients using narcotics, depolarizing and non-depolarizing muscle relaxants, anticholinesterases, propofol, and inhalational agents.

—Questionable agents are benzodiazepines and ketamine.

Methohexital and renal dysfunction

—Renal dysfunction has not been demonstrated to cause significant changes in pharmacokinetics or pharmacodynamics of benzodiazepines, narcotics, barbiturates, or propofol.

—In patients with renal dysfunction, the above drugs may appear to have an increase in duration or intensity. This has been explained as a response to the systemic effects of renal dysfunction rather than specific effects on the metabolism of theses drugs.

—Some muscle relaxants are significantly affected by renal failure.

Methohexital Interactions with Patient Drugs
Methohexital and monoamine oxidase inhibitors (isocarboxazid, phenelzine, selegilene, tranylcypromine)

—Barbiturates given to a patient receiving monoamine oxidase inhibitors may have a prolonged effect resulting in delayed awakening.

METHOXAMINE (Vasoxyl)

Classification and indications

—Methoxamine is a synthetic sympathomimetic amine, similar to phenylephrine.

—It is indicated for the management of hypotension when fluid therapy, patient positioning, or other specific corrective action (such as using inotropes for cardiogenic shock) is ineffective or contraindicated.

Pharmacology

—Methoxamine is an alpha adrenergic receptor agonist. At high doses, there also may be some beta blockade.

—Cardiovascular effects include an increase in systolic and diastolic blood pressure resulting from the increase in peripheral resistance.

—Bradycardia usually occurs and is a result of increased vagal tone secondary to the rise in blood pressure.

—Unlike phenylephrine, coronary and pulmonary arteries are not constricted.

—Renal vessels are constricted by methoxamine and blood flow may be decreased if there is hypovolemia or if hypertension is induced. Otherwise, renal blood flow and urine output is normally increased by the increase in blood pressure.

—Onset of action is almost immediate after intravenous administration and within 15–20 minutes of intramuscular administration.

—Elimination of methoxamine is by unknown mechanisms.

Dose
Adults:

—Intravenous: 3–5 mg IV or by slow infusion (35–40 mg in 250-mL D5W).

—Intramuscular: 5–20 mg (usually 10–15 mg).
Children:
—Intravenous: 0.08 mg/kg slowly IV.
—Intramuscular: 0.25 mg/kg.

Methoxamine Interactions with Anesthesia Drugs
Methoxamine and methylergonovine
—Oxytocics (oxytocin, ergonovine, methylergonovine) may interact with vasopressors to produce hypertension, which is more likely to be severe in patients with a predisposition to hypertension.
—The use of an intramuscular or intravenous ergot alkaloid (such as IM methylergonovine) either preceded or followed by a vasopressor may result in severe hypertension. The safest method of administering an oxytocic is a dilute intravenous infusion of oxytocin.

Methoxamine and oxytocin
—Severe hypertension has been reported in patients given oxytocin who had received a prophylactic vasoconstrictor up to 4 hours previously for a caudal block.
—This interaction is more likely to occur in patients with existing mild hypertension and who receive an ergot alkaloid (such as methylergonovine) rather than a dilute solution of oxytocin.

Methoxamine and phentolamine
—The pressor effects of vasopressors can be blunted in patients receiving alpha blockers.
—Norepinephrine and metaraminol stimulate mainly beta 1 (cardiac stimulation) and alpha receptors. When norepinephrine is given to patients on alpha blockers, the beta 1 stimulation may produce some increase in blood pressure. Hypotension is unlikely because of minimal beta 2 agonism.

Methoxamine Interactions with Diseases
Methoxamine and hyperthyroidism, thyrotoxicosis
—Agents that stimulate the sympathetic nervous system (such as metaraminol) may have exaggerated effects in patients with hyperthyroidism. Although most evident in untreated patients, even patients receiving treatment for excess thyroid hormone may demonstrate this response.
—Excess thyroid hormone causes stimulation of metabolism of most body tissues. As a result, cardiac output increases by 50% or more to remove the extra metabolic by-products.

Also, direct stimulatory effects on the myocardium at even slightly elevated thyroid hormone levels cause tachycardia and increased contractility.

—At higher thyroid hormone levels, myocardial depression may occur as a result of excess demands or a direct myocardial depression.

Methoxamine and pheochromocytoma

—The pressor effects of vasopressors can be blunted in patients receiving alpha blockers.

—Norepinephrine and metaraminol stimulate mainly beta 1 (cardiac stimulation) and alpha receptors. When norepinephrine is given to patients on alpha blockers, the beta 1 stimulation may produce some increase in blood pressure. Hypotension is unlikely because of minimal beta 2 agonism.

Methoxamine and pregnancy

—Ephedrine, mephentermine, and metaraminol are the preferred agents for treatment of hypotension in pregnancy.

—The above agents have both alpha and beta agonist activity and are not associated with reduced placental blood flow.

—Phenylephrine, norepinephrine, angiotensin, and methoxamine are predominantly alpha adrenergic agents that act peripherally and can cause uterine artery vasoconstriction and placental hypoperfusion.

Methoxamine Interactions with Patient Drugs

Methoxamine and alpha adrenergic blockers (doxazasin, phenoxybenzamine, phentolamine, prazosin, terazosin)

—The pressor effects of vasopressors can be blunted in patients receiving alpha blockers.

—Norepinephrine and metaraminol stimulate mainly beta 1 (cardiac stimulation) and alpha receptors. When norepinephrine is given to patients on alpha blockers, the beta 1 stimulation may produce some increase in blood pressure. Hypotension is unlikely because of minimal beta 2 agonism.

Methoxamine and ergot alkaloids (dihydroergotamine, ergonovine, ergotamine tartrate, methylergonovine)

—Ergot alkaloids may interact with vasopressors to produce hypertension, which is more likely to be severe in patients with a predisposition to hypertension.

—Because of possibly additive vasoconstrictive effects, the administration of vasopressors to patients receiving ergot alkaloids may produce unexpected degrees of hypertension.

Methoxamine and guanadrel, guanethidine

—Patients receiving guanethidine and guanadrel can have an exaggerated hypertensive response to norepinephrine and other direct-acting catecholamines such as phenylephrine, dobutamine, and epinephrine.

—Indirect-acting catecholamines, such as ephedrine, metaraminol, mephentermine, and dopamine, may have fewer pressor effects than expected.

—Guanethidine and guanadrel deplete intraneuronal norepinephrine in postganglionic sympathetic neurons and in this way may diminish the response of indirect-acting catecholamines while sensitizing adrenergic receptors to direct-acting amines.

Methoxamine and monoamine oxidase inhibitors (isocarboxazid, phenelzine, selegilene, tranylcypromine)

—Indirect-acting vasopressors (ephedrine, mephentermine, and metaraminol) act by releasing intraneuronal monoamines such as dopamine and norepinephrine. This is the explanation of the hypertensive crises seen when patients receiving monamine oxidase (MAO) inhibitors are given these vasopressors.

—Direct-acting vasopressors such as phenylephrine, epinephrine, norepinephrine, and dobutamine may be potentiated by MAO inhibitors and should be used in smaller amounts than normally used.

—Dopamine has both direct and indirect actions and must be used with caution (perhaps one tenth the normal dose).

Methoxamine and oxytocin

—Oxytocin administration has been associated with severe hypertension in patients who had received a prophylactic vasoconstrictor up to 4 hours previously for a caudal block.

—Severe hypertension is more likely to occur in patients with existing mild hypertension and in those patients who receive an ergot alkaloid (such as methylergonovine) rather than a dilute solution of oxytocin.

Methoxamine and ritodrine, terbutaline

—Ritodrine and terbutaline, beta 2 agonists, may potentiate other sympathomimetic agents.

—The mechanism of this interaction is probably related to the beta 1 adrenergic stimulation that can be seen with administration of these drugs.

METHYLERGONOVINE (Methergine)

Classification and indications
—Methylergonovine is an ergot alkaloid.
—It is used in obstetrics to treat or prevent hemorrhage either postpartum or postabortion.

Pharmacology
—Both ergonovine and methylergonovine directly stimulate contractions of uterine muscle. For this reason, they are useful in controlling bleeding from a hypotonic uterus postpartum or postabortion.
—The cardiovascular effects of these agents can be significant. Vasoconstriction occurs as a result of alpha adrenergic stimulation and blockade of the reuptake of norepinephrine.
—Although ergonovine and methylergonovine mainly cause vasoconstriction of the venous system, arterial vasoconstriction can occur, resulting in hypertension.
—Significant interactions can occur with vasoactive agents (phenylephrine, dopamine, etc.), resulting in severe hypertension.

Dose
—IM: 0.2 mg IM every 2–4 hours as necessary, up to 1.0 mg.
—IV: 0.2 mg IV slowly over 1 minute. Because of potential hypertensive reactions, this route of administration should only be used in cases of severe uterine bleeding.
—Oral: Following parenteral administration, 0.2–0.4 mg PO may be given every 6–12 hours for up to 7 days.

Methylergonovine Interactions with Anesthesia Drugs
Methylergonovine and vasopressors (ephedrine, epinephrine, metaraminol, methoxamine, norepinephrine, phenylephrine)
—Oxytocics (oxytocin, ergonovine, methylergonovine) may interact with vasopressors to produce hypertension, which is more likely to be severe in patients with a predisposition to hypertension.
—The use of an intramuscular or intravenous ergot alkaloid (such as IM methylergonovine) either preceded or followed by a vasopressor may result in severe hypertension. The

safest method of administering an oxytocic is a dilute intravenous infusion of oxytocin.

Methylergonovine Interactions with Diseases

Methylergonovine and hypertension

—Patients with hypertension are at highest risk for severe hypertensive reactions to ergot alkaloids such as methylergonovine.

—If stimulation of uterine muscle tone is necessary in these patients, a dilute solution of oxytocin may be preferable.

Methylergonovine and PIH (pregnancy-induced hypertension), preeclampsia/eclampsia, toxemia

—Patients with hypertension are at highest risk for severe hypertensive reactions to ergot alkaloids such as methylergonovine.

—If stimulation of uterine muscle tone is necessary in these patients, a dilute solution of oxytocin may be preferable.

METOCURINE (Metubine)

Classification and indications

—Metocurine is a non-depolarizing neuromuscular blocker. It is a derivative of tubocurarine and shares many of its properties.

—Although it has been used for skeletal muscle relaxation for intubation and during surgery, it has been replaced by newer agents. It can be used as a defasciculating agent in small doses prior to use of succinylcholine.

Pharmacology

—Metocurine competes with acetylcholine at the neuromuscular junction of skeletal muscle by binding to acetylcholine receptors.

—Pharmacologic effects are very similar to those of tubocurarine. Histamine release is probably less than that of curare, but is significant and may result in hypotension.

—Intubation doses of metocurine (0.3–0.4 mg/kg) have a clinical duration of about 60–120 minutes.

—Elimination is through renal excretion, with no hepatic metabolism.

Dose

—Intubation: 0.3–0.4 mg/kg.

—Maintenance: 0.05–0.1 mg/kg.

Metocurine Interactions with Anesthesia Drugs

Metocurine and calcium channel blockers (diltiazem, nicardipine, nifedipine, verapamil)

—Calcium channel blockers have been associated with prolongation of neuromuscular blockade from non-depolarizing agents.

—This interaction is probably related to the depletion of intracellular calcium associated with chronic therapy. This can result in a decrease in acetylcholine release at the neuromuscular junction.

Metocurine and inhalational anesthetics (desflurane, enflurane, halothane, isoflurane, sevoflurane)

—Desflurane, enflurane, halothane, isoflurane, and sevoflurane can significantly potentiate neuromuscular blockade, depending on the neuromuscular blocker used. Nitrous oxide has minimal effects.

—Tubocurarine and pancuronium are potentiated the most by inhalational agents, whereas atracurium and vecuronium are intensified significantly less.

—Potentiation by inhalational agents occurs through depression of spinal cord reflexes as well as effects at or distal to the neuromuscular junction.

Metocurine and diphenylhydantoin, phenytoin

—Patients on chronic phenytoin therapy may be resistant to non-depolarizing muscle blockade. The studies involved metocurine and vecuronium but may involve other nondepolarizing agents.

—The mechanism of this interaction is not known.

—Acute infusions of phenytoin may prolong non-depolarizing blockade. This was studied prospectively in a small number of patients who received a 10 mg/kg loading dose of phenytoin during steady-state muscle blockade with vecuronium. They had significant potentiation of their neuromuscular block compared to control patients.

Metocurine and furosemide

—Furosemide may potentiate neuromuscular blockade from tubocurarine and succinylcholine. This is based on a case report of several patients given furosemide and tubocurarine during surgery and on animal studies.

—The implication for this interaction for other neuromuscular blocking drugs is uncertain and the mechanism is not known.

Metocurine and lidocaine
—Most local anesthetics can block neuromuscular transmission from non-depolarizing agents as well as depolarizing muscle relaxants. Of clinical significance to the anesthesiologist, lidocaine, given as a 50- to 100- mg bolus or even by infusion, can significantly increase a non-depolarizer block or a phase II block from succinylcholine.

Metocurine and procainamide
—Procainamide can potentiate muscle relaxation from non-depolarizing agents. This is probably a result of decreased acetylcholine release at the neuromuscular junction caused by procainamide.

Metocurine and quinidine
—Quinidine, procainamide, propranolol, and most local anesthetics have been shown to enhance the neuromuscular blockade from depolarizing and non-depolarizing agents.

—A number of well-documented cases have illustrated the ability of these agents, when given in the immediate postoperative period, to convert subclinical muscle weakness from neuromuscular blocking drugs into significant muscle weakness requiring reintubation.

Metocurine and succinylcholine
—Prior administration of succinylcholine has been shown to potentiate neuromuscular blockade of some non-depolarizing agents.

—Although this interaction has been documented with pancuronium, it was not seen with doxacurium and may not be a consistent finding with non-depolarizing agents.

Metocurine Interactions with Diseases
Metocurine and advanced age
—Prolonged duration of neuromuscular blockade can be seen in older patients with several non-depolarizing agents including doxacurium, mivacurium, and rocuronium.

—In some cases, delayed onset of muscle relaxation also occurs. This has been attributed to decreased perfusion of the neuromuscular junction as a result of advanced age.

Metocurine and burns
—Patients with burn injuries are susceptible to a life-threatening hyperkalemic response to succinylcholine and can have marked resistance to non-depolarizing muscle relaxants.

—Both of these altered responses to neuromuscular blocking agents have been attributed to proliferation of extrajunctional acetylcholine receptors, similar to that in the patient with a denervation injury.

—Resistance to non-depolarizing agents appears to increase with larger area burns and in fact may not be significant in patients with less than 30% body surface area burns. In addition to proliferation of extrajunctional acetylcholine receptors, this abnormal response is probably also related to the increased metabolic rate and hepatic and renal clearance seen in burn patients. Doses of non-depolarizing agents may need to be increased by as much as 300%.

—Duration of this resistance usually is 2 months following the injury but has been reported in a patient 463 days after the burn.

Metocurine and cirrhosis, liver disease

—Prolonged neuromuscular blockade in patients with liver disease can be seen with doxacurium, mivacurium, vecuronium, pancuronium, rocuronium, and tubocurarine.

—This interaction is complex and may be due to decreased clearance, decreased hepatic uptake of the agent, or decreased synthesis of enzymes important for degradation of the neuromuscular blocker. An example of the latter is prolongation of mivacurium's duration of action as a result of decreased plasma cholinesterase from severe liver disease.

—Because of the increased volume of distribution of many drugs seen in patients with liver disease, initial doses of muscle relaxants may need to be larger than in healthy patients. Once neuromuscular blockade is achieved, recovery may be prolonged.

Metocurine and Eaton–Lambert syndrome

—Patients with Eaton–Lambert syndrome are very sensitive to both depolarizing and non-depolarizing neuromuscular blockade.

—This disorder is similar to myasthenia gravis and patients complain of skeletal muscle weakness, but it is usually associated with carcinoma (especially small cell tumors of the lung).

—If the diagnosis is known or suspected prior to surgery, reduced doses of muscle relaxants should be used. However, sometimes the diagnosis is first made when a patient has surgery for a lung tumor and has an unexpected, prolonged neuromuscular block.

—Anticholinesterases are unreliable in reversing muscle weakness.

Metocurine and hyperthyroidism, thyrotoxicosis

—Muscle weakness is commonly seen with hyperthyroidism and affects proximal muscles, usually sparing respiratory function. In some cases, myopathy is the dominant feature of thyroid hormone excess and can resemble myasthenia. Lower doses of muscle relaxants may be indicated.

Metocurine and hypokalemia

—Hypokalemia appears to potentiate the effects of neuromuscular blockade from non-depolarizing agents.

—The interaction is probably due to hyperpolarization of the muscle endplate and, therefore, resistance to depolarization. Hyperpolarization would more likely occur with more acute changes in potassium concentration because the potassium losses would be from the extracellular compartment rather than from intracellular sites.

—Chronic hypokalemia is more likely to be associated with potassium depletion from both extra- and intracellular compartments with no significant change in transmembrane potential. As a result, significant effects on neuromuscular blockade would be less likely.

Metocurine and hypothermia

—Non-depolarizing muscle blockade is prolonged by hypothermia. This interaction is a result of an effect on the neuromuscular blocking agents themselves rather than on the anticholinesterases used to reverse the neuromuscular blocking agents.

—Hypothermia appears to prolong the effect of the non-depolarizing agents by several mechanisms, including delayed metabolism into inactive metabolites as well as delayed excretion via the urinary and biliary routes.

Metocurine and malignant hyperthermia

—Anesthetic agents considered safe for use in patients with known or suspected susceptibility for developing malignant hyperthermia (MH) include propofol, barbiturates, etomidate, ketamine, non-depolarizing neuromuscular blocking agents, narcotics, benzodiazepines, droperidol, epinephrine, norepinephrine, and anticholinesterases.

—Nitrous oxide is probably safe in the susceptible patient based on repeated use in MH-susceptible humans and swine.

—Local or regional anesthesia with either amide (such as lidocaine) or ester (such as procaine) anesthetics is now considered safe for MH-susceptible patients.

Metocurine and myasthenia gravis

—Patients with myasthenia gravis are very sensitive to neuromuscular blockade from non-depolarizing agents.

—This is probably a result of decreased acetylcholine receptors from autoimmune destruction associated with myasthenia gravis.

—Although these patients are treated with the same or similar anticholinesterases used to antagonize muscle blockade, sensitivity (not resistance) to neuromuscular blockade is seen clinically.

Metocurine and neuromuscular disease (amyotrophic lateral sclerosis, multiple sclerosis, syringomyelia)

—Patients with a wide variety of neuromuscular disorders may be more resistant than normal patients to the effects of non-depolarizing neuromuscular blockers.

—This includes patients with disuse atrophy of the muscles (such as bedridden patients with chronic disease) as well as patients with upper or lower motor neuron disease such as amyotrophic lateral sclerosis, multiple sclerosis, or syringomyelia.

—Disuse or denervation of muscle results in production of extrajunctional acetylcholine receptors on the muscle membrane. These receptors are less easily blocked by non-depolarizing agents but are activated by lower concentrations of depolarizing drugs (succinylcholine).

—When these receptors, which can be scattered over a large surface of the muscle, are depolarized by succinylcholine, ion flow takes place through the receptor channel. Large amounts of potassium may exit the muscle cell, causing hyperkalemia.

—Despite initial resistance to blockade, such patients may demonstrate prolonged neuromuscular weakness as a result of decreased muscle strength and mass.

Metocurine and PIH (pregnancy-induced hypertension), preeclampsia/eclampsia, toxemia

—Patients with hypertensive disorders of pregnancy may require treatment with antihypertensives such as trimethaphan or magnesium sulfate (for preeclampsia/eclampsia). These medications can have significant interactions with anesthetic agents such as succinylcholine, non-depolarizing neuromuscular blocking agents, or calcium channel blockers.

—Neuromuscular blockade produced by both depolarizing and non-depolarizing agents can be potentiated in patients receiving magnesium sulfate. The mechanisms involved include a decreased amount of acetylcholine released by the nerve impulse at the motor nerve terminal and a decrease in the depolarizing action of acetylcholine on the muscle.

Metocurine Interactions with Patient Drugs
Metocurine and antibiotics

—A number of antibiotics have significant interactions with neuromuscular blocking agents.

—These include the aminoglycosides (amikacin, gentamicin, kanamycin, neomycin, paromomycin, netilmicin, neomycin, streptomycin, tobramycin), as well as polymyxin B, colistin, amphotericin B, clindamycin, bacitracin, and lincomycin.

—All of the above antibiotics may potentiate non-depolarizing agents, but some (aminoglycosides, amphotericin B, clindamycin, colistin) can also potentiate succinylcholine blockade.

—These antibiotics potentiate neuromuscular blockade by different mechanisms, making management of these problems difficult. Although treatment with anticholinesterases or calcium has been recommended, results are inconsistent.

Metocurine and amphotericin B

—Prolonged neuromuscular blockade can occur with depolarizing and non-depolarizing agents in patients receiving amphotericin B.

—The mechanism for this interaction is thought to be associated with the hypokalemia that can be caused by amphotericin B therapy.

Metocurine and beta blockers, propranolol

—Beta blockers may potentiate non-depolarizing neuromuscular blocking agents. This interaction has been reported between propranolol and tubocurarine.

—Other beta blockers are also capable of causing weakness in patients with myasthenia gravis, but the mechanism or significance of these interactions is unclear.

Metocurine and calcium channel blockers (amlodipine, bepridil, diltiazem, felodipine, isradipine, lidoflazine, nicardipine, nimodipine, nisoldipine, nitrendipine, verapamil)

—Calcium channel blockers have been associated with prolongation of neuromuscular blockade from non-depolarizing agents.

—This interaction is probably related to the depletion of intracellular calcium associated with chronic therapy. This can result in a decrease in acetylcholine release at the neuromuscular junction.

Metocurine and diphenylhydantoin, phenytoin

—Patients on chronic phenytoin therapy may be resistant to non-depolarizing muscle blockade. The studies involved metocurine and vecuronium, but may involve other nondepolarizing agents.

—The mechanism of this interaction is not known.

—Acute infusions of phenytoin may prolong non-depolarizing blockade. This was studied prospectively in a small number of patients who received a 10 mg/kg loading dose of phenytoin during steady-state muscle blockade with vecuronium. They had significant potentiation of their neuromuscular block compared to control patients.

Metocurine and lidocaine

—Most local anesthetics can block neuromuscular transmission from non-depolarizing agents as well as depolarizing muscle relaxants. Of clinical significance to the anesthesiologist, lidocaine, given as a 50- to 100-mg bolus or even by infusion, can significantly increase a non-depolarizer block or a phase II block from succinylcholine.

Metocurine and lithium

—Lithium has been reported to increase the duration of both non-depolarizing and depolarizing neuromuscular blocking drugs.

—The mechanism of this interaction is unknown and the clinical significance of this interaction is uncertain.

Metocurine and magnesium sulfate

—Neuromuscular blockade produced by both depolarizing and non-depolarizing agents can be potentiated in patients receiving magnesium sulfate. The mechanisms involved include a decreased amount of acetylcholine released by the nerve impulse at the motor nerve terminal and a decrease in the depolarizing action of acetylcholine on the muscle.

Metocurine and mexilitene
—Mexilitene, like lidocaine and most local anesthetics, can potentiate neuromuscular blockade from depolarizing and non-depolarizing agents.

Metocurine and procainamide
—Procainamide can potentiate muscle relaxation from non-depolarizing agents. This is probably a result of decreased acetylcholine release at the neuromuscular junction caused by procainamide.

Metocurine and quinidine
—Quinidine and quinine can potentiate muscle relaxation from both depolarizing and non-depolarizing agents.
—The mechanism of this interaction is a curare-like action at the myoneural junction. Also, plasma pseudo-cholinesterase is inhibited by quinidine (and quinine), resulting in possible prolongation of muscle relaxation from succinylcholine.

Metocurine and tocainide
—Tocainide, an orally active form of lidocaine, can potentiate both depolarizing and non-depolarizing neuromuscular blockade. This is a property of most local anesthetics as well as a number of other medications.

MIDAZOLAM (Versed)

Classification and indications
—Midazolam is a benzodiazepine.
—It is indicated for use as a preoperative sedative, for intraoperative use as part of a general anesthetic, or for conscious sedation.

Pharmacology
—Benzodiazepines apparently exert some of their effects through GABA (gamma aminobutyric acid), but the exact mechanism of action is not known.
—Absorption after intramuscular injection is reliable and rapid with lorazepam and midazolam, but not with other benzodiazepines.
—Onset of sedative, anxiolytic, and anticonvulsant action is from 1 to 5 minutes after intravenous administration. Duration varies from 15 minutes to 1 hour for chlor-

diazepoxide and diazepam, <2 hours for midazolam, and 12–24 hours after IV lorazepam.

—Because benzodiazepines are metabolized in the liver, patients with liver disease can experience prolonged effects from usual doses. Also, geriatric patients may have prolonged elimination times.

Dose

—For preoperative sedation:

  —Adults: 70–80 μg/kg (up to 5 mg) 30–60 minutes before surgery. Patients who are >60 years, sicker, or receiving other sedatives or narcotics should receive lower doses.

  —Children: 50–75 μg/kg orally with some liquid (15 mL grape juice) 30 minutes before surgery.

—Conscious sedation:

  —Bolus: 1–2.5 mg intravenously. Patients who are >60 years, sicker, or receiving other sedatives or narcotics should receive lower doses.

  —Induction of general anesthesia: 150–300 μg/kg, depending on the patient's age, severity of disease, or presence of other sedatives or narcotics.

Midazolam Interactions with Diseases

Midazolam and advanced age

—Elderly patients may have decreased requirements for benzodiazepines.

—The exact mechanism for this response is controversial but may be related to decreased metabolism of this class of drugs. Alternatively, some elderly patients may be more sensitive to the CNS effects of these medications.

Midazolam and alcohol—acute intoxication

—Patients who are acutely intoxicated with alcohol (including chronic alcoholics) usually demonstrate increased sensitivity to general anesthesia.

—Although the precise mechanism of interactions are not agreed on, it appears that alcohol intoxication has additive CNS depression with barbiturates, benzodiazepines, and narcotics, as well as inhalational agents.

Midazolam and alcohol—chronic abuse

—Chronic abuse of alcohol has complex and incompletely understood effects on a patient's response to anesthetic agents. In general, these patients tend to be more tolerant (in a nonintoxicated state) to barbiturates, benzodiazepines, narcotics, and inhalational agents.

—Exceptions to this generalization include the alcoholic patient with a cardiomyopathy who may demonstrate increased sensitivity to myocardial depression from inhalational agents.

—Also, the patient with severe liver disease may have impaired ability to metabolize succinylcholine due to decreased levels of plasma pseudocholinesterase.

Midazolam and cerebral edema, intracranial hypertension

—Most intravenous anesthetics cause a reduction in cerebral blood flow (CBF) and intracranial pressure (ICP) or have no effect on ICP. Although this effect is primarily from depression of cerebral metabolic rate (CMR), in some cases a direct vasoconstriction occurs.

—The exception to the above is ketamine, which causes an increased CMR and CBF with an increase in ICP.

—All of the narcotics, as well as barbiturates, etomidate, benzodiazepines, and propofol, have been associated with a reduction or maintenance of ICP during anesthesia.

Midazolam and cirrhosis, liver disease

—The benzodiazepines are metabolized extensively in the liver and patients with cirrhosis will demonstrate more prolonged effects of this class of drugs.

Midazolam and malignant hyperthermia

—Anesthetic agents considered safe for use in patients with known or suspected susceptibility for developing malignant hyperthermia (MH) include propofol, barbiturates, etomidate, ketamine, non-depolarizing neuromuscular blocking agents, narcotics, benzodiazepines, droperidol, epinephrine, norepinephrine, and anticholinesterases.

—Nitrous oxide is probably safe in the susceptible patient based on repeated use in MH-susceptible humans and swine.

—Local or regional anesthesia with either amide (such as lidocaine) or ester (such as procaine) anesthetics is now considered safe for MH-susceptible patients.

Midazolam and porphyria

—Benzodiazepines are considered to be questionable triggering agents for porphyria. This is based on their ability to provoke attacks of porphyria in rat models, though use in humans has not been associated with this reaction.

—Not all of the porphyrias have significance for the anesthesiologist. Three of the four hepatic porphyrias (acute intermittent, variegate, hereditary coproporphyria) and none of the erythropoietic porphyrias are associated with neurologic symptoms that can be triggered by certain medications: barbiturates, etomidate, and corticosteroids.

—Benzodiazepines and etomidate are considered to be questionable triggering agents, whereas safe anesthetics are inhalational agents, narcotics, muscle relaxants, anticholinesterases, and propofol.

Midazolam and pregnancy

—Benzodiazepines may cause damage to the fetus, especially during the first trimester of pregnancy.

—Retrospective studies of chlordiazepoxide and diazepam have shown an increased risk of congenital malformations when administered to pregnant patients in their first trimester of pregnancy.

—Administration of preoperative benzodiazepines for obstetric procedures (such as caesarean sections) may produce CNS depression in neonates.

Midazolam and renal dysfunction

—Renal dysfunction has not been demonstrated to cause significant changes in pharmacokinetics or pharmacodynamics of benzodiazepines, narcotics (with the possible exception of butorphanol), barbiturates, or propofol.

—In patients with renal dysfunction, the above drugs may appear to have an increase in duration or intensity. This has been explained as a response to the systemic effects of renal dysfunction rather than specific effects on the metabolism of theses drugs.

—Some muscle relaxants are significantly affected by renal failure.

Midazolam Interactions with Patient Drugs

Midazolam and diphenylhydantoin, phenytoin

—Benzodiazepines, when given to a patient on chronic diphenylhydantoin therapy, may cause an increased serum level of diphenylhydantoin. This may be due to a decrease in the metabolism of diphenylhydantoin caused by benzodiazepines.

—The half-life of benzodiazepines can be decreased in patients on chronic diphenylhydantoin therapy.

Midazolam and erythromycin

—Erythromycin may potentiate and prolong the effects of midazolam. This effect has been documented in both a controlled study and a case report of orally administered midazolam.

—The interaction can apparently occur with both oral and intravenous erythromycin and, in the case report, the intravenous erythromycin can alter midazolam pharmacokinetics even when given shortly following the midazolam.

—Erythromycin may alter midazolam metabolism by interfering with the cytochrome P450 isoenzyme that affects midazolam metabolism.

MIVACURIUM (Mivacron)

Classification and indications

—Mivacurium is a non-depolarizing neuromuscular blocking agent.

—It is indicated for skeletal muscle relaxation for intubation and during surgery.

Pharmacology

—Mivacurium competes with acetylcholine for binding at the acetylcholine receptor at the neuromuscular junction of skeletal muscle.

—Histamine release occurs with doses greater than 0.2 mg/kg and may result in decreases in mean arterial blood pressure. This effect may be reduced by slow injection of mivacurium over 30–60 seconds.

—Doses of 0.25 mg/kg can produce intubating conditions within 1.5–2 minutes with a duration of about 25 minutes (25% recovery of twitch height).

—Repeated dosing or infusion for up to 2.5 hours has not been associated with cumulative muscle blockade.

—Elimination of mivacurium is a result of hydrolysis by plasma cholinesterase. Reduced levels of this enzyme can be seen in patients with inherited defects of plasma cholinesterase as well as patients with severe liver disease.

—These patients can experience duration of blockade from mivacurium about three times that of healthy patients.

—Patients with renal disease will have a duration of muscle blockade about 1.5 times that of normal patients.

—Elderly patients may have a 15–20% prolongation in muscle blockade compared to young patients.

—Children (age 2–12) have a faster onset of blockade and a shorter duration of action.

Dose

—Intubation: 0.15–0.3 mg/kg

—Infusion: Average dose is 6–7 µg/kg/min.

Mivacurium Interactions with Anesthesia Drugs

Mivacurium and calcium channel blockers (diltiazem, nicardipine, nifedipine, verapamil)

—Calcium channel blockers have been associated with prolongation of neuromuscular blockade from non-depolarizing agents.

—This interaction is probably related to the depletion of intracellular calcium associated with chronic therapy. This can result in a decrease in acetylcholine release at the neuromuscular junction.

Mivacurium and inhalational anesthetics (desflurane, enflurane, halothane, isoflurane, sevoflurane)

—Desflurane, enflurane, halothane, isoflurane, and sevoflurane can significantly potentiate neuromuscular blockade, depending on the neuromuscular blocker used. Nitrous oxide has minimal effects.

—Tubocurarine and pancuronium are potentiated the most by inhalational agents, whereas atracurium and vecuronium are intensified significantly less.

—Potentiation by inhalational agents occurs through depression of spinal cord reflexes as well as effects at or distal to the neuromuscular junction.

Mivacurium and diphenylhydantoin, phenytoin

—Patients on chronic phenytoin therapy may be resistant to non-depolarizing muscle blockade. The studies involved metocurine and vecuronium but may involve other non-depolarizing agents.

—The mechanism of this interaction is not known.

—Acute infusions of phenytoin may prolong non-depolarizing blockade. This was studied prospectively in a small number of patients who received a 10 mg/kg loading dose of phenytoin during steady-state muscle blockade with vecuronium. They had significant potentiation of their neuromuscular block compared to control patients.

Mivacurium and furosemide

—Furosemide may potentiate neuromuscular blockade from tubocurarine and succinylcholine.

—This is based on a case report of several patients given furosemide and tubocurarine during surgery and on animal studies.

—The implication for this interaction for other neuromuscular blocking drugs is uncertain and the mechanism is not known.

Mivacurium and lidocaine

—Most local anesthetics can block neuromuscular transmission from non-depolarizing agents as well as depolarizing muscle relaxants. Of clinical significance to the anesthesiologist, lidocaine, given as a 50- to 100-mg bolus or even by infusion, can significantly increase a non-depolarizer block or a phase II block from succinylcholine.

Mivacurium and procainamide

—Procainamide can potentiate muscle relaxation from non-depolarizing ,agents. This is probably a result of decreased acetylcholine release at the neuromuscular junction caused by procainamide.

Mivacurium and quinidine

—Quinidine, procainamide, propranolol, and most local anesthetics have been shown to enhance the neuromuscular blockade from depolarizing and non-depolarizing agents.

—A number of well-documented cases have illustrated the ability of these agents, when given in the immediate postoperative period, to convert subclinical muscle weakness from neuromuscular blocking drugs into significant muscle weakness requiring reintubation.

Mivacurium and succinylcholine

—Prior administration of succinylcholine has been shown to potentiate neuromuscular blockade of some non-depolarizing agents.

—Although this interaction has been documented with pancuronium, it was not seen with doxacurium and may not be a consistent finding with non-depolarizing agents.

Mivacurium Interactions with Diseases

Mivacurium and advanced age

—Prolonged duration of neuromuscular blockade can be seen in older patients with several different non-depolarizing agents including doxacurium, mivacurium, and rocuronium.

—In some cases, delayed onset of muscle relaxation also occurs. This has been attributed to decreased perfusion of the neuromuscular junction as a result of advanced age.

Mivacurium and burns

—Patients with burn injuries are susceptible to a life-threatening hyperkalemic response to succinylcholine and can have marked resistance to non-depolarizing muscle relaxants.

—Both of these altered responses to neuromuscular blocking agents have been attributed to proliferation of extrajunctional acetylcholine receptors, similar to the patient with a denervation injury.

—Resistance to non-depolarizing agents appears to increase with larger area burns and, in fact, may not be significant in patients with <30% body surface area burns. In addition to proliferation of extrajunctional acetylcholine receptors, this abnormal response is probably also related to the increased metabolic rate and hepatic and renal clearance seen in burn patients. Doses of non-depolarizing agents may need to be increased by as much as 300%.

—Duration of this resistance usually is 2 months following the injury but has been reported in a patient 463 days after the burn.

Mivacurium and cirrhosis, liver disease

—Prolonged neuromuscular blockade in patients with liver disease can be seen with doxacurium, mivacurium, vecuronium, pancuronium, rocuronium, and tubocurarine.

—This interaction is complex and may be due to decreased clearance, decreased hepatic uptake of the agent, or decreased synthesis of enzymes important for degradation of the neuromuscular blocker. An example of the latter is prolongation of mivacurium's duration of action as a result of decreased plasma cholinesterase from severe liver disease.

—Because of the increased volume of distribution of many drugs seen in patients with liver disease, initial doses of muscle relaxants may need to be larger than in healthy patients. Once neuromuscular blockade is achieved, recovery may be prolonged.

Mivacurium and Eaton–Lambert syndrome

—Patients with Eaton–Lambert syndrome are very sensitive to both depolarizing and non-depolarizing neuromuscular blockade.

—This disorder is similar to myasthenia gravis and patients complain of skeletal muscle weakness, but it is usually associated with carcinoma (especially small cell tumors of the lung).

—If the diagnosis is known or suspected prior to surgery, reduced doses of muscle relaxants should be used, but sometimes the diagnosis is first made when a patient has surgery for a lung tumor and has an unexpected, prolonged neuromuscular block.

—Anticholinesterases are unreliable in reversing muscle weakness.

Mivacurium and hyperthyroidism, thyrotoxicosis

—Muscle weakness is commonly seen with hyperthyroidism and affects proximal muscles, usually sparing respiratory function. In some cases, myopathy is the dominant feature of thyroid hormone excess and can resemble myasthenia. Lower doses of muscle relaxants may be indicated.

Mivacurium and hypokalemia

—Hypokalemia appears to potentiate the effects of neuromuscular blockade from non-depolarizing agents.

—The interaction is probably due to hyperpolarization of the muscle endplate and, therefore, resistance to depolarization. Hyperpolarization would more likely occur with more acute changes in potassium concentration since the potassium losses would be from the extracellular compartment rather than from intracellular sites.

—Chronic hypokalemia is more likely to be associated with potassium depletion from both extra- and intracellular compartments with no significant change in transmembrane potential. As a result, significant effects on neuromuscular blockade would be less likely.

Mivacurium and hypothermia

—Non-depolarizing muscle blockade is prolonged by hypothermia. This interaction is a result of an effect on the neuromuscular blocking agents themselves rather than on the anticholinesterases used to reverse the neuromuscular blocking agents.

—Hypothermia appears to prolong the effect of the non-depolarizing agents by several mechanisms, including delayed metabolism into inactive metabolites as well as delayed excretion via the urinary and biliary routes.

Mivacurium and malignant hyperthermia

—Anesthetic agents considered safe for use in patients with known or suspected susceptibility for developing malignant hyperthermia (MH) include propofol, barbiturates, etomidate, ketamine, non-depolarizing neuromuscular blocking agents, narcotics, benzodiazepines, droperidol, epinephrine, norepinephrine, and anticholinesterases.

—Nitrous oxide is probably safe in the susceptible patient based on repeated use in MH-susceptible humans and swine.

—Local or regional anesthesia with either amide (such as lidocaine) or ester (such as procaine) anesthetics is now considered safe for MH-susceptible patients.

Mivacurium and myasthenia gravis

—Patients with myasthenia gravis are very sensitive to neuromuscular blockade from non-depolarizing agents.

—This is probably a result of decreased acetylcholine receptors from autoimmune destruction associated with myasthenia gravis.

—Although these patients are treated with the same or similar anticholinesterases used to antagonize muscle blockade, sensitivity (not resistance) to neuromuscular blockade is seen clinically.

Mivacurium and neuromuscular disease (amyotrophic lateral sclerosis, multiple sclerosis, syringomyelia)

—Patients with a wide variety of neuromuscular disorders may be more resistant than normal patients to the effects of non-depolarizing neuromuscular blockers.

—This includes patients with disuse atrophy of the muscles (such as bedridden patients with chronic disease) as well as patients with upper or lower motor neuron disease such as amyotrophic lateral sclerosis, multiple sclerosis, or syringomyelia.

—Disuse or denervation of muscle results in production of extrajunctional acetylcholine receptors on the muscle membrane. These receptors are less easily blocked by non-depolarizing agents but are activated by lower concentrations of depolarizing drugs (succinylcholine).

—When these receptors, which can be scattered over a large surface of the muscle, are depolarized by succinylcholine, ion flow takes place through the receptor channel. Large amounts of potassium may exit the muscle cell causing hyperkalemia.

—Despite initial resistance to blockade, such patients may demonstrate prolonged neuromuscular weakness as a result of decreased muscle strength and mass.

Mivacurium and PIH (pregnancy-induced hypertension), preeclampsia/eclampsia, toxemia

—Patients with hypertensive disorders of pregnancy may require treatment with antihypertensives such as trimethaphan or magnesium sulfate (for preeclampsia/eclampsia). These medications can have significant interactions with anesthetic agents such as succinylcholine, non-depolarizing neuromuscular blocking agents, or calcium channel blockers.

—Neuromuscular blockade produced by both depolarizing and non-depolarizing agents can be potentiated in patients receiving magnesium sulfate. The mechanisms involved include a decreased amount of acetylcholine released by the nerve impulse at the motor nerve terminal and a decrease in the depolarizing action of acetylcholine on the muscle.

Mivacurium Interactions with Patient Drugs

Mivacurium and antibiotics

—A number of antibiotics have significant interactions with neuromuscular blocking agents.

—These include the aminoglycosides (amikacin, gentamicin, kanamycin, neomycin, paromomycin, netilmicin, neomycin, streptomycin, tobramycin), as well as polymyxin B, colistin, amphotericin B, clindamycin, bacitracin, and lincomycin.

—All of the above antibiotics may potentiate non-depolarizing agents, but some (aminoglycosides, amphotericin B, clindamycin, colistin) can also potentiate succinylcholine blockade.

—These antibiotics potentiate neuromuscular blockade by different mechanisms, making management of these problems difficult. Although treatment with anticholinesterases or calcium has been recommended, results are inconsistent.

Mivacurium and amphotericin B

—Prolonged neuromuscular blockade can occur with depolarizing and non-depolarizing agents in patients receiving amphotericin B.

—The mechanism for this interaction is thought to be associated with the hypokalemia that can be caused by amphotericin B therapy.

Mivacurium and beta blockers, propranolol

—Beta blockers may potentiate non-depolarizing neuromuscular blocking agents. This interaction has been reported between propranolol and tubocurarine.

—Other beta blockers are also capable of causing weakness in patients with myasthenia gravis, but the mechanism or significance of these interactions is unclear.

Mivacurium and calcium channel blockers (amlodipine, bepridil, diltiazem, felodipine, isradipine, lidoflazine, nicardipine, nimodipine, nisoldipine, nitrendipine, verapamil)

—Calcium channel blockers have been associated with prolongation of neuromuscular blockade from non-depolarizing agents.

—This interaction is probably related to the depletion of intracellular calcium associated with chronic therapy. This can result in a decrease in acetylcholine release at the neuromuscular junction.

Mivacurium and diphenylhydantoin, phenytoin

—Patients on chronic phenytoin therapy may be resistant to non-depolarizing muscle blockade. The studies involved metocurine and vecuronium but may involve other non-depolarizing agents.

—The mechanism of this interaction is not known.

—Acute infusions of phenytoin may prolong non-depolarizing blockade. This was studied prospectively in a small number of patients who received a 10 mg/kg loading dose of phenytoin during steady-state muscle blockade with vecuronium. They had significant potentiation of their neuromuscular block compared to control patients.

Mivacurium and lidocaine

—Most local anesthetics can block neuromuscular transmission from non-depolarizing agents as well as depolarizing muscle relaxants. Of clinical significance to the anesthesiologist, lidocaine, given as a 50- to 100-mg bolus or even by infusion, can significantly increase a non-depolarizer block or a phase II block from succinylcholine.

Mivacurium and lithium
—Lithium has been reported to increase the duration of both non-depolarizing and depolarizing neuromuscular blocking drugs.
—The mechanism of this interaction is unknown and the clinical significance of this interaction is uncertain.

Mivacurium and magnesium sulfate
—Neuromuscular blockade produced by both depolarizing and non-depolarizing agents can be potentiated in patients receiving magnesium sulfate. The mechanisms involved include a decreased amount of acetylcholine released by the nerve impulse at the motor nerve terminal and a decrease in the depolarizing action of acetylcholine on the muscle.

Mivacurium and mexilitene
—Mexilitene, like lidocaine and most local anesthetics, can potentiate neuromuscular blockade from depolarizing and non-depolarizing agents.

Mivacurium and procainamide
—Procainamide can potentiate muscle relaxation from non-depolarizing agents. This is probably a result of decreased acetylcholine release at the neuromuscular junction caused by procainamide.

Mivacurium and quinidine
—Quinidine and quinine can potentiate muscle relaxation from both depolarizing and nondepolarizing agents.
—The mechanism of this interaction is a curare-like action at the myoneural junction. Also, plasma pseudocholinesterase is inhibited by quinidine (and quinine), resulting in possible prolongation of muscle relaxation from succinylcholine.

Mivacurium and tocainide
—Tocainide, an orally active form of lidocaine, can potentiate both depolarizing and non-depolarizing neuromuscular blockade. This is a property of most local anesthetics as well as a number of other medications.

MORPHINE (Astramorph, Duramorph, Infumorph)

Classification and indications
—Morphine is an opium alkaloid derived from the poppy plant (heroin is a derivative of morphine).

—It is indicated for analgesia or preoperative sedation. As a preservative-free formulation, it is used in the epidural or subarachnoid space for analgesia.

Pharmacology

—Morphine, like other narcotics, exerts its analgesic effects through opioid receptors in the CNS (brain and spinal cord).

—Although narcotics used in anesthesia are potent analgesics, there is controversy about the level of amnesia induced with even large doses of narcotics. To avoid awareness during anesthesia, use of other anesthetic agents (benzodiazepines, inhalation agents, etc.) is recommended.

—Somatosensory evoked potentials (SEPs) are not significantly affected by narcotics.

—Although there is some controversy about increases in intracranial pressure from opioids, in general, opioids cause slight decreases in cerebral blood flow, metabolic rate, and intracranial pressure.

—Cardiovascular effects of morphine include hypotension, which results from histamine release (causing arteriolar dilation) and venodilation. Bradycardia, especially after rapid administration, probably results from decreased central sympathetic outflow and/or central vagal stimulation.

—Like other narcotics, morphine causes respiratory depression and reduced hypoxic ventilatory drive.

—Muscle rigidity, particularly of the chest wall, has been associated with rapid administration of narcotics. The mechanism of this action is not clear, but older patients seem more prone to this response. It has also been associated most frequently with alfentanil.

—Muscle rigidity can occur not only during induction but also on emergence from anesthesia or, rarely, hours after the last opioid dose.

—Onset of analgesia following intravenous morphine is within minutes, with an elimination half-life of 2–4 hours.

—Correlation of elimination half-life with clinical duration is unpredictable. In the case of morphine, clinical duration is about 4 hours, whereas that of meperidine is approximately 2–4 hours.

—For comparison, the elimination half-lives of fentanyl, sufentanil, and alfentanil are 219, 164, and 90 minutes, respectively.

—Epidural injection of morphine results in prolonged (up to 20 hours) levels in the cerebrospinal fluid (CSF). Peak CSF concentrations occur after about 60–90 minutes following epidural injection of morphine.

—Subarachnoid (intrathecal) injection of morphine requires much lower doses for analgesia than other routes because of the lack of meningeal barriers with intrathecal dosing.

—Correlation of elimination half-life with clinical duration is unpredictable. In the case of IV morphine, clinical duration is about 4 hours, whereas that of meperidine is approximately 2–4 hours.

—For comparison, the elimination half-lives of fentanyl, sufentanil, and alfentanil are 219, 164, and 90 minutes, respectively.

—Elimination of morphine is mainly a result of hepatic metabolism.

Dose

—Intravenous:

—Adults:

—Bolus: 2–5 mg IV slowly every 5 minutes as necessary to control pain.

—Infusion: 0.8–10 mg/hr IV. Chronic pain patients usually require much higher doses.

—Children: 0.05–0.1 mg/kg (up to 15 mg) IV slowly every 2–4 hours.

—Epidural:

—Bolus: 5 mg (usual adult dose).

—Infusion: 0.5 mg/hr (usual adult dose).

—Subarachnoid: 0.1–0.3 mg.

Morphine Interactions with Anesthesia Drugs

Morphine and clonidine

—Clonidine has been shown to potentiate narcotics and reduce the MAC of inhaled anesthetics.

—This effect may be related to clonidine's inhibition of the sympathetic outflow from the vasomotor center in the medulla (clonidine is a central alpha 2 receptor agonist, which results in inhibition of CNS sympathetic centers).

Morphine and esmolol

—Coadministration of esmolol and morphine has resulted in significant increases (up to almost 50%) in steady-state levels of esmolol, but not morphine.

Morphine and naloxone
—Use of naloxone in postoperative patients for reversal of respiratory depression has resulted in cases of pulmonary edema in some cases.
—The etiology of this interaction is not completely understood.

Morphine Interactions with Diseases
Morphine and advanced age
—Elderly patients may require lower doses of narcotics than younger adults.
—This may be a result of reduced metabolism of this class of drugs or represent an increased brain sensitivity to narcotics as a result of aging.

Morphine and alcohol—acute intoxication
—Patients who are acutely intoxicated with alcohol (including chronic alcoholics) usually demonstrate increased sensitivity to general anesthesia.
—Although the precise mechanism of interactions are not agreed on, it appears that alcohol intoxication has additive CNS depression with barbiturates, benzodiazepines, and narcotics, as well as inhalational agents.

Morphine and alcohol—chronic abuse
—Chronic abuse of alcohol has complex and incompletely understood effects on a patient's response to anesthetic agents. In general, these patients tend to be more tolerant (in a nonintoxicated state) to barbiturates, benzodiazepines, narcotics, and inhalational agents.
—Exceptions to this generalization include the alcoholic patient with a cardiomyopathy who may demonstrate increased sensitivity to myocardial depression from inhalational agents.
—Also, the patient with severe liver disease may have impaired ability to metabolize succinylcholine due to decreased levels of plasma pseudocholinesterase.

Morphine and cerebral edema, intracranial hypertension
—Most intravenous anesthetics cause a reduction in cerebral blood flow (CBF) and intracranial pressure (ICP) or have no effect on ICP. Although this effect is primarily from depression of cerebral metabolic rate (CMR), in some cases a direct vasoconstriction occurs.
—The exception to the above is ketamine, which causes an increased CMR and CBF with an increase in ICP.

—All the narcotics, as well as barbiturates, etomidate, benzo-diazepines, and propofol, have been associated with a reduction or maintenance of ICP during anesthesia.

Morphine and herpes simplex

—There are several reports of patients receiving epidural morphine who developed reactivation of herpes labialis (oral herpes; herpes simplex virus, type 1).

—In addition, several studies suggested a possible central triggering mechanism for this interaction, though no definite relationship has been proven.

—The original case report involved children who had received subarachnoid morphine.

—There is some controversy about this since activation of HSV can result from other causes including infections, fever, emotional or physical stress, and surgery.

—Also a high percentage of herpes-infected women experience recurrence in the peripartum period even without having received epidural or intrathecal narcotics.

Morphine and malignant hyperthermia

—Anesthetic agents considered safe for use in patients with known or suspected susceptibility for developing malignant hyperthermia (MH) include propofol, barbiturates, etomidate, ketamine, non-depolarizing neuromuscular blocking agents, narcotics, benzodiazepines, droperidol, epinephrine, norepinephrine, and anticholinesterases.

—Nitrous oxide is probably safe in the susceptible patient based on repeated use in MH-susceptible humans and swine.

—Local or regional anesthesia with either amide (such as lidocaine) or ester (such as procaine) anesthetics is now considered safe for MH-susceptible patients.

Morphine and porphyria

—Narcotics are considered safe anesthetics for use in porphyrias.

—Not all of the porphyrias have significance for the anesthesiologist. Three of the four hepatic porphyrias (acute intermittent, variegate, hereditary coproporphyria) and none of the erythropoietic porphyrias are associated with neurologic symptoms that can be triggered by certain medications: barbiturates, etomidate, and corticosteroids.

—Benzodiazepines and etomidate are considered to be questionable triggering agents, while safe anesthetics are inhalational agents, narcotics, muscle relaxants, anticholinester-ases, and propofol.

Morphine and pregnancy

—Reactivation of oral herpes simplex virus (HSV-1) in post-caesarean section patients has been associated with admin-istration of epidural or intrathecal morphine. There is apparently no association with recurrence of genital her-pes.

—There is some controversy about this because activation of HSV can result from other causes including infections, fever, emotional or physical stress, and surgery. Also a high percentage of herpes-infected women experience recurrence in the peripartum period even without having received epidural or intrathecal narcotics.

Morphine and renal dysfunction

—Renal dysfunction has not been demonstrated to cause sig-nificant changes in pharmacokinetics or pharmacodynamics of benzodiazepines, narcotics (with the possible exception of butorphanol), barbiturates, or propofol.

—In patients with renal dysfunction, the above drugs may appear to have an increase in duration or intensity. This has been explained as a response to the systemic effects of renal dysfunction rather than specific effects on the metabolism of theses drugs.

—Some muscle relaxants are significantly affected by renal failure.

Morphine Interactions with Patient Drugs

Morphine and cimetidine

—Cimetidine may potentiate narcotics, causing greater respi-ratory depression and sedation than expected. This may be related to the alteration of hepatic metabolism of narcotics produced by cimetidine.

—This effect is seen less with morphine than other narcotics and is probably related to the fact that morphine undergoes a different metabolic process than some other narcotics such as fentanyl or meperidine.

—Ranitidine is not associated with this interaction.

Morphine and clonidine

—Clonidine has been shown to potentiate narcotics and reduce the MAC of inhaled anesthetics.

—This effect may be related to clonidine's inhibition of the sympathetic outflow from the vasomotor center in the medulla (clonidine is a central alpha 2 receptor agonist, which results in inhibition of CNS sympathetic centers).

NALBUPHINE (Nubain)

Classification and indications
—Nalbuphine is a synthetic narcotic agonist–antagonist.
—It is indicated for relief of moderate to severe pain and is also used as part of a general anesthetic.

Pharmacology
—Nalbuphine is thought to exert its narcotic agonist activity by interaction with the kappa receptor and its antagonist activity via the mu receptors of the CNS.
—Onset of analgesia occurs within 2–3 minutes after intravenous administration and lasts for 3–6 hours.
—Like buprenorphine, nalubphine may cause spasm of the sphincter of Oddi.
—Elimination of nalbuphine is a dependent on hepatic metabolism and renal excretion.

Dose
—Intravenous dose:
—For use as part of a general anesthetic: 0.3–3.0 mg/kg on induction followed by 0.25–0.5 mg/kg IV as needed

Nalbuphine Interactions with Diseases

Nalbuphine and advanced age
—Elderly patients may require lower doses of narcotics than younger adults.
—This may be a result of reduced metabolism of this class of drugs or represent an increased brain sensitivity to narcotics as a result of aging.

Nalbuphine and alcohol—acute intoxication
—Patients who are acutely intoxicated with alcohol (including chronic alcoholics) usually demonstrate increased sensitivity to general anesthesia.
—Although the precise mechanism of interactions is not agreed on, it appears that alcohol intoxication has additive CNS depression with barbiturates, benzodiazepines, and narcotics, as well as inhalational agents.

Nalbuphine and cerebral edema, intracranial hypertension
—Most intravenous anesthetics cause a reduction in cerebral blood flow (CBF) and intracranial pressure (ICP) or have

no effect on ICP. Although this effect is primarily from depression of cerebral metabolic rate (CMR), in some cases a direct vasoconstriction occurs.

—The exception to the above is ketamine, which causes an increased CMR and CBF with an increase in ICP.

—All of the narcotics, as well as barbiturates, etomidate, benzodiazepines, and propofol, have been associated with a reduction or maintenance of ICP during anesthesia.

Nalbuphine and malignant hyperthermia

—Anesthetic agents considered safe for use in patients with known or suspected susceptibility for developing malignant hyperthermia (MH) include propofol, barbiturates, etomidate, ketamine, non-depolarizing neuromuscular blocking agents, narcotics, benzodiazepines, droperidol, epinephrine, norepinephrine, and anticholinesterases.

—Nitrous oxide is probably safe in the susceptible patient based on repeated use in MH-susceptible humans and swine.

—Local or regional anesthesia with either amide (such as lidocaine) or ester (such as procaine) anesthetics is now considered safe for MH-susceptible patients.

Nalbuphine and narcotic dependence

—Nalbuphine has both narcotic agonist and antagonist properties. Patients who are dependent on low doses of morphine (60 mg daily) demonstrate withdrawal symptoms when given nalbuphine.

—Patients addicted to other narcotics (such as methadone) may also experience withdrawal symptoms when given a narcotic agonist/antagonist (butorphanol, buprenorphine, nalbuphine).

Nalbuphine and porphyria

—Narcotics are considered safe anesthetics for use in porphyrias.

—Not all of the porphyrias have significance for the anesthesiologist. Three of the four hepatic porphyrias (acute intermittent, variegate, hereditary coproporphyria) and none of the erythropoietic porphyrias are associated with neurologic symptoms that can be triggered by certain medications: barbiturates, etomidate, and corticosteroids.

—Benzodiazepines and etomidate are considered to be questionable triggering agents, whereas safe anesthetics are inhalational agents, narcotics, muscle relaxants, anticholinesterases, and propofol.

Nalbuphine and renal dysfunction
—Renal dysfunction has not been demonstrated to cause significant changes in pharmacokinetics or pharmacodynamics of benzodiazepines, narcotics (with the possible exception of butorphanol), barbiturates, or propofol.

—In patients with renal dysfunction, the above drugs may appear to have an increase in duration or intensity. This has been explained as a response to the systemic effects of renal dysfunction rather than specific effects on the metabolism of theses drugs.

—Some muscle relaxants are significantly affected by renal failure.

Nalbuphine Interactions with Patient Drugs
Nalbuphine and methadone
—Patients who are physically dependent on methadone or other narcotics may experience withdrawal symptoms when given a narcotic with agonist/antagonist properties. This includes buprenorphine, butorphenol, and nalbuphine.

NALOXONE (Narcan)

Classification and indications
—Naloxone is an opiate antagonist.

—It is indicated for reversal of the respiratory depression produced by narcotics.

Pharmacology
—Naloxone is a virtually pure narcotic antagonist with no significant agonist properties, even at 10 times the normal therapeutic dose.

—The precise mechanism of action is unclear, though it is believed that naloxone probably is a competitive inhibitor at the opiate receptors.

—Onset of action following intravenous administration is in 1–2 minutes. A dose of 0.4 mg has a duration of about 45 minutes in an average adult (70 kg). The reported half-life is 60–90 minutes in adults and 3 hours in neonates.

—Because the duration of action of naloxone is shorter than some narcotics, renarcotization can occur in some situations.

—Cases of pulmonary edema, hypertension, and ventricular arrhythmias have occurred in postoperative patients receiving naloxone. The precise etiology of these reactions is not known.

—Elimination of naloxone is a result of rapid metabolism by the liver.

Dose

—For postoperative narcotic-induced respiratory depression:

—Adults:

—Bolus: 0.1–0.2 mg IV initially, repeated at 3- to 5-minute intervals as necessary.

—Infusion: 4 µg/kg/hr.

—Children: 5–10 µg/kg/dose, repeated at 3- to 5-minute intervals.

Naloxone Interactions with Anesthesia Drugs

Naloxone and clonidine

—Naloxone can reverse the antihypertensive effects of clonidine. Also, it may precipitate the exaggerated hypertensive response seen from sudden withdrawal of clonidine in patients on chronic therapy with the drug.

Naloxone and meperidine

—Cases of pulmonary edema, hypertension, and ventricular arrhythmias have occurred in postoperative patients receiving naloxone for reversal of respiratory depression induced by narcotics. The precise etiology of these reactions is not known.

—A patient who receives multiple doses of meperidine over a prolonged period will accumulate a metabolite called normeperidine, which is a CNS stimulant with few analgesic qualities. When naloxone is used in such patients, the result of reversing the primarily CNS depressant effect of meperidine may be seizure activity.

Naloxone and narcotics (alfentanil, fentanyl, morphine, sufentanil)

—Cases of pulmonary edema, hypertension, and ventricular arrhythmias have occurred in postoperative patients receiving naloxone for reversal of respiratory depression induced by narcotics. The precise etiology of these reactions is not known.

Naloxone Interactions with Diseases

Naloxone and narcotic dependence

—Naloxone can precipitate withdrawal symptoms in patients who are physically dependent on narcotics.

Naloxone Interactions with Patient Drugs

Naloxone and meperidine

—Cases of pulmonary edema, hypertension, and ventricular arrhythmia have occurred in postoperative patients receiving naloxone for reversal of respiratory depression induced by narcotics. The precise etiology of these reactions is not known.

—A patient who receives multiple doses of meperidine over a prolonged period will accumulate a metabolite called normeperidine, which is a CNS stimulant with little analgesic qualities. When naloxone is used in such patients, the result of reversing the primarily CNS depressant effect of meperidine may be seizure activity.

Naloxone and methadone

—Naloxone reverses the respiratory depression as well as the analgesic effects of narcotics, including methadone. In patients who are receiving methadone for treatment of narcotic addiction, naloxone can precipitate withdrawal symptoms.

Naloxone and morphine

—Use of naloxone in postoperative patients for reversal of respiratory depression has resulted in pulmonary edema in some cases.

—The etiology of this interaction is not completely understood.

NEOSTIGMINE (Prostigmin)

Classification and indications

—Neostigmine is a synthetic parasympathomimetic agent.

—It is indicated for use as a reversal agent for non-depolarizing neuromuscular blocking agents (competitive inhibitors of acetylcholine). It is also used for testing for myasthenia gravis and has been used in the treatment of supraventricular tachycardias.

Pharmacology

—Neostigmine inhibits the destruction of acetylcholine by binding reversibly to acetylcholinesterase. As a result, acetylcholine accumulates at cholinergic synapses (such as the neuromuscular junction and the sinus node).

—Speed of reversal of the anticholinesterases depends on several factors, including depth of muscle blockade, neuromuscular blocker used, and dose and type of anticholinesterase.

—In general, onset of action is fastest with edrophonium, followed by neostigmine and pyridostigmine.

—At moderate levels of neuromuscular blockade (<twitch depression), neostigmine, edrophonium, and pyridostigmine

are about equivalent in their ability to induce reversal. When muscle blockade is profound (>90% twitch depression), edrophonium is not as effective as neostigmine.

—Pyridostigmine has the longest duration of action. Although edrophonium was thought to have a very short duration of action, studies with edrophonium doses of 0.5–1.0 mg/kg demonstrate a similar duration between edrophonium and neostigmine.

—Cardiac effects of parasympathomimetic agents, such as the anticholinesterases, result in bradycardia. To antagonize these responses, reversal agents are usually administered with either atropine or glycopyrrolate.

—Because of the rapid onset of edrophonium, atropine is usually recommended for coadministration, whereas glycopyrrolate (which is also slower in onset) is used for the slower onset of neostigmine and pyridostigmine.

Dose

—For reversal of neuromuscular blockade: neostigmine, 0.04–0.07 mg/kg with glycopyrrolate, 7–15 µg/kg.

Neostigmine Interactions with Anesthesia Drugs
Neostigmine and succinylcholine

—Neostigmine, edrophonium, pyridostigmine, and any other anticholinesterase can significantly prolong the duration of neuromuscular blockade from succinylcholine.

—Since these medications are nonspecific anticholinesterases, they also inhibit plasma pseudocholinesterase and therefore delay metabolism of succinylcholine.

—The exact amount of time necessary to prevent this interaction after administering an anticholinesterase is not known. Because the duration of action of neostigmine is 50–90 minutes, this may be a minimum interval to avoid this interaction.

Neostigmine Interactions with Diseases
Neostigmine and acidosis

—Alterations of the normal acid–base status may result in difficulty reversing non-depolarizing neuromuscular blockade.

—Respiratory acidosis ($pCO_2 > 50$) and metabolic alkalosis have been shown to prevent adequate reversal of pancuronium neuromuscular block. This interaction appears to be complex and is incompletely understood, but is probably related to changes in electrolytes and intracellular pH rather than simple changes in acid–base measurements.

Neostigmine and Eaton–Lambert syndrome

—Anticholinesterases are unreliable in reversing the muscle relaxation of non-depolarizing agents in patients with Eaton–Lambert syndrome.

—Patients with this syndrome may experience prolonged neuromuscular blockade with both non-depolarizing and depolarizing agents.

Neostigmine and hypocalcemia

—Reversal of neuromuscular blockade can be impaired in the presence of hypocalcemia.

—Stimulation of a motor nerve causes a nerve action potential that allows entry of calcium into the nerve ending. The calcium appears to cause release of acetylcholine from vesicles in the nerve ending into the neuromuscular junction, resulting in endplate depolarization.

—In the presence of inadequate ionized calcium, less acetylcholine is released, impairing the ability of acetylcholinesterase inhibitors to overcome the competitive blockade of acetylcholine receptors by neuromuscular blocking agents.

Neostigmine and hypokalemia

—Reversal of neuromuscular blockade in patients with hypokalemia may be more difficult. Although this has been demonstrated in animal studies, there is some controversy about the clinical importance of hypokalemia in reversal of muscle blockade in humans.

—Hypokalemia, particularly acute hypokalemia, can potentiate non-depolarizing neuromuscular blockers.

Neostigmine and hypothermia

—Non-depolarizing muscle blockade is prolonged by hypothermia. This interaction is a result of an effect on the neuromuscular blocking agents themselves rather than on the anticholinesterases used to reverse the neuromuscular blocking agents.

—Hypothermia appears to prolong the effect of the non-depolarizing agents by several mechanisms, including delayed metabolism into inactive metabolites as well as delayed excretion via the urinary and biliary routes.

Neostigmine and malignant hyperthermia

—Anesthetic agents considered safe for use in patients with known or suspected susceptibility for developing malignant hyperthermia (MH) include propofol, barbiturates, etomidate, ketamine, non-depolarizing neuromuscular blocking

agents, narcotics, benzodiazepines, droperidol, epinephrine, norepinephrine, and anticholinesterases.

—Nitrous oxide is probably safe in the susceptible patient based on repeated use in MH-susceptible humans and swine.

—Local or regional anesthesia with either amide (such as lidocaine) or ester (such as procaine) anesthetics is now considered safe for MH-susceptible patients.

Neostigmine and myasthenia gravis

—Reversal of a non-depolarizing blockade in patients with myasthenia gravis is controversial. Because patients are treated chronically with anticholinesterases, anticholinesterase inhibition is already nearly maximized.

—Conservative recommendations are to not use anticholinesterases for reversal of muscle blockade but rather to allow spontaneous recovery.

NICARDIPINE (Cardene)

Classification and indications

—Nicardipine is a calcium channel blocker.

—It is indicated for the management of hypertension.

Pharmacology

—Depolarization of cardiac and smooth muscle cells is associated with ion movement (sodium, calcium, potassium, chloride) through ion channels. These channels are voltage-gated, meaning that they are opened and closed according to changes in transmembrane potentials.

—With depolarization, there is rapid movement of sodium through "fast channels," whereas calcium moves much more slowly through "slow channels." It is by interfering with calcium movement through these slow calcium channels that calcium channel blockers mainly exert their effects.

—Some of the calcium channel blockers have more pronounced effects on cardiac conduction (verapamil, diltiazem), whereas others have greater effects on vascular smooth muscle resulting in lower blood pressure and coronary vasodilation (nifedipine, nicardipine).

—A negative inotropic effect (decreased myocardial contractility) is associated mainly with verapamil but can also be seen with diltiazem and nicardipine.

—Because nicardipine is dependent on hepatic metabolism and renal excretion, use of nicardipine in these patients may require use of lower doses.

Dose
—Intravenous dose:
—Initial infusion: Begin at 5.0 mg/hr. Rate may be increased by 2.5 mg/hr every 5–15 minutes up to 15 mg/hr.
—Once blood pressure is controlled, recommended infusion rate is about 3.0 mg/hr. This may be continued and adjusted as long as necessary.

Nicardipine Interactions with Anesthesia Drugs
Nicardipine and calcium chloride, calcium gluconate
—Calcium may antagonize some effects of calcium channel blockers.
—In some patients, intravenous calcium has reduced the hypotensive effects of nifedipine but not its ability to prevent angina. In other cases, calcium has caused a return of an arrhythmia that had been controlled with a calcium channel blocker.
—Since the response to calcium may not be completely predictable in patients treated with calcium channel blockers, caution should be used when using intravenous calcium in such patients.

Nicardipine and muscle relaxants (atracurium, doxacurium, gallamine, metocurine, mivacurium, pancuronium, pipercuronium, rocuronium, tubocurarine, vecuronium)
—Calcium channel blockers have been associated with prolongation of neuromuscular blockade from non-depolarizing agents.
—This interaction is probably related to the depletion of intracellular calcium associated with chronic therapy. This can result in a decrease in acetylcholine release at the neuromuscular junction.

Nicardipine Interactions with Diseases
Nicardipine and autonomic dysfunction, Shy–Drager syndrome
—Patients whose autonomic nervous system responses are impaired by disease (Shy–Drager) or medications (beta blockers) may be unable to adequately compensate for vasodilation or negative inotropic and chronotropic effects of calcium channel blockers.
—In these patients, exaggerated hypotension or bradycardia may be seen with calcium channel blockers.

—Nicardipine would be more likely to be associated with hypotension than either bradycardia or myocardial depression, which would be more often seen with verapamil.

Nicardipine and cerebral edema, intracranial hypertension

—Most systemic vasodilators (nitroglycerin, nitroprusside, hydralazine, calcium channel blockers, and adenosine) can produce cerebrovascular vasodilation as well. As a result, cerebral blood volume is either maintained or increased even though systemic blood pressure is decreased.

—Trimethaphan, a ganglionic blocker, usually will not increase cerebral blood volume because ganglionic blockade normally does not cause vasodilation of the cerebral circulation.

Nicardipine and congestive heart failure

—Some calcium channel blockers have negative inotropic activity (decreased myocardial contractility) and can worsen or precipitate congestive heart failure.

—Verapamil should be avoided in patients with impaired ventricular function. Although diltiazem and nicardipine have a less potent negative inotropic effect than verapamil, they should be used cautiously in patients with decreased ventricular function.

—Nifedipine appears to have only slight negative inotropic actions.

Nicardipine and PIH (pregnancy-induced hypertension). preeclampsia/eclampsia, toxemia

—Calcium channel blockers should be used cautiously in patients who have pregnancy-induced hypertension (preeclampsia, eclampsia, toxemia).

—Such patients are likely to be treated with magnesium sulfate which, combined with calcium channel blockers, can cause profound hypotension.

Nicardipine Interactions with Patient Drugs
Nicardipine and flecainide

—Flecainide can cause decreased myocardial contractility, particularly at the onset of intravenous therapy. Patients most significantly affected are those with compromised left ventricular function (ejection fraction <30%).

—Beta blockers and some calcium channel blockers may have added negative inotropic effects with flecainide.

—Verapamil has more negative inotropic effect than diltiazem, nicardipine, or nifedipine.

Nicardipine and magnesium sulfate

—Magnesium potentiates the effect of calcium channel blockers; the combination may result in profound hypotension.

Nicardipine and rifampin

—Patients taking rifampin require significantly higher doses of calcium channel blockers. This interaction has been documented with verapamil, diltiazem, and nifedipine.

—The studies done demonstrated the increased requirement for both oral and intravenous forms of the calcium channel blockers, but requirements were higher for patients taking oral medications.

—The mechanisms of this interaction include an increased metabolism and reduced protein binding of the calcium channel blockers by rifampin.

NIFEDIPINE (Adalat, Procardia)

Classification and indications

—Nifedipine is a calcium channel blocker.

—It is indicated for management of angina and hypertension.

Pharmacology

—Depolarization of cardiac and smooth muscle cells is associated with ion movement (sodium, calcium, potassium, chloride) through ion channels. These channels are voltage-gated, meaning they are opened and closed according to changes in transmembrane potentials.

—With depolarization, there is rapid movement of sodium through fast channels, whereas calcium moves much more slowly through "slow channels." It is by interfering with calcium movement through these slow calcium channels that calcium channel blockers mainly exert their effects.

—Some of the calcium channel blockers have more pronounced effects on cardiac conduction (verapamil, diltiazem), whereas others have greater effects on vascular smooth muscle, resulting in lower blood pressure and coronary vasodilation (nifedipine, nicardipine).

—Because nifedipine is dependent on hepatic metabolism and renal excretion, use of nifedipine in patients with hepatic or renal dysfunction may result in prolonged effects.

Dose

—For perioperative hypertension: Liquid-filled capsules (10 mg) may be administered sublingually (by puncturing with a needle and squeezing the contents sublingually).

Nifedipine Interactions with Anesthesia Drugs

Nifedipine and calcium chloride, calcium gluconate

—Calcium may antagonize some effects of calcium channel blockers.

—In some patients, intravenous calcium has reduced the hypotensive effects of nifedipine but not its ability to prevent angina. In other cases, calcium has caused a return of an arrhythmia that had been controlled with a calcium channel blocker.

—Since the response to calcium may not be completely predictable in patients treated with calcium channel blockers, caution should be used when using intravenous calcium in such patients.

Nifedipine and muscle relaxants (atracurium, doxacurium, gallamine, metocurine, mivacurium, pancuronium, pipercuronium, rocuronium, tubocurarine, vecuronium)

—Calcium channel blockers have been associated with prolongation of neuromuscular blockade from non-depolarizing agents.

—This interaction is probably related to the depletion of intracellular calcium associated with chronic therapy. This can result in a decrease in acetylcholine release at the neuromuscular junction.

Nifedipine Interactions with Diseases

Nifedipine and autonomic dysfunction, Shy–Drager syndrome

—Patients whose autonomic nervous system responses are impaired by disease (Shy–Drager) or medications (beta blockers) may be unable to adequately compensate for vasodilation or negative inotropic and chronotropic effects of calcium channel blockers.

—In these patients, exaggerated hypotension or bradycardia may be seen with calcium channel blockers.

—Nifedipine would be more likely to be associated with hypotension than either bradycardia or myocardial depression, which would be more often seen with verapamil.

Nifedipine and cerebral edema, intracranial hypertension

—Most systemic vasodilators (nitroglycerin, nitroprusside, hydralazine, calcium channel blockers, and adenosine) can produce cerebrovascular vasodilation as well. As a result, cerebral blood volume is either maintained or increased even though systemic blood pressure is decreased.

—Trimethaphan, a ganglionic blocker, usually will not increase cerebral blood volume because ganglionic blockade normally does not cause vasodilation of the cerebral circulation.

Nifedipine and congestive heart failure

—Some calcium channel blockers have negative inotropic activity (decreased myocardial contractility) and can worsen or precipitate congestive heart failure.

—Verapamil should be avoided in patients with impaired ventricular function. Although diltiazem and nicardipine have less potent negative inotropic effect than verapamil, they should be used cautiously in patients with decreased ventricular function.

—Nifedipine appears to have only slight negative inotropic actions.

Nifedipine and PIH (pregnancy-induced hypertension), preeclampsia/eclampsia, toxemia

—Calcium channel blockers should be used cautiously in patients who have pregnancy-induced hypertension (preeclampsia, eclampsia, toxemia).

—Such patients are likely to be treated with magnesium sulfate which, combined with calcium channel blockers, can cause profound hypotension.

Nifedipine Interactions with Patient Drugs

Nifedipine and flecainide

—Flecainide can cause decreased myocardial contractility, particularly at the onset of intravenous therapy. Patients most significantly affected are those with compromised left ventricular function (ejection fraction <30%).

—Beta blockers and some calcium channel blockers may have added negative inotropic effects with flecainide.

—Verapamil has more negative inotropic effect than diltiazem, nicardipine, or nifedipine.

Nifedipine and magnesium sulfate

—Magnesium potentiates the effect of calcium channel blockers and the combination may result in profound hypotension.

Nifedipine and mefloquine

—Mefloquine is a derivative of quinine and has rarely been associated with bradycardia and prolonged QT interval. Beta blockers and calcium channel blockers should be used with caution in patients on this medication.

Nifedipine and rifampin

—Patients taking rifampin require significantly higher doses of calcium channel blockers. This interaction has been documented with verapamil, diltiazem, and nifedipine.

—The studies that were done demonstrated the increased requirement for both oral and intravenous forms of the calcium channel blockers, but requirements were higher for patients taking oral medications.

—The mechanisms of this interaction include an increased metabolism and reduced protein binding of the calcium channel blockers by rifampin.

NITROGLYCERIN (Nitro-Bid, Nitrostat, Tridil)

Classification and indications

—Nitroglycerin is an organic nitrate that in its undiluted form as a powder is a powerful explosive.

—It is indicated for the management of angina and in its intravenous form also for perioperative control of blood pressure and congestive heart failure.

Pharmacology

—Nitrates produce vasodilation through an unknown mechanism.

—Dilation of both venous capacitance vessels and arterioles results in decreased preload as well as afterload reduction. The effect on the venous system is usually greater than on the arterial side.

—Increased myocardial oxygen consumption from the reflex increases in heart rate seen with nitroglycerin are offset by the decreased ventricular preload, afterload, and wall tension.

—Effects on the coronary system include coronary arterial dilation or, in the case of total occlusion, redistribution of coronary blood flow resulting in improved perfusion of ischemic myocardium. Preferential increases in subendocardial flow are also associated with nitroglycerin use.

—Cerebrovascular dilation from nitroglycerin or nitroprusside can have detrimental or beneficial effects on cerebral perfusion, depending on the clinical situation. In the setting of elevated intracranial pressure and hypertension, nitroglycerin may decrease arterial pressure but increase cerebral blood flow and thus raise intracranial pressure (with a resultant decrease in cerebral perfusion pressure).

—When nitroglycerin or nitroprusside are used for induced hypotension for surgery, cerebrovascular dilation may maintain cerebral perfusion in the setting of decreased arterial pressure.

—Following intravenous administration, nitroglycerin has an almost immediate onset. Rapid termination of effects is a result of hepatic metabolism.

—Absorption of nitroglycerin is also very rapid via nasal inhalation (amyl nitrite) and in the sublingual form. Transcutaneous and oral absorption are slower in onset and of longer duration.

Dose

—Intravenous infusion: Approximately 0.25 to 7.5 µg/kg/min. Dose must be titrated to blood pressure and/or pulmonary artery or occlusion pressures.

—Sublingual: 0.2, 0.3, or 0.4 mg SL every 5 minutes for three doses to relieve angina.

—2% NTG ointment: 1/2 to 2 in. every 4–6 hours for angina.

—Isosorbide dinitrate
  —Sublingual: 2.5 to 10 mg SL every 2–4 hours for angina.
  —Oral: 5–40 mg PO every 6 hours.
  —Transdermal patch: 1 patch (2.5–22.4 mg) once daily.

Nitroglycerin Interactions with Anesthesia Drugs

Nitroglycerin and heparin

—Nitroglycerin infusions have been shown in several studies to increase requirements of heparin to maintain anticoagulation. However, this effect was demonstrated in long-term infusions over a 72-hour period or more. In studies of 1–2 hours, no interaction was found.

Nitroglycerin and pancuronium

—Nitroglycerin can reportedly potentiate the neuromuscular blockade from pancuronium. Other depolarizing agents and succinylcholine apparently do not interact with nitroglycerin.

Nitroglycerin Interactions with Diseases
Nitroglycerin and cerebral edema, intracranial hypertension
—Most systemic vasodilators (nitroglycerin, nitroprusside, hydralazine, calcium channel blockers, and adenosine) can produce cerebrovascular vasodilation as well. As a result, cerebral blood volume is either maintained or increased even though systemic blood pressure is decreased.

—Trimethaphan, a ganglionic blocker, usually will not increase cerebral blood volume because ganglionic blockade normally does not cause vasodilation of the cerebral circulation.

NITROPRUSSIDE (Nipride, Nitropress)

Classification and indications
—Nitroprusside is a systemic vasodilator.

—It is indicated for the short-term management of hypertension, for temporary lowering of blood pressure for surgical procedures, or to increase cardiac output in patients with cardiac failure (by decreasing preload and/or afterload).

Pharmacology
—Nitroprusside lowers blood pressure by dilation of arterioles and venules. This appears to be a result of a direct action on vascular smooth muscle.

—In patients with cardiac dysfunction and decreased cardiac output, reduction in preload and/or afterload by nitroprusside may improve cardiac output.

—Heart rate is usually minimally affected but may decrease in patients as cardiac performance improves. In hypertensive patients, there may be a slight increase in heart rate with administration of nitroprusside.

—Nitroprusside may cause some dilation of coronary arteries.

—Cerebrovascular dilation from nitroglycerin or nitroprusside can have detrimental or beneficial effects on cerebral perfusion, depending on the clinical situation. In the setting of elevated intracranial pressure and hypertension, nitroglycerin may decrease arterial pressure but increase cerebral blood flow and thus raise intracranial pressure (with a resultant decrease in cerebral perfusion pressure).

—Toxicity of nitroprusside is related to accumulation of cyanide, which results from the breakdown of nitroprusside in the blood. Cyanide binds to cytochrome oxidase in the tissues and interferes with electron transport. As a result, cells are unable to utilize oxygen and tissue hypoxia occurs.

—A suggested limit for acute administration is 1.5 mg/kg total dose and for chronic administration, 8 µg/kg/min.

—Laboratory evidence of cyanide toxicity includes metabolic acidosis in the presence of normal oxygen tension in the blood.

—Treatment of cyanide toxicity includes:

—Discontinuation of nitroprusside infusion.

—Amyl nitrite inhalation for 15–30 seconds each minute in awake patients until intravenous sodium nitrite is available.

—3% sodium nitrite infusion of 4–6 mg/kg. The nitrites produce methemoglobinemia, which binds the cyanide, producing cyanomethemoglobinemia.

—Thiosulfate solution, 150–200 mg/kg of a 10% or 25% solution (normal adult dose is 50 mL of a 25% solution). Thiosulfate provides additional binding sites for cyanide and the thiocyanate is excreted by the kidneys.

—Onset of hypotensive effect is within 30 seconds and peak hypotensive effect is within 2 minutes. The blood pressure returns to normal within about 3 minutes. Unlike nitroglycerin, nitroprusside may be associated with a rebound phenomenon following discontinuation.

—Elimination of nitroprusside is a result of interaction with membrane-bound sulfhydryl groups in the vascular walls and red blood cells. This interaction produces cyanide (which is metabolized in the liver) and nitric acid.

Dose

—Adults: 0.3–10 µg/kg/min of a solution of nitroprusside 50 mg in 250, 500, or 1000 mL D5W. Acute administration should not exceed a total dose of 1.5 mg/kg.

—Children: Dissolve 15 mg/kg of nitroprusside in 250 mL D5W. Then the rate in µg/kg/min will equal ml/hr (such as 5 mL/hr = 5 µg/kg/min). Dosage range is 0.5–10 µg/kg/min.

Nitroprusside Interactions with Anesthesia Drugs
Nitroprusside and clonidine

—Severe hypotension developed in several patients who had been receiving nitroprusside and immediately after were given clonidine.

—Apparently, the mechanism involved is one of additive hypotensive effects of the two medications.

Nitroprusside and diltiazem

—The combination of diltiazem and nitroprusside may reduce significantly the dose of nitroprusside required to lower arterial pressure.

—In a study of 20 patients to assess the interaction of these two medications, intravenous infusions of diltiazem reduced by up to 50% the dose of nitroprusside required to achieve a certain level of arterial blood pressure.

Nitroprusside Interactions with Diseases

Nitroprusside and cerebral edema, intracranial hypertension

—Most systemic vasodilators (nitroglycerin, nitroprusside, hydralazine, calcium channel blockers, and adenosine) can produce cerebrovascular vasodilation as well. As a result, cerebral blood volume is either maintained or increased even though systemic blood pressure is decreased.

—Trimethaphan, a ganglionic blocker, usually will not increase cerebral blood volume because ganglionic blockade normally does not cause vasodilation of the cerebral circulation.

NITROUS OXIDE

Classification and indications

—Nitrous oxide is an inhalational anesthetic.

—It is indicated for use as a general anesthetic but must be supplemented with other agents (other inhalational agents, narcotics, propofol infusions, etc.).

Pharmacology

—Nitrous oxide has a MAC of about 105% but can only be delivered at a maximum concentration of 75% to prevent hypoxia. Therefore, other agents must be used to maintain general anesthesia.

—Combination of nitrous oxide with other inhalational agents reduces the MAC of these agents.

—The solubility of nitrous oxide in blood is low (blood/gas solubility is 0.47) compared to halothane (blood/gas solubility of 2.3), enflurane (blood/gas solubility of 1.9), and isoflurane (blood/gas solubility of 1.4).

—Low blood solubility causes a rapid accumulation of nitrous oxide in the alveoli and a high concentration delivered to the brain. For this reason, the onset of effects and reversal of effects from nitrous oxide are very rapid.

—All inhalational agents depress myocardial contractility in a dose-dependent manner. The order of myocardial depression from most to least is enflurane > halothane > isoflurane >> nitrous oxide.

—Decreased cardiac contractility may result in decreased cardiac output, especially in the patient with a diseased myocardium. However, it also produces an indirect stimulation of the sympathetic nervous system that may increase the systemic vascular resistance, maintaining blood pressure. Unless invasive monitoring is used, the decreased myocardial function may not be noticed.

—When nitrous oxide is combined with narcotics, the myocardial depressant effects of nitrous oxide may be potentiated.

—Nitrous oxide can cause increases in cerebral blood flow. The extent of this effect depends on other agents used for anesthesia. When administered alone, significant increases in intracranial pressure (ICP) occur with nitrous oxide. When nitrous oxide is used with or following intravenous agents (barbiturates, propofol), the increase in cerebral blood flow may be attenuated or eliminated.

—The effect of nitrous oxide on cerebral blood flow when combined with other inhalational agents is controversial. A number of studies have demonstrated an increase in cerebral blood flow when nitrous oxide is added to volatile anesthetics.

—However, anesthesia for the patient with elevated ICP usually involves intravenous agents, hyperventilation, and other methods for reducing ICP. In most cases, therefore, nitrous oxide is unlikely to significantly increase ICP. When ICP is a persistent problem, though, nitrous oxide should be suspected of contributing to the elevated pressure, and its elimination should be considered.

—Nitrous oxide is a relatively weak anesthetic and does not significantly depress the ventilatory response to hypocarbia at a concentration of 50%. Also, the combination of nitrous oxide with other potent inhalational anesthetics decreases the MAC and the respiratory depression of the more potent agent.

Dose

—General anesthesia: Nitrous oxide 50–75% with oxygen. Because this is <1 MAC, it must be combined with other intravenous agents or inhalational agents for general anesthesia.

Nitrous Oxide Interactions with Anesthesia Drugs
Nitrous oxide and clonidine
—Clonidine has been shown to reduce the MAC of inhaled and opioid anesthetics.

—This effect may be related to clonidine's inhibition of the sympathetic outflow from the vasomotor center in the medulla (clonidine is a central alpha 2 receptor agonist, which results in inhibition of CNS sympathetic centers).

Nitrous Oxide Interactions with Diseases
Nitrous oxide and air embolism
—Nitrous oxide can result in rapid expansion of gas- or air-filled cavities in the anesthetized patient. For this reason, it should not be administered to patients with a pneumothorax, acute intestinal obstruction, or patients at significant risk for air embolism.

—Additionally, for patients having surgery for retinal detachment, where sulfahexafluoride gas, nitrogen, or a combination is injected into the vitreous cavity, use of nitrous oxide could produce unwanted expansion or pressure in the eye. The same is true for patients having tympanoplasty.

—Because nitrous oxide is used in high concentrations (50–70%) and is 35 times more soluble in blood than is nitrogen, nitrous oxide will enter an air-containing cavity, causing expansion or increase in pressure. This effect cannot be offset by displacement of nitrogen (comprising 78% of air) because of nitrogen's low solubility.

Nitrous oxide and alcohol—acute intoxication
—Patients who are acutely intoxicated with alcohol (including chronic alcoholics) usually demonstrate increased sensitivity to general anesthesia.

—Although the precise mechanism of interactions is not agreed on, it appears that alcohol intoxication has additive CNS depression with barbiturates, benzodiazepines, and narcotics, as well as inhalational agents.

Nitrous oxide and alcohol—chronic abuse
—Chronic abuse of alcohol has complex and incompletely understood effects on a patient's response to anesthetic agents. In general, these patients tend to be more tolerant (in a nonintoxicated state) to barbiturates, benzodiazepines, narcotics, and inhalational agents.

—Exceptions to this generalization include the alcoholic patient with a cardiomyopathy who may demonstrate increased sensitivity to myocardial depression from inhalational agents.

—Also, the patient with severe liver disease may have impaired ability to metabolize succinylcholine due to decreased levels of plasma pseudocholinesterase.

Nitrous oxide and cerebral edema, intracranial hypertension

—All commonly used inhalational volatile anesthetics (halothane > enflurane > isoflurane) cause an increased cerebral blood flow (CBF). Less is known about sevoflurane and desflurane, but they are believed to have effects similar to those of isflurane. Nitrous oxide has minimal effects on CBF.

—The volatile anesthetics, although they depress cerebral metabolic rate, cause cerebrovascular dilation that results in increased CBF. Hyperventilation to a $PaCO_2$ between 25 and 35 mm Hg will effectively prevent increased CBF from isoflurane, but not the other volatile anesthetics.

Nitrous oxide and hepatitis

—All forms of anesthesia, including general, regional, and nitrous-narcotic, are associated with postoperative liver function test abnormalities. The exact mechanism of this reaction is not known but is likely related to reduced liver blood flow from anesthesia and surgery.

—The presence of hepatitis or any liver disease has been shown to increase the morbidity and mortality in patients receiving anesthesia. The mechanism of this increase in morbidity and mortality is not clear but is most likely related to changes in hepatic blood flow as a result of anesthesia and surgery.

—Because there is no known method of avoiding exacerbation of pre-existing liver disease by anesthesia, most recommendations are to postpone surgery in patients suspected of having acute hepatitis.

—There is no evidence that enflurane, isoflurane, desflurane, or sevoflurane is hepatotoxic. Halothane, however, can occasionally cause fulminant hepatic necrosis in both adults and children. A milder form of hepatotoxicity is also seen with halothane anesthesia.

Nitrous oxide and intestinal obstruction

—Nitrous oxide can result in rapid expansion of gas- or air-filled cavities in the anesthetized patient. For this reason, it should not be administered to patients with a pneumothorax, acute intestinal obstruction, or those at significant risk for air embolism.

— Additionally, for patients having surgery for retinal detachment, where sulfahexafluoride gas, nitrogen, or a combination is injected into the vitreous cavity, use of nitrous oxide could produce unwanted expansion or pressure in the eye. The same is true for patients having tympanoplasty.

— Because nitrous oxide is used in high concentrations (50–70%) and is 35 times more soluble in blood than is nitrogen, nitrous oxide will enter an air-containing cavity, causing expansion or increase in pressure. This effect cannot be offset by displacement of nitrogen (comprising 78% of air) because of nitrogen's low solubility.

Nitrous oxide and malignant hyperthermia

— Nitrous oxide is probably safe in the susceptible patient based on repeated use in MH-susceptible humans and swine.

— Anesthetic agents considered safe for use in patients with known or suspected susceptibility for developing malignant hyperthermia (MH) include propofol, barbiturates, etomidate, ketamine, non-depolarizing neuromuscular blocking agents, narcotics, benzodiazepines, droperidol, epinephrine, norepinephrine, and anticholinesterases.

— Local or regional anesthesia with either amide (such as lidocaine) or ester (such as procaine) anesthetics is now considered safe for MH-susceptible patients.

Nitrous oxide and pneumothorax

— Nitrous oxide can result in rapid expansion of gas- or air-filled cavities in the anesthetized patient. For this reason, it should not be administered to patients with a pneumothorax, acute intestinal obstruction, or patients at significant risk for air embolism.

— Additionally, for patients having surgery for retinal detachment, where sulfahexafluoride gas, nitrogen, or a combination is injected into the vitreous cavity, use of nitrous oxide could produce unwanted expansion or pressure in the eye. The same is true for patients having tympanoplasty.

— Because nitrous oxide is used in high concentrations (50–70%) and is 35 times more soluble in blood than is nitrogen, nitrous oxide will enter an air-containing cavity, causing expansion or increase in pressure. This effect cannot be offset by displacement of nitrogen (comprising 78% of air) because of nitrogen's low solubility.

Nitrous oxide and porphyria

—Inhalational agents are considered to be safe for use in patients with porphyria, as are narcotics, depolarizing and non-depolarizing muscle relaxants, etomidate, anticholinesterases, and propofol.

—Barbiturates are contraindicated in three of the four hepatic porphyrias (acute intermittent porphyria, variegate porphyria, and hereditary coproporphyria). Porphyria cutanea tarda and the erythropoietic porphyrias are not exacerbated by barbiturates.

—It is theorized that barbiturates can provoke an attack of porphyria by inducing the enzyme aminolevulinic acid synthetase, which results in synthesis of more porphyrin compounds and their precursors.

Nitrous oxide and pulmonary air cysts

—Nitrous oxide can result in rapid expansion of gas- or air-filled cavities in the anesthetized patient. For this reason, it should not be administered to patients with a pneumothorax, acute intestinal obstruction, pulmonary air cysts, or patients at significant risk for air embolism.

—Additionally, for patients having surgery for retinal detachment, where sulfahexafluoride gas, nitrogen, or a combination is injected into the vitreous cavity, use of nitrous oxide could produce unwanted expansion or pressure in the eye. The same is true for patients having tympanoplasty.

—Because nitrous oxide is used in high concentrations (50–70%) and is 35 times more soluble in blood than is nitrogen, nitrous oxide will enter an air-containing cavity, causing expansion or increase in pressure. This effect cannot be offset by displacement of nitrogen (comprising 78% of air) because of nitrogen's low solubility.

Nitrous oxide and pulmonary hypertension

—Use of nitrous oxide is controversial in patients with elevated pulmonary vascular pressure.

—Although some studies have shown no significant effect of nitrous oxide in patients with pulmonary hypertension, others demonstrate that nitrous oxide is capable of producing pulmonary vasoconstriction.

Nitrous oxide and retinal detachment

—Nitrous oxide can result in rapid expansion of gas- or air-filled cavities in the anesthetized patient. For this reason, it should not be administered to patients with a pneumothorax, acute intestinal obstruction, or patients at significant risk for air embolism.

—Additionally, for patients having surgery for retinal detachment, where sulfahexafluoride gas, nitrogen, or a combination is injected into the vitreous cavity, use of nitrous oxide could produce unwanted expansion or pressure in the eye. The same is true for patients having tympanoplasty.

—Because nitrous oxide is used in high concentrations (50–70%) and is 35 times more soluble in blood than is nitrogen, nitrous oxide will enter an air-containing cavity, causing expansion or increase in pressure. This effect cannot be offset by displacement of nitrogen (comprising 78% of air) because of nitrogen's low solubility.

NOREPINEPHRINE (Levophed)

Classification and indications

—Norepinephrine is an endogenous catecholamine that is the chemical mediator of postganglionic adrenergic nerves. It also accounts for 10–20% of the catecholamines in the adrenal medulla.

—It is indicated for the management of hypotension from cardiac decompensation or sepsis when patient positioning or fluid therapy is impractical, ineffective, or contraindicated.

Pharmacology

—Norepinephrine stimulates both alpha and beta receptors, but in different ratios than does epinephrine.

—Whereas epinephrine has prominent beta 2 (bronchodilation) effects, norepinephrine has little effect on the beta 2 receptors. Norepinephrine has prominent alpha receptor effects and beta 1 (cardiac) effects similar to those of epinephrine.

—Cardiac effects of norepinephrine are a result of beta 1 stimulation producing an increase in contractility and stroke volume. Although a positive chronotropic effect occurs, it is outweighed by vagal tone resulting from increased blood pressure. As a result, cardiac output may remain unchanged or decrease.

—Increased blood pressure is a result of alpha adrenergic stimulation. Vasoconstriction of most vascular beds includes kidney, liver, mesentery, and skeletal muscle (unlike epinephrine).

—Glomerular filtration rate is usually maintained unless vasoconstriction is excessive, or if hypovolemia or hypotension is not corrected.

—Metabolism of norepinephrine occurs in the liver and other tissues.

Dose

—Adults: Intravenous infusion of a solution of 4 µg/ml of norepinephrine at 8–12 µg/min.

—Children: 0.1 µg/kg/min initial dose.

Norepinephrine Interactions with Anesthesia Drugs

Norepinephrine and beta blockers (esmolol, labetalol, propranolol)

—Use of esmolol for treatment of supraventricular tachycardia may have undesirable effects in some patients; specifically, in patients requiring cardiovascular support with agents that are both inotropic and vasoconstrictive (dopamine, epinephrine, norepinephrine), blockade of beta receptors may result in decreased cardiac contractility in the face of systemic vasoconstriction, resulting in cardiac failure.

Norepinephrine and cocaine

—Cocaine may potentiate the vasopressor responses to sympathomimetic agents.

—The mechanism of this interaction involves the inhibition of reuptake of catecholamines by cocaine. This property probably accounts for the vasoconstriction caused by cocaine use.

—Cardiovascular symptoms of hypertension, arrhythmias, and tachycardia from cocaine use are related to both central and sympathetic nervous system effects of cocaine.

Norepinephrine and inhalational anesthetics (enflurane, desflurane, halothane, isoflurane, sevoflurane)

—Halothane and, to a lesser extent, isoflurane and ethrane reduce the threshold for arrhythmias from epinephrine and norepinephrine. The mechanism of this "sensitization" of the myocardium to these sympathomimetic amines includes an increase in automaticity and changes in depolarization.

—Although exact numbers are not agreed on, a general guideline for safe administration of epinephrine based on some

clinical studies is to use no more than 10 mL of 1:100,000
(1 µg/mL) epinephrine solution every 10 minutes with a
limit of 30 mL/hour. with isoflurane or ethrane, a slightly
larger amount can probably be used.

Norepinephrine and methylergonovine

—Oxytocics (oxytocin, ergonovine, methylergonovine) may
interact with vasopressors to produce hypertension, which
is more likely to be severe in patients with a predisposition
to hypertension.

—The use of an intramuscular or intravenous ergot alkaloid
(such as IM methylergonovine) either preceded or followed
by a vasopressor may result in severe hypertension. The
safest method of administering an oxytocic is a dilute intravenous infusion of oxytocin.

Norepinephrine and oxytocin

—Severe hypertension has been reported in patients given
oxytocin who had received a prophylactic vasoconstrictor
up to 4 hours previously for a caudal block.

—This interaction is more likely to occur in patients with
existing mild hypertension and those who receive an ergot
alkaloid (such as methylergonovine) rather than a dilute
solution of oxytocin.

Norepinephrine and phentolamine

—The pressor effects of vasopressors can be blunted in
patients receiving alpha blockers.

—Norepinephrine and metaraminol stimulate mainly beta 1
(cardiac stimulation) and alpha receptors. When norepinephrine is given to patients on alpha blockers, the beta 1 stimulation may produce some increase in blood pressure.
Hypotension is unlikely because of minimal beta 2 agonism.

Norepinephrine Interactions with Diseases

Norepinephrine and hyperthyroidism, thyrotoxicosis

—Agents that stimulate the sympathetic nervous system (catecholamines, ephedrine, phenylephrine, dopram, ketamine)
may have exaggerated effects in patients with hyperthyroidism. Although most evident in untreated patients, even
patients receiving treatment for excess thyroid hormone
may demonstrate this response.

—Excess thyroid hormone causes stimulation of metabolism
of most body tissues. As a result, cardiac output increases by
50% or more to remove the extra metabolic byproducts.
Also, direct stimulatory effects on the myocardium at even

slightly elevated thyroid hormone levels causes tachycardia and increased contractility.

—At higher thyroid hormone levels, myocardial depression may occur as a result of excess demands or a direct myocardial depression.

Norepinephrine and malignant hyperthermia

—Anesthetic agents considered safe for use in patients with known or suspected susceptibility for developing malignant hyperthermia (MH) include propofol, barbiturates, etomidate, ketamine, non-depolarizing neuromuscular blocking agents, narcotics, benzodiazepines, droperidol, epinephrine, norepinephrine, and anticholinesterases.

—Nitrous oxide is probably safe in the susceptible patient based on repeated use in MH-susceptible humans and swine.

—Local or regional anesthesia with either amide (such as lidocaine) or ester (such as procaine) anesthetics is now considered safe for MH-susceptible patients.

Norepinephrine and pheochromocytoma

—The pressor effects of vasopressors can be blunted in patients receiving alpha blockers.

—Norepinephrine and metaraminol stimulate mainly beta 1 (cardiac stimulation) and alpha receptors. When norepinephrine is given to patients on alpha blockers, the beta 1 stimulation may produce some increase in blood pressure. Hypotension is unlikely because of minimal beta 2 agonism.

Norepinephrine and pregnancy

—Ephedrine, mephentermine, and metaraminol are the preferred agents for treatment of hypotension in pregnancy.

—The above agents have both alpha and beta agonist activity and are not associated with reduced placental blood flow.

—Phenylephrine, norepinephrine, angiotensin, and methoxamine are predominantly alpha adrenergic agents that act peripherally and can cause uterine artery vasoconstriction and placental hypoperfusion.

Norepinephrine Interactions with Patient Drugs
Norepinephrine and alpha adrenergic blockers (doxazasin, phenoxybenzamine, phentolamine, prazosin, terazosin)

—The pressor effects of vasopressors can be blunted in patients receiving alpha blockers.

—Norepinephrine and metaraminol stimulate mainly beta 1 (cardiac stimulation) and alpha receptors. When norepinephrine is given to patients on alpha blockers, the beta 1 stimulation may produce some increase in blood pressure. Hypotension is unlikely because of minimal beta 2 agonism.

Norepinephrine and ergot alkaloids (dihydroergotamine, ergonovine, ergotamine tartrate, methylergonovine)

—Ergot alkaloids may interact with vasopressors to produce hypertension, which is more likely to be severe in patients with a predisposition to hypertension.

—Because of possibly additive vasoconstrictive effects, the administration of vasopressors to patients receiving ergot alkaloids may produce unexpected degrees of hypertension.

Norepinephrine and guanadrel, guanethidine

—Patients receiving guanethidine and guanadrel can have an exaggerated hypertensive response to norepinephrine and other direct-acting catecholamines such as phenylephrine, dobutamine, and epinephrine.

—Indirect-acting catecholamines, such as ephedrine, metaraminol, mephentermine, and dopamine, may have fewer pressor effects than expected.

—Guanethidine and guanadrel deplete intraneuronal norepinephrine in postganglionic sympathetic neurons and in this way may diminish the response of indirect-acting catecholamines while sensitizing adrenergic receptors to direct-acting amines.

Norepinephrine and monoamine oxidase inhibitors (isocarboxazid, phenelzine, selegilene, tranylcypromine)

—Indirect-acting vasopressors (ephedrine, mephentermine, and metaraminol) act by releasing intraneuronal monoamines such as dopamine and norepinephrine. This is the explanation of the hypertensive crises seen when patients receiving monamine oxidase inhibitors are given these vasopressors.

—Direct-acting vasopressors such as phenylephrine, epinephrine, norepinephrine, and dobutamine may be potentiated by MAO inhibitors and should be used in smaller amounts than normally used.

—Dopamine has both direct and indirect actions and must be used with caution (perhaps one-tenth the normal dose).

Norepinephrine and oxytocin

—Oxytocin administration has been associated with severe hypertension in patients who had received a prophylactic vasoconstrictor up to 4 hours previously for a caudal block.

—Severe hypertension is more likely to occur in patients with existing mild hypertension and in those who receive an ergot alkaloid (such as methylergonovine) rather than a dilute solution of oxytocin.

Norepinephrine and ritodrine, terbutaline

—Ritodrine and terbutaline, beta 2 agonists, may potentiate other sympathomimetic agents.

—The mechanism of this interaction is probably related to the beta 1 adrenergic stimulation that can be seen with administration of these drugs.

OXYTOCIN (Pitocin, Syntocinon)

Classification and indications

—Oxytocin is a hormone that is secreted by the hypothalamus and stored in the posterior pituitary gland (as well as vasopressin). In medical practice, the oxytocin used is a synthetic form.

—It is indicated for obstetrical use as a stimulant for uterine contractions to induce or augment labor, or to help control postpartum bleeding and expulsion of the uterus.

Pharmacology

—Oxytocin causes increased contraction of the uterus. This effect is most pronounced in the patient in labor, as opposed to patients in early pregnancy when large amounts of oxytocin are required to increase uterine tone.

—Cardiovascular effects include vasodilation, including renal, coronary, and cerebral vessels. If oxytocin is used in very large amounts, there may be a drop in blood pressure with a reflex tachycardia and increased cardiac output.

—Following intravenous administration, onset of increased uterine tone is almost immediate and lasts for about 1 hour.

—Severe hypertension has been reported in patients given oxytocin who had received a prophylactic vasoconstrictor up to 4 hours previously for a caudal block.

—This interaction is more likely to occur in patients with existing mild hypertension and who receive an ergot alkaloid (such as methylergonovine), rather than a dilute solution of oxytocin.

—It is because of the above interaction that the administration of prophylactic vasopressors for regional anesthesia in obstetrics is no longer recommended.

—Elimination of oxytocin is accomplished rapidly by the liver and kidneys.

Dose

—Postpartum: 20–40 mU/min (20 units in 1000 mL at about 100 mL/hr).

Oxytocin Interactions with Anesthesia Drugs

Oxytocin and vasopressors (ephedrine, epinephrine, metaraminol, methoxamine, norepinephrine, phenylephrine)

—Severe hypertension has been associated with administration of oxytocin to patients who had received a prophylactic vasoconstrictor up to 4 hours previously for a caudal block.

—This interaction is more likely to be seen in patients with underlying mild hypertension and in those receiving an ergot alkaloid (such as methylergonovine) rather than a dilute solution of oxytocin.

PANCURONIUM (Pavulon)

Classification and indications

—Pancuronium is a non-depolarizing neuromuscular blocking agent.

—It is indicated for skeletal muscle relaxation for intubation or during surgery.

Pharmacology

—Pancuronium competes with acetylcholine at the neuromuscular junction of skeletal muscle by binding to acetylcholine receptors.

—After a dose of 0.08 mg/kg, adequate relaxation for intubation occurs within 2–3 minutes and has a clinical duration (reversal to 25% of twitch height) of 40–120 minutes.

—Pancuronium causes an increase in heart rate that results from a vagolytic effect and some sympathetic stimulation (catecholamine release, decreased reuptake of catecholamines).

—Elimination of pancuronium depends on both renal excretion and hepatic metabolism. Because renal elimination is the main route of excretion, patients with renal dysfunction may have prolonged effects from pancuronium.

—Patients with hepatobiliary disease may have initial resistance to muscle relaxation (due to increased volume of distribution) but may show prolonged elimination and effects due to delayed metabolism.

Dose

—Intubation: 0.06–0.1 mg/kg.

—Maintenance: 0.01 mg/kg as necessary to maintain relaxation.

Pancuronium Interactions with Anesthesia Drugs

Pancuronium and calcium channel blockers (diltiazem, nicardipine, nifedipine, verapamil)

—Calcium channel blockers have been associated with prolongation of neuromuscular blockade from non-depolarizing agents.

—This interaction is probably related to the depletion of intracellular calcium associated with chronic therapy. This can result in a decrease in acetylcholine release at the neuromuscular junction.

Pancuronium and inhalational anesthetics (desflurane, enflurane, halothane, isoflurane, sevoflurane)

—Desflurane, enflurane, halothane, isoflurane, and sevoflurane can significantly potentiate neuromuscular blockade, depending on the neuromuscular blocker used. Nitrous oxide has minimal effects.

—Tubocurarine and pancuronium are potentiated the most by inhalational agents, whereas atracurium and vecuronium are intensified significantly less.

—Potentiation by inhalational agents occurs through depression of spinal cord reflexes as well as effects at or distal to the neuromuscular junction.

Pancuronium and diphenylhydantoin, phenytoin

—Patients on chronic phenytoin therapy may be resistant to non-depolarizing muscle blockade. The studies involved metocurine and vecuronium but may involve other nondepolarizing agents.

—The mechanism of this interaction is not known.

—Acute infusions of phenytoin may prolong non-depolarizing blockade. This was studied prospectively in a small number of patients who received a 10 mg/kg loading dose of phenytoin during steady-state muscle blockade with vecuronium. They had significant potentiation of their neuromuscular block compared to control patients.

Pancuronium and furosemide

—Furosemide may potentiate neuromuscular blockade from tubocurarine and succinylcholine.

—This is based on a case report of several patients given furosemide and tubocurarine during surgery and on animal studies.

—The implication for this interaction for other neuromuscular blocking drugs is uncertain and the mechanism is not known.

Pancuronium and lidocaine

—Most local anesthetics can block neuromuscular transmission from non-depolarizing agents as well as depolarizing muscle relaxants. Of clinical significance to the anesthesiologist, lidocaine, given as a 50- to 100-mg bolus or even by infusion, can significantly increase a non-depolarizer block or a phase II block from succinylcholine.

Pancuronium and procainamide

—Procainamide can potentiate muscle relaxation from non-depolarizing agents. This is probably a result of decreased acetylcholine release at the neuromuscular junction caused by procainamide.

Pancuronium and quinidine

—Quinidine, procainamide, propranolol, and most local anesthetics have been shown to enhance the neuromuscular blockade from depolarizing and non-depolarizing agents.

—A number of well-documented cases have illustrated the ability of these agents, when given in the immediate postoperative period, to convert subclinical muscle weakness from neuromuscular blocking drugs into significant muscle weakness requiring reintubation.

Pancuronium and succinylcholine

—Prior administration of succinylcholine has been shown to potentiate neuromuscular blockade of some non-depolarizing agents.

—Although this interaction has been documented with pancuronium, it was not seen with doxacurium and may not be a consistent finding with non-depolarizing agents.

Pancuronium Interactions with Diseases
Pancuronium and advanced age
—Prolonged duration of neuromuscular blockade can be seen in older patients with several different non-depolarizing agents including doxacurium, mivacurium, and rocuronium.
—In some cases, delayed onset of muscle relaxation also occurs. This has been attributed to decreased perfusion of the neuromuscular junction as a result of advanced age.
Pancuronium and burns
—Patients with burn injuries are susceptible to a life-threatening hyperkalemic response to succinylcholine and can have marked resistance to non-depolarizing muscle relaxants.
—Both of these altered responses to neuromuscular blocking agents have been attributed to proliferation of extrajunctional acetylcholine receptors, similar to that in the patient with a denervation injury.
—Resistance to non-depolarizing agents appears to increase with larger area burns and in fact may not be significant in patients with <30% body surface area burns. In addition to proliferation of extrajunctional acetylcholine receptors, this abnormal response is probably also related to the increased metabolic rate and hepatic and renal clearance seen in burn patients. Doses of non-depolarizing agents may need to be increased by as much as 300%.
—Duration of this resistance usually is 2 months following the injury but has been reported in a patient 463 days after the burn.
Pancuronium and cirrhosis, liver disease
—Prolonged neuromuscular blockade in patients with liver disease can be seen with doxacurium, mivacurium, vecuronium, pancuronium, rocuronium, and tubocurarine.
—This interaction is complex and may be due to decreased clearance, decreased hepatic uptake of the agent, or decreased synthesis of enzymes important for degradation of the neuromuscular blocker. An example of the latter is the prolongation of mivacurium's duration of action as a result of decreased plasma cholinesterase from severe liver disease.
—Because of the increased volume of distribution of many drugs seen in patients with liver disease, initial doses of muscle relaxants may need to be larger than in healthy

patients. Once neuromuscular blockade is achieved, recovery may be prolonged.

Pancuronium and Eaton–Lambert syndrome

—Patients with Eaton–Lambert syndrome are very sensitive to both depolarizing and non-depolarizing neuromuscular blockade.

—This disorder is similar to myasthenia gravis and patients complain of skeletal muscle weakness, but it is usually associated with carcinoma (especially small cell tumors of the lung).

—If the diagnosis is known or suspected prior to surgery, reduced doses of muscle relaxants should be used, but sometimes the diagnosis is first made when a patient has surgery for a lung tumor and has an unexpected, prolonged neuromuscular block.

—Anticholinesterases are unreliable in reversing muscle weakness.

Pancuronium and hyperthyroidism, thyrotoxicosis

—Muscle weakness is commonly seen with hyperthyroidism and affects proximal muscles, usually sparing respiratory function. In some cases, myopathy is the dominant feature of thyroid hormone excess and can resemble myasthenia. Lower doses of muscle relaxants may be indicated.

Pancuronium and hypokalemia

—Hypokalemia appears to potentiate the effects of neuromuscular blockade from non-depolarizing agents.

—The interaction is probably due to hyperpolarization of the muscle endplate and, therefore, resistance to depolarization. Hyperpolarization would more likely occur with more acute changes in potassium concentration because the potassium losses would be from the extracellular compartment rather than from intracellular sites.

—Chronic hypokalemia is more likely to be associated with potassium depletion from both extra- and intracellular compartments with no significant change in transmembrane potential. As a result, significant effects on neuromuscular blockade would be less likely.

Pancuronium and hypothermia

—Non-depolarizing muscle blockade is prolonged by hypothermia. This interaction is a result of an effect on the neuromuscular blocking agents themselves rather than on the anticholinesterases used to reverse the neuromuscular blocking agents.

—Hypothermia appears to prolong the effect of the non-depolarizing agents by several mechanisms, including delayed metabolism into inactive metabolites as well as delayed excretion via the urinary and biliary routes.

Pancuronium and malignant hyperthermia

—Anesthetic agents considered safe for use in patients with known or suspected susceptibility for developing malignant hyperthermia (MH) include propofol, barbiturates, etomidate, ketamine, non-depolarizing neuromuscular blocking agents, narcotics, benzodiazepines, droperidol, epinephrine, norepinephrine, and anticholinesterases.

—Nitrous oxide is probably safe in the susceptible patient based on repeated use in MH-susceptible humans and swine.

—Local or regional anesthesia with either amide (such as lidocaine) or ester (such as procaine) anesthetics is now considered safe for MH-susceptible patients.

Pancuronium and myasthenia gravis

—Patients with myasthenia gravis are very sensitive to neuromuscular blockade from non-depolarizing agents.

—This is probably a result of decreased acetylcholine receptors from autoimmune destruction associated with myasthenia gravis.

—Although these patients are treated with the same or similar anticholinesterases used to antagonize muscle blockade, sensitivity (not resistance) to neuromuscular blockade is seen clinically.

Pancuronium and neuromuscular disease (amyotrophic lateral sclerosis, multiple sclerosis, syringomyelia)

—Patients with a wide variety of neuromuscular disorders may be more resistant than normal patients to the effects of non-depolarizing neuromuscular blockers.

—This includes patients with disuse atrophy of the muscles (such as bedridden patients with chronic disease) as well as patients with upper or lower motor neuron disease such as amyotrophic lateral sclerosis, multiple sclerosis, or syringomyelia.

—Disuse or denervation of muscle results in production of extrajunctional acetylcholine receptors on the muscle membrane. These receptors are less easily blocked by non-depolarizing agents but are activated by lower concentrations of depolarizing drugs (succinylcholine).

—When these receptors, which can be scattered over a large surface of the muscle, are depolarized by succinylcholine, ion flow takes place through the receptor channel. Large amounts of potassium may exit the muscle cell, causing hyperkalemia.

—Despite initial resistance to blockade, such patients may demonstrate prolonged neuromuscular weakness as a result of decreased muscle strength and mass.

Pancuronium and PIH (pregnancy-induced hypertension), preeclampsia/eclampsia, toxemia

—Patients with hypertensive disorders of pregnancy may require treatment with antihypertensives such as trimethaphan or magnesium sulfate (for preeclampsia/eclampsia). These medications can have significant interactions with anesthetic agents such as succinylcholine, non-depolarizing neuromuscular blocking agents, or calcium channel blockers.

—Neuromuscular blockade produced by both depolarizing and non-depolarizing agents can be potentiated in patients receiving magnesium sulfate. The mechanisms involved include a decreased amount of acetylcholine released by the nerve impulse at the motor nerve terminal and a decrease in the depolarizing action of acetylcholine on the muscle.

Pancuronium Interactions with Patient Drugs

Pancuronium and antibiotics

—A number of antibiotics have significant interactions with neuromuscular blocking agents. These include the aminoglycosides (amikacin, gentamicin, kanamycin, neomycin, paromomycin, netilmicin, neomycin, streptomycin, tobramycin), as well as polymyxin B, colistin, amphotericin B, clindamycin, bacitracin, and lincomycin.

—All of the above antibiotics may potentiate non-depolarizing agents, but some (aminoglycosides, amphotericin B, clindamycin, colistin) can also potentiate succinylcholine blockade.

—These antibiotics potentiate neuromuscular blockade by different mechanisms, making management of these problems difficult. Although treatment with anticholinesterases or calcium has been recommended, results are inconsistent.

Pancuronium and amphotericin B
—Prolonged neuromuscular blockade can occur with depolarizing and non-depolarizing agents in patients receiving amphotericin B.
—The mechanism for this interaction is thought to be associated with the hypokalemia that can be caused by amphotericin B therapy.

Pancuronium and beta blockers, propranolol
—Beta blockers may potentiate non-depolarizing neuromuscular blocking agents. This interaction has been reported between propranolol and tubocurarine.
—Other beta blockers are also capable of causing weakness in patients with myasthenia gravis, but the mechanism or significance of these interactions is unclear.

Pancuronium and calcium channel blockers (amlodipine, bepridil, diltiazem, felodipine, isradipine, lidoflazine, nicardipine, nimodipine, nisoldipine, nitrendipine, verapamil)
—Calcium channel blockers have been associated with prolongation of neuromuscular blockade from non-depolarizing agents.
—This interaction is probably related to the depletion of intracellular calcium associated with chronic therapy. This can result in a decrease in acetylcholine release at the neuromuscular junction.

Pancuronium and diphenylhydantoin, phenytoin
—Patients on chronic phenytoin therapy may be resistant to non-depolarizing muscle blockade. The studies involved metocurine and vecuronium but may involve other non-depolarizing agents.
—The mechanism of this interaction is not known.
—Acute infusions of phenytoin may prolong non-depolarizing blockade. This was studied prospectively in a small number of patients who received a 10 mg/kg loading dose of phenytoin during steady-state muscle blockade with vecuronium. They had significant potentiation of their neuromuscular block compared to control patients.

Pancuronium and lidocaine
—Most local anesthetics can block neuromuscular transmission from non-depolarizing agents as well as depolarizing muscle relaxants. Of clinical significance to the anesthesiologist, lidocaine, given as a 50- to 100-mg bolus or even by

infusion, can significantly increase a non-depolarizer block or a phase II block from succinylcholine.

Pancuronium and lithium

—Lithium has been reported to increase the duration of both non-depolarizing and depolarizing neuromuscular blocking drugs.

—The mechanism of this interaction is unknown and the clinical significance of this interaction is uncertain.

Pancuronium and magnesium sulfate

—Neuromuscular blockade produced by both depolarizing and non-depolarizing agents can be potentiated in patients receiving magnesium sulfate. The mechanisms involved include a decreased amount of acetylcholine released by the nerve impulse at the motor nerve terminal and a decrease in the depolarizing action of acetylcholine on the muscle.

Pancuronium and mexilitene

—Mexilitene, like lidocaine and most local anesthetics, can potentiate neuromuscular blockade from depolarizing and non-depolarizing agents.

Pancuronium and nitroglycerin

—Nitroglycerin can reportedly potentiate the neuromuscular blockade from pancuronium. Other depolarizing agents and succinylcholine apparently do not interact with nitroglycerin.

Pancuronium and procainamide

—Procainamide can potentiate muscle relaxation from non-depolarizing agents. This is probably a result of decreased acetylcholine release at the neuromuscular junction caused by procainamide.

Pancuronium and quinidine

—Quinidine and quinine can potentiate muscle relaxation from both depolarizing and non-depolarizing agents.

—The mechanism of this interaction is a curare-like action at the myoneural junction. Also, plasma pseudocholinesterase is inhibited by quinidine (and quinine), resulting in possible prolongation of muscle relaxation from succinylcholine.

Pancuronium and tocainide

—Tocainide, an orally active form of lidocaine, can potentiate both depolarizing and non-depolarizing neuromuscular blockade. This is a property of most local anesthetics as well as a number of other medications.

PHENTOLAMINE (Regitine)
Classification
—Phentolamine is an alpha adrenergic receptor blocker.
—It is indicated for the treatment of hypertension associated with pheochromocytoma.

Pharmacology
—Phentolamine competitively inhibits both alpha 1 and alpha 2 adrenergic receptors
—Alpha 1 blockade results in arterial and venous vasodilation and a decrease in cardiac preload and afterload.
—Alpha 2 receptors are mainly in the cerebral cortex and medulla and stimulation of these receptors results in inhibition of sympathetic outflow. There are, however, some alpha 2 receptors located in the peripheral nervous system, but their exact function is not clear.
—Blockade of alpha 2 receptors may account partly for the tachycardia that can be associated with use of phentolamine or phenoxybenzamine.
—Significant interactions with anesthetics can occur with patients who are receiving alpha blocking agents. Blockade of alpha 1 receptors can result in unresponsiveness to vasopressors, depending on the vasopressor being used.
—In patients receiving alpha 1 blockers, the response to vasopressors that are primarily alpha agonists (phenylephrine and methoxamine) can be suppressed.
—Vasopressors that stimulate both alpha and beta receptors can interact with alpha 1 blockers in different ways, depending on the amount of alpha and beta agonist activity.
—Epinephrine at lower doses stimulates beta receptors more than alpha receptors. When epinephrine is used to treat patients receiving alpha blockers, hypotension may occur due to the vasodilating effect from epinephrine's prominent beta 2 stimulation.
—Norepinephrine differs from epinephrine by stimulating mainly beta 1 and alpha receptors rather than beta 2 receptors. When norepinephrine is given to patients on alpha blockers, the beta 1 stimulation may produce some increase in blood pressure. Hypotension is unlikely because of minimal beta 2 agonism. Metaraminol may have similar effects.
—Ephedrine and mephentermine are likely to have interactions similar to those of epinephrine with patients receiving alpha

blockers. These agents have significant beta 2 stimulation along with beta 1 and alpha adrenergic activity.

Dose

—Preoperatively: 5 mg IV or IM 1 or 2 hours prior to surgery.

—Intraoperatively: 5 mg IV as necessary to control blood pressure.

Phentolamine Interactions with Anesthesia Drugs

Phentolamine and vasopressors (ephedrine, epinephrine, metaraminol, methoxamine, norepinephrine, phenylephrine)

—Blockade of alpha 1 receptors can result in unresponsiveness to vasopressors, depending on the vasopressor being used.

—Ephedrine and mephentermine have significant beta 2 stimulation along with beta 1 and alpha adrenergic activity. As a result, it is possible that hypotension could worsen in patients on alpha blockers given ephedrine due to the unopposed vasodilation resulting from beta 2 stimulation.

—Although good documentation of this interaction is scarce, this is similar to the response that can be seen with epinephrine.

—Because norepinephrine has beta 1 activity, it is more likely to be effective in treating hypotension in patients on alpha blockers.

PHENYLEPHRINE

Classification and indications

—Phenylephrine is a sympathomimetic amine.

—It is indicated for the management of hypotension from shock or spinal anesthesia when fluid therapy or patient positioning is either ineffective or contraindicated. It is also used as a topical vasoconstrictor in areas such as the nasal mucosa.

Pharmacology

—Phenylephrine is predominantly an alpha adrenergic receptor agonist. Although at very high doses it may cause some beta 1 stimulation (increased heart rate and contractility), there is no beta 2 effect (bronchodilation, skeletal muscle vasodilation).

—Cardiac effects of phenylephrine are primarily a result of peripheral vasoconstriction, resulting in increased systolic and diastolic blood pressure. Bradycardia usually occurs and is a consequence of vagal tone in response to increased blood pressure.

—Vasoconstriction affects the coronary arteries (unlike methoxamine) and pulmonary system. The increased blood pressure may offset coronary constriction and result in increased coronary blood flow.

—Renal vasoconstriction may result in decreased glomerular filtration rate unless hypovolemia is corrected or if hypertension is induced with phenylephrine.

—Elimination of phenylephrine is a result of metabolism by the liver (monoamine oxidase) and by tissue uptake.

Dose

—Adults:

—Intravenous: 40–100 μg/dose or by infusion starting at 10–20 μg/min.

—Intramuscular or subcutaneous: 1- to 10-mg/dose every 1–2 hours as needed.

—Children:

—Intravenous: 5–20 μg/kg/dose or by infusion at 0.1–0.5 μg/kg/minute.

—Intramuscular or subcutaneous: 0.1 mg/kg/dose every 1–2 hours as needed.

Phenylephrine Interactions with Anesthesia Drugs

Phenylephrine and beta blockers (esmolol, labetalol, propranolol)

—Phenylephrine produces mostly alpha stimulation and in patients who are receiving beta blockers has been associated with exaggerated hypertensive responses. This is due to the unopposed vasoconstriction from beta blockade. A similar response is seen with epinephrine.

—This interaction is more likely to occur with nonselective beta blockers such as propranolol, nadolol, timolol, or pindolol.

Phenylephrine and cocaine

—Cocaine may potentiate the vasopressor responses to sympathomimetic agents.

—The mechanism of this interaction involves the inhibition of reuptake of catecholamines by cocaine. This property probably accounts for the vasoconstriction caused by cocaine use.

—Cardiovascular symptoms of hypertension, arrhythmias, and tachycardia from cocaine use are related to both central and sympathetic nervous system effects of cocaine.

Phenylephrine and methylergonovine

—Oxytocics (oxytocin, ergonovine, methylergonovine) may interact with vasopressors to produce hypertension, which is more likely to be severe in patients with a predisposition to hypertension.

—The use of an intramuscular or intravenous ergot alkaloid (such as IM methylergonovine) either preceded or followed by a vasopressor may result in severe hypertension. The safest method of administering an oxytocic is a dilute intravenous infusion of oxytocin.

Phenylephrine and oxytocin

—Severe hypertension has been reported in patients given oxytocin who had received a prophylactic vasoconstrictor up to 4 hours previously for a caudal block.

—This interaction is more likely to occur in patients with existing mild hypertension and who receive an ergot alkaloid (such as methylergonovine) rather than a dilute solution of oxytocin.

Phenylephrine and phentolamine

—In patients receiving alpha 1 blockers, the response to vasopressors that are primarily alpha agonists (phenylephrine and methoxamine) can be suppressed.

—Because norepinephrine has beta 1 activity, it is more likely to be effective in treating hypotension in patients on alpha blockers.

Phenylephrine Interactions with Diseases

Phenylephrine and hyperthyroidism, thyrotoxicosis

—Agents that stimulate the sympathetic nervous system (catecholamines, ephedrine, phenylephrine, dopram, ketamine) may have exaggerated effects in patients with hyperthyroidism. Although most evident in untreated patients, even patients receiving treatment for excess thyroid hormone may demonstrate this response.

—Excess thyroid hormone causes stimulation of metabolism of most body tissues. As a result, cardiac output increases by 50% or more to remove the extra metabolic byproducts. Also, direct stimulatory effects on the myocardium at even slightly elevated thyroid hormone levels causes tachycardia and increased contractility.

—At higher thyroid hormone levels, myocardial depression may occur as a result of excess demands or a direct myocardial depression.

Phenylephrine and pheochromocytoma

—In patients receiving alpha 1 blockers, the response to vasopressors which are primarily alpha agonists (phenylephrine and methoxamine) can be suppressed.

—Because norepinephrine has beta 1 activity, it is more likely to be effective in treating hypotension in patients on alpha blockers.

Phenylephrine and pregnancy

—Ephedrine, mephentermine, and metaraminol are the preferred agents for treatment of hypotension in pregnancy.

—The above agents have both alpha and beta agonist activity and are not associated with reduced placental blood flow.

—Phenylephrine, norepinephrine, angiotensin, and methoxamine are predominantly alpha adrenergic agents that act peripherally and can cause uterine artery vasoconstriction and placental hypoperfusion.

Phenylephrine Interactions with Patient Drugs

Phenylephrine and alpha adrenergic blockers (doxazasin, phenoxybenzamine, phentolamine, prazosin, terazosin

—In patients receiving alpha 1 blockers, the response to vasopressors that are primarily alpha agonists (phenylephrine and methoxamine) can be suppressed.

—Because norepinephrine has beta 1 activity, it is more likely to be effective in treating hypotension in patients on alpha blockers.

Phenylephrine and beta blockers (acebutolol, atenolol, betaxolol, carteolol, labetalol, levobunolol, metoprolol, nadolol, penbutolol, pindolol, propranolol, timolol)

—Phenylephrine produces mostly alpha stimulation and in patients who are receiving beta blockers has been associated with exaggerated hypertensive responses. This is due to the unopposed vasoconstriction from beta blockade. A similar response is seen with epinephrine.

—This interaction is more likely to occur with nonselective beta blockers such as propranolol, nadolol, timolol, or pindolol.

Phenylephrine and ergot alkaloids (dihydroergotamine, ergonovine, ergotamine tartrate, methylergonovine)

—Ergot alkaloids may interact with vasopressors to produce hypertension, which is more likely to be severe in patients with a predisposition to hypertension.

—Because of possibly additive vasoconstrictive effects, the administration of vasopressors to patients receiving ergot alkaloids may produce unexpected degrees of hypertension.

Phenylephrine and guanadrel, guanethidine

—Patients receiving guanethidine and guanadrel can have an exaggerated hypertensive response to norepinephrine and other direct-acting catecholamines such as phenylephrine, dobutamine, and epinephrine.

—Indirect-acting catecholamines, such as ephedrine, metaraminol, mephentermine, and dopamine, may have fewer pressor effects than expected.

—Guanethidine and guanadrel deplete intraneuronal norepinephrine in postganglionic sympathetic neurons, and in this way may diminish the response of indirect-acting catecholamines while sensitizing adrenergic receptors to direct-acting amines.

Phenylephrine and monoamine oxidase inhibitors (isocarboxazid, phenelzine, selegilene, tranylcypromine)

—Indirect-acting vasopressors (ephedrine, mephentermine, and metaraminol) act by releasing intraneuronal monoamines such as dopamine and norepinephrine. This is the explanation of the hypertensive crises seen when patients receiving monamine oxidase (MAO) inhibitors are given these vasopressors.

—Direct-acting vasopressors such as phenylephrine, epinephrine, norepinephrine, and dobutamine may be potentiated by MAO inhibitors and should be used in smaller amounts than normally used.

—Dopamine has both direct and indirect actions and must be used with caution (perhaps one-tenth the normal dose).

Phenylephrine and oxytocin

—Oxytocin administration has been associated with severe hypertension in patients who had received a prophylactic vasoconstrictor up to 4 hours previously for a caudal block.

—Severe hypertension is more likely to occur in patients with existing mild hypertension and in those patients who receive an ergot alkaloid (such as methylergonovine) rather than a dilute solution of oxytocin.

Phenylephrine and ritodrine, terbutaline
—Ritodrine and terbutaline, beta 2 agonists, may potentiate other sympathomimetic agents.
—The mechanism of this interaction is probably related to the beta 1 adrenergic stimulation that can be seen with administration of these drugs.

PIPECURONIUM (Arduan)

Classification and indications
—Pipecuronium is a non-depolarizing neuromuscular blocker that is a derivative of pancuronium.
—It is used for skeletal muscle relaxation during intubation and for maintenance of muscle relaxation during general anesthesia and surgery.

Pharmacology
—Pipecuronium competes with acetylcholine at the neuromuscular junction of skeletal muscle by binding to acetylcholine receptors.
—After a dose of 0.08–0.1 mg/kg, intubating conditions are achieved in 1–3 minutes with a clinical duration (reversal to 25% of twitch height) of 40–120 minutes, which is similar to pancuronium.
—Unlike pancuronium, pipecuronium is not vagolytic and therefore does not result in increased heart rate. Also, there is no significant release of histamine. As a result, cardiovascular stability is maintained.
—Elimination of pipecuronium is primarily excreted in the urine. It undergoes no metabolism. Patients with renal dysfunction will experience prolonged effects.

Dose
—Intubation: 0.08–0.12 mg/kg.
—Maintenance: 0.005–0.01 mg/kg.

Pipecuronium Interactions with Anesthesia Drugs
Pipecuronium and calcium channel blockers (diltiazem, nicardipine, nifedipine, verapamil)
—Calcium channel blockers have been associated with prolongation of neuromuscular blockade from non-depolarizing agents.
—This interaction is probably related to the depletion of intracellular calcium associated with chronic therapy. This

can result in a decrease in acetylcholine release at the neuromuscular junction.

Pipecuronium and inhalational anesthetics (desflurane, enflurane, halothane, isoflurane, sevoflurane)

—Desflurane, enflurane, halothane, isoflurane, and sevoflurane can significantly potentiate neuromuscular blockade, depending on the neuromuscular blocker used. Nitrous oxide has minimal effects.

—Tubocurarine and pancuronium are potentiated the most by inhalational agents, while atracurium and vecuronium are intensified significantly less.

—Potentiation by inhalational agents occurs through depression of spinal cord reflexes as well as effects at or distal to the neuromuscular junction.

Pipecuronium and diphenylhydantoin, phenytoin

—Patients on chronic phenytoin therapy may be resistant to non-depolarizing muscle blockade. The studies involved metocurine and vecuronium but may involve other non-depolarizing agents.

—The mechanism of this interaction is not known.

—Acute infusions of phenytoin may prolong non-depolarizing blockade. This was studied prospectively in a small number of patients who received a 10 mg/kg loading dose of phenytoin during steady-state muscle blockade with vecuronium. They had significant potentiation of their neuromuscular block compared to control patients.

Pipecuronium and furosemide

—Furosemide may potentiate neuromuscular blockade from tubocurarine and succinylcholine. This is based on a case report of several patients given furosemide and tubocurarine during surgery and on animal studies.

—The implication for this interaction for other neuromuscular blocking drugs is uncertain and the mechanism is not known.

Pipecuronium and lidocaine

—Most local anesthetics can block neuromuscular transmission from non-depolarizing agents as well as depolarizing muscle relaxants. Of clinical significance to the anesthesiologist, lidocaine, given as a 50- to 100-mg bolus or even by infusion, can significantly increase a non-depolarizer block or a phase II block from succinylcholine.

Pipecuronium and procainamide

—Procainamide can potentiate muscle relaxation from non-depolarizing agents. This is probably a result of decreased acetylcholine release at the neuromuscular junction caused by procainamide.

Pipecuronium and quinidine

—Quinidine, procainamide, propranolol, and most local anesthetics have been shown to enhance the neuromuscular blockade from depolarizing and non-depolarizing agents.

—A number of well-documented cases have illustrated the ability of these agents, when given in the immediate post-operative period, to convert subclinical muscle weakness from neuromuscular blocking drugs into significant muscle weakness requiring reintubation.

Pipecuronium and succinylcholine

—Prior administration of succinylcholine has been shown to potentiate neuromuscular blockade of some non-depolarizing agents.

—Although this interaction has been documented with pancuronium, it was not seen with doxacurium and may not be a consistent finding with non-depolarizing agents.

Pipecuronium Interactions with Diseases

Pipecuronium and advanced age

—Prolonged duration of neuromuscular blockade can be seen in older patients with several different non-depolarizing agents, including doxacurium, mivacurium, and rocuronium.

—In some cases, delayed onset of muscle relaxation also occurs. This has been attributed to decreased perfusion of the neuromuscular junction as a result of advanced age.

Pipecuronium and burns

—Patients with burn injuries are susceptible to a life-threatening hyperkalemic response to succinylcholine and can have marked resistance to non-depolarizing muscle relaxants.

—Both of these altered responses to neuromuscular blocking agents have been attributed to proliferation of extrajunctional acetylcholine receptors, similar to that in the patient with a denervation injury.

—Resistance to non-depolarizing agents appears to increase with larger area burns and in fact may not be significant in patients with <30% body surface area burns. In addition to proliferation of extrajunctional acetylcholine receptors, this abnormal response is probably also related to the increased metabolic rate and hepatic and renal clearance seen in burn patients. Doses of non-depolarizing agents may need to be increased by as much as 300%.

—Duration of this resistance usually is 2 months following the injury but has been reported in a patient 463 days after the burn.

Pipecuronium and cirrhosis, liver disease

—Prolonged neuromuscular blockade in patients with liver disease can be seen with doxacurium, mivacurium, vecuronium, pancuronium, rocuronium, and tubocurarine.

—This interaction is complex and may be due to decreased clearance, decreased hepatic uptake of the agent, or decreased synthesis of enzymes important for degradation of the neuromuscular blocker. An example of the latter is prolongation of mivacurium's duration of action as a result of decreased plasma cholinesterase from severe liver disease.

—Because of the increased volume of distribution of many drugs seen in patients with liver disease, initial doses of muscle relaxants may need to be larger than in healthy patients. Once neuromuscular blockade is achieved, recovery may be prolonged.

Pipecuronium and Eaton–Lambert syndrome

—Patients with Eaton–Lambert syndrome are very sensitive to both depolarizing and non-depolarizing neuromuscular blockade.

—This disorder is similar to myasthenia gravis and patients complain of skeletal muscle weakness, but it is usually associated with carcinoma (especially small cell tumors of the lung).

—If the diagnosis is known or suspected prior to surgery, reduced doses of muscle relaxants should be used, but sometimes the diagnosis is first made when a patient has surgery for a lung tumor and has an unexpected, prolonged neuromuscular block.

—Anticholinesterases are unreliable in reversing muscle weakness.

Pipecuronium and hyperthyroidism, thyrotoxicosis

—Muscle weakness is commonly seen with hyperthyroidism and affects proximal muscles, usually sparing respiratory function. In some cases, myopathy is the dominant feature of thyroid hormone excess and can resemble myasthenia. Lower doses of muscle relaxants may be indicated.

Pipecuronium and hypokalemia

—Hypokalemia appears to potentiate the effects of neuro-muscular blockade from non-depolarizing agents.

—The interaction is probably due to hyperpolarization of the muscle endplate and, therefore, resistance to depolarization. Hyperpolarization would more likely occur with more acute changes in potassium concentration because the potassium losses would be from the extracellular compartment rather than from intracellular sites.

—Chronic hypokalemia is more likely to be associated with potassium depletion from both extra- and intracellular compartments with no significant change in transmembrane potential. As a result, significant effects on neuro-muscular blockade would be less likely.

Pipecuronium and hypothermia

—Non-depolarizing muscle blockade is prolonged by hypo-thermia. This interaction is a result of an effect on the neuromuscular blocking agents themselves rather than on the anticholinesterases used to reverse the neuromuscular blocking agents.

—Hypothermia appears to prolong the effect of the non-depolarizing agents by several mechanisms, including delayed metabolism into inactive metabolites as well as delayed excretion via the urinary and biliary routes.

Pipecuronium and malignant hyperthermia

—Anesthetic agents considered safe for use in patients with known or suspected susceptibility for developing malignant hyperthermia (MH) include propofol, barbiturates, etomi-date, ketamine, non-depolarizing neuromuscular blocking agents, narcotics, benzodiazepines, droperidol, epinephrine, norepinephrine, and anticholinesterases.

—Nitrous oxide is probably safe in the susceptible patient based on repeated use in MH-susceptible humans and swine.

—Local or regional anesthesia with either amide (such as lido-caine) or ester (such as procaine) anesthetics is now consid-ered safe for MH-susceptible patients.

Pipecuronium and myasthenia gravis

—Patients with myasthenia gravis are very sensitive to neuro-muscular blockade from non-depolarizing agents.

—This is probably a result of decreased acetylcholine receptors from autoimmune destruction associated with myasthenia gravis.

—Although these patients are treated with the same or similar anticholinesterases used to antagonize muscle blockade, sensitivity (not resistance) to neuromuscular blockade is seen clinically.

Pipecuronium and neuromuscular disease (amyotrophic lateral sclerosis, multiple sclerosis, syringomyelia)

—Patients with a wide variety of neuromuscular disorders may be more resistant than normal patients to the effects of non-depolarizing neuromuscular blockers.

—This includes patients with disuse atrophy of the muscles (such as bedridden patients with chronic disease) as well as patients with upper or lower motor neuron disease such as amyotrophic lateral sclerosis, multiple sclerosis, or syringomyelia.

—Disuse or denervation of muscle results in production of extrajunctional acetylcholine receptors on the muscle membrane. These receptors are less easily blocked by non-depolarizing agents but are activated by lower concentrations of depolarizing drugs (succinylcholine).

—When these receptors, which can be scattered over a large surface of the muscle, are depolarized by succinylcholine, ion flow takes place through the receptor channel. Large amounts of potassium may exit the muscle cell, causing hyperkalemia.

—Despite initial resistance to blockade, such patients may demonstrate prolonged neuromuscular weakness as a result of decreased muscle strength and mass.

Pipecuronium and PIH (pregnancy-induced hypertension), preeclampsia/eclampsia, toxemia

—Patients with hypertensive disorders of pregnancy may require treatment with antihypertensives such as trimethaphan or magnesium sulfate (for preeclampsia/eclampsia). These medications can have significant interactions with anesthetic agents such as succinylcholine, non-depolarizing neuromuscular blocking agents, or calcium channel blockers.

—Neuromuscular blockade produced by both depolarizing and non-depolarizing agents can be potentiated in patients receiving magnesium sulfate. The mechanisms involved include a decreased amount of acetylcholine released by the nerve impulse at the motor nerve terminal and a decrease in the depolarizing action of acetylcholine on the muscle.

Pipecuronium Interactions with Patient Drugs

Pipecuronium and antibiotics

—A number of antibiotics have significant interactions with neuromuscular blocking agents. These include the aminoglycosides (amikacin, gentamicin, kanamycin, neomycin, paromomycin, netilmicin, neomycin, streptomycin, tobramycin), as well as polymyxin B, colistin, amphotericin B, clindamycin, bacitracin, and lincomycin.

—All of the above antibiotics may potentiate non-depolarizing agents, but some (aminoglycosides, amphotericin B, clindamycin, colistin) can also potentiate succinylcholine blockade.

—These antibiotics potentiate neuromuscular blockade by different mechanisms, making management of these problems difficult. Although treatment with anticholinesterases or calcium has been recommended, results are inconsistent.

Pipecuronium and amphotericin B

—Prolonged neuromuscular blockade can occur with depolarizing and non-depolarizing agents in patients receiving amphotericin B.

—The mechanism for this interaction is thought to be associated with the hypokalemia that can be caused by amphotericin B therapy.

Pipecuronium and beta blockers, propranolol

—Beta blockers may potentiate non-depolarizing neuromuscular blocking agents. This interaction has been reported between propranolol and tubocurarine.

—Other beta blockers are also capable of causing weakness in patients with myasthenia gravis, but the mechanism or significance of these interactions is unclear.

Pipecuronium and calcium channel blockers (amlodipine, bepridil, diltiazem, felodipine, isradipine, lidoflazine, nicardipine, nimodipine, nisoldipine, nitrendipine, verapamil)

—Calcium channel blockers have been associated with prolongation of neuromuscular blockade from non-depolarizing agents.

—This interaction is probably related to the depletion of intracellular calcium associated with chronic therapy. This can result in a decrease in acetylcholine release at the neuromuscular junction.

Pipecuronium and diphenylhydantoin, phenytoin

—Patients on chronic phenytoin therapy may be resistant to non-depolarizing muscle blockade. The studies involved metocurine and vecuronium but may involve other non-depolarizing agents.

—The mechanism of this interaction is not known.

—Acute infusions of phenytoin may prolong non-depolarizing blockade. This was studied prospectively in a small number of patients who received a 10 mg/kg loading dose of phenytoin during steady-state muscle blockade with vecuronium. They had significant potentiation of their neuromuscular block compared to control patients.

Pipecuronium and lidocaine

—Most local anesthetics can block neuromuscular transmission from non-depolarizing agents as well as depolarizing muscle relaxants. Of clinical significance to the anesthesiologist, lidocaine, given as a 50- to 100-mg bolus or even by infusion, can significantly increase a non-depolarizer block or a phase II block from succinylcholine.

Pipecuronium and lithium

—Lithium has been reported to increase the duration of both non-depolarizing and depolarizing neuromuscular blocking drugs.

—The mechanism of this interaction is unknown and the clinical significance of this interaction is uncertain.

Pipecuronium and magnesium sulfate

—Neuromuscular blockade produced by both depolarizing and non-depolarizing agents can be potentiated in patients receiving magnesium sulfate. The mechanisms involved include a decreased amount of acetylcholine released by the nerve impulse at the motor nerve terminal and a decrease in the depolarizing action of acetylcholine on the muscle.

Pipecuronium and mexilitene

—Mexilitene, like lidocaine and most local anesthetics, can potentiate neuromuscular blockade from depolarizing and non-depolarizing agents.

Pipecuronium and procainamide

—Procainamide can potentiate muscle relaxation from non-depolarizing agents. This is probably a result of decreased acetylcholine release at the neuromuscular junction caused by procainamide.

Pipecuronium and quinidine
—Quinidine and quinine can potentiate muscle relaxation from both depolarizing and non-depolarizing agents.

—The mechanism of this interaction is a curare-like action at the myoneural junction. Also, plasma pseudocholinesterase is inhibited by quinidine (and quinine), resulting in possible prolongation of muscle relaxation from succinylcholine.

Pipecuronium and tocainide
—Tocainide, an orally active form of lidocaine, can potentiate both depolarizing and non-depolarizing neuromuscular blockade. This is a property of most local anesthetics as well as a number of other medications.

PROCAINAMIDE (Pronestyl)

Classification and indications
—Procainamide is a class IA antiarrhythmic agents (as are quinidine and lidocaine).

—It is indicated for the management of atrial and ventricular arrhythmias.

Pharmacology
—Cardiac conduction effects from procainamide include an increased refractory period of the atria, ventricles, and the His-Purkinje fibers. Also, there is decreased automaticity and excitability of these tissues.

—Conduction can be more rapid through the atrioventricular node, so that ventricular response to atrial tachyarrhythmias may be increased unless AV conduction is blocked first by other means (digoxin).

—At toxic levels, procainamide may cause prolonged AV conduction times, even producing AV block. This can be manifested as a widened QRS, prolonged QT and PR, and increasing AV block.

—In patients with impaired ventricular function, procainamide may worsen contractility.

—Elimination of procainamide is highly dependent on adequate renal function and patients with renal disease may show toxicity earlier than normal patients.

Dose
—Adults:
  —Bolus: 100 mg/min IV up to a total of 1 g (usual dose 500–600 mg).
  —Infusion: 1–6 mg/min. IV or 0.02–0.08 mg/kg/min.
—Children:
  —Bolus: 3–6 mg/kg IV (maximum dose 100 mg) IV.
  —Infusion: 0.02–0.08 mg/kg/min IV.

Procainamide Interactions with Anesthesia Drugs

Procainamide and muscle relaxants (atracurium, doxacurium, gallamine, metocurine, mivacurium, pancuronium, pipercuronium, rocuronium, tubocurarine, vecuronium)

—Procainamide can potentiate muscle relaxation from non-depolarizing agents. This is probably a result of decreased acetylcholine release at the neuromuscular junction caused by procainamide.

Procainamide Interactions with Diseases

Procainamide and atrial fibrillation or flutter

—Quinidine and procainamide (class IA antiarrhythmics) can cause an increased ventricular response in some patients with atrial fibrillation or flutter.
—Although class IA antiarrhythmics depress conduction through the atrioventricular (AV) node, they can also have a vagolytic effect that offsets this effect and can result in increased conduction through the AV node. This is more pronounced with quinidine than with procainamide.
—In patients with atrial fibrillation, a decreased conduction time (increased rate of conduction) through the AV node would result in a more rapid ventricular rate.
—Because of quinidine's depressant effect on atrial conduction, patients with atrial flutter may experience a decreased atrial rate, but the increased conduction rate through the AV node may offset this effect with a net increase in the ventricular rate.
—Both quinidine and procainamide can be effective for management of these arrhythmias, but prior digitalization or treatment with verapamil or beta blockers is recommended to avoid increased AV conduction.

Procainamide and heart block (second, third degree)

—Procainamide should not be used for treatment of tachyarrhythmias in patients with second- or third-degree AV block unless a pacemaker is in place.

—Class IA antiarrhythmics such as procainamide can depress atrioventricular conduction as well as nodal and Purkinje fiber automaticity. Therefore, while its ability to suppress excitability in most cardiac tissues and inhibit ectopic pacemaker activity make procainamide useful in treating atrial and ventricular tachyarrhythmias, patients with these arrhythmias overlying an AV block may become severely bradycardic or asystolic if treated with class IA antiarrhythmic agents.

Procainamide and myasthenia gravis

—Patients receiving anticholinesterase drugs for myasthenia gravis can have exacerbation of muscle weakness if given procainamide or quinidine.

—This is related to the ability of these drugs to enhance neuromuscular blockade from depolarizing and non-depolarizing agents.

—Lidocaine and propranolol would also be expected to have this interaction but appear to be safe for use in myasthenics.

Procainamide and renal dysfunction

—Elimination of procainamide is very dependent on adequate renal function and patients with renal disease can show toxicity from procainamide earlier than normal patients.

—Up to 70% of a procainamide dose can be eliminated unchanged in the urine. Hepatic metabolism converts procainamide to *N*-acetylprocainamide, which has slightly different properties from the parent compound but can cause toxicity at high levels.

—In patients with renal disease, more procainamide is converted to *N*-acetylprocainamide, which can accumulate to toxic levels.

Procainamide and sick sinus syndrome

—Patients with sick sinus syndrome can experience supraventricular tachyarrhythmias. The diseased sinus nodes of these patients appear to be very sensitive to depression by, among other things, class IA antiarrhythmics (quinidine, procainamide, disopyramide) and treatment of arrhythmias in patients with sick sinus syndrome can result in severe sinus bradycardia or asystole.

Procainamide and Wolf–Parkinson–White syndrome

—Verapamil, diltiazem, digitalis, beta blockers, and lidocaine should not be used to acutely treat wide complex tachyarrhythmias associated with the Wolf–Parkinson–White syndrome.

—In tachyarrhythmias with wide QRS complexes, antegrade conduction must be assumed to be taking place via accessory paths. Conduction through these paths can be accelerated by verapamil, diltiazem, digitalis, lidocaine, or propranolol. Intravenous procainamide is the treatment of choice.

—If the QRS complex is narrow, indicating antegrade conduction via normal conduction paths, treatment can be with agents that slow conduction through the AV node: verapamil, propranolol, digitalis, procainamide, or diltiazem.

Procainamide Interactions with Patient Drugs
Procainamide and ambenonium chloride

—Patients receiving cholinergic medications for myasthenia gravis may experience worsening muscle weakness with administration of procainamide.

—Procainamide, in addition to acting as an antagonist to the neuromuscular effects of cholinergic medications, has neuromuscular blocking properties.

Procainamide and amiodarone

—Amiodarone increases refractoriness and slows conduction in most cardiac tissue. A number of medications, including class I antiarrhythmics (such as lidocaine or procainamide), calcium channel blockers, and beta blockers, which have similar effects, can precipitate severe bradycardia when given to a patient taking amiodarone.

—A case was reported of a patient with sick sinus syndrome on amiodarone who developed profound sinus bradycardia after local anesthesia with lidocaine.

Procainamide and neostigmine, pyridostigmine bromide

—Patients receiving cholinergic medications for myasthenia gravis may experience worsening muscle weakness with administration of procainamide.

—Procainamide, in addition to acting as an antagonist to the neuromuscular effects of cholinergic medications, has neuromuscular blocking properties.

PROCAINE (Anuject, Novocain, Ravocaine)

Classification and indications

—Procaine is an ester-type local anesthetic.

—It is used for infiltration anesthesia or for peripheral and sympathetic nerve blocks.

Pharmacology
—Like all local anesthetics, procaine prevents the generation and conduction of nerve impulses by blocking the normal increase in sodium permeability that accompanies depolarization of nerve axons.

—Onset of action is about 2–3 minutes and has a duration of about 1 hour.

—Metabolism is a result of the action of plasma pseudocholinesterase (like succinylcholine).

—Patients with deficiencies of plasma pseudocholinesterase have been reported to experience toxicity from normal doses of procaine. Although chloroprocaine is also metabolized by this enzyme, there are no reports of similar toxicity.

Dose
—Infiltration anesthesia: 350–600 mg of procaine either as a 0.25% or a 0.5% solution.

—Nerve block: Maximum dose is 1 g of a 0.5% or 1% solution.

Procaine Interactions with Diseases
Procaine and malignant hyperthermia
—Local or regional anesthesia with either amide (such as lidocaine) or ester (such as procaine) anesthetics is now considered safe for MH-susceptible patients.

—Anesthetic agents considered safe for use in patients with known or suspected susceptibility for developing malignant hyperthermia include propofol, barbiturates, etomidate, ketamine, non-depolarizing neuromuscular blocking agents, narcotics, benzodiazepines, droperidol, epinephrine, norepinephrine, and anticholinesterases.

—Nitrous oxide is probably safe in the susceptible patient based on repeated use in MH-susceptible humans and swine.

Procaine Interactions with Patient Drugs
Procaine and echothiophate
—Echothiophate, an antagonist of plasma pseudocholinesterase, may interact with procaine to cause procaine toxicity.

—Because procaine depends on pseudocholinesterase for its metabolism, reduced activity of this enzyme could lead to toxicity. Although patients with inherited deficiencies of plasma cholinesterase have been reported to experience severe toxicity with procaine, there is no documentation of this reaction with echothiophate.

PROPOFOL (Diprivan)
Classification and indications
—Propofol, an alkylphenol, is an intravenous anesthetic agent. It consists of propofol, soybean oil, glycerol, and purified egg lecithin.

—It is indicated for use as an induction agent for general anesthesia, or for intravenous sedation either during surgery or in the intensive care unit. It is also used as an infusion for anesthesia during surgery combined with narcotics, benzodiazepines, and/or inhalational agents.

Pharmacology
—Propofol, like thiopental and etomidate, is believed to induce hypnosis through its effect on the GABA receptors. Gamma aminobutyric acid (GABA) is the main inhibitory neurotransmitter in the central nervous system (CNS) and propofol enhances its activity.

—CNS effects of propofol include a decrease in intracranial pressure and cerebral metabolic rate, but with decreases in cerebral perfusion pressure. In patients with elevated ICP, this may be undesirable.

—Although propofol has anticonvulsant properties, there are reports of convulsions following its administration, in some cases up to 6 days later. Some of these patients had no previous history of seizures.

—Cardiac effects of propofol include a reduction in cardiac output, stroke volume, and systemic vascular resistance. There also appears to be a decrease in myocardial contractility, which is probably dose-dependent.

—Onset of hypnosis occurs rapidly following intravenous administration (<1 minute) and has a duration of about 5–10 minutes.

—Termination of the effect of propofol is a result of redistribution and elimination. Hepatic or renal disease has little effect on the kinetics of propofol.

Dose
—Induction: 1–2.5 mg/kg IV. Reduced dosage should be used in older patients (>50 years).

—Maintenance of general anesthesia: 80–150 µg/kg/min, combined with an opiate and/or nitrous oxide or a volatile anesthetic.

—Sedation: 10–50 µg/kg/min alone or combined with an opiate.

Propofol Interactions with Diseases

Propofol and advanced age

—A reduced induction dose is recommended for thiopental, etomidate, and propofol in most elderly patients.

—Reduction in the dose requirements for these drugs may be a result of a decreased volume of distribution, decreased elimination, or a combination of effects brought about by aging.

Propofol and alcohol—acute intoxication

—Patients who are acutely intoxicated with alcohol (including chronic alcoholics) usually demonstrate increased sensitivity to general anesthesia.

—Although the precise mechanisms of interactions are not agreed on, it appears that alcohol intoxication has additive CNS depression with barbiturates, benzodiazepines, and narcotics, as well as inhalational agents.

Propofol and alcohol—chronic abuse

—Chronic abuse of alcohol has complex and incompletely understood effects on a patient's response to anesthetic agents. In general, these patients tend to be more tolerant (in a nonintoxicated state) to barbiturates, benzodiazepines, narcotics, inhalational agents, and, probably, propofol.

—Exceptions to this generalization include the alcoholic patient with a cardiomyopathy who may demonstrate increased sensitivity to myocardial depression from inhalational agents.

Propofol and cerebral edema, intracranial hypertension

—Most intravenous anesthetics cause a reduction in cerebral blood flow (CBF) and intracranial pressure (ICP) or have no effect on ICP. Although this effect is primarily from depression of cerebral metabolic rate (CMR), in some cases a direct vasoconstriction occurs.

—The exception to the above is ketamine, which causes an increased CMR and CBF with an increase in ICP.

—All of the narcotics, as well as barbiturates, etomidate, benzodiazepines, and propofol have been associated with a reduction or maintenance of ICP during anesthesia.

Propofol and epilepsy

—There are several reports of seizure activity or opisthotonus (tetanic spasm of back and neck) in postoperative patients who had received propofol. The mechanism of this adverse reaction is unknown, and the reaction very rare.

—The seizures or opisthotonus have been transient in most patients but lasted for 1–3 weeks in two European patients.

Propofol and hypothermia

—Hypothermia can have significant effects on propofol plasma levels.

—Plasma levels of propofol, when administered as a constant infusion, have been shown to be increased by as much as 30% in patients with hypothermia to 34°C.

Propofol and malignant hyperthermia

—Anesthetic agents considered safe for use in patients with known or suspected susceptibility for developing malignant hyperthermia (MH) include propofol, barbiturates, etomidate, ketamine, non-depolarizing neuromuscular blocking agents, narcotics, benzodiazepines, droperidol, epinephrine, norepinephrine, and anticholinesterases.

—Nitrous oxide is probably safe in the susceptible patient, based on repeated use in MH-susceptible humans and swine.

—Local or regional anesthesia with either amide (such as lidocaine) or ester (such as procaine) anesthetics is now considered safe for MH-susceptible patients.

Propofol and porphyria

—Use of propofol is considered to be probably safe for use in patients with porphyria, as are narcotics, depolarizing and non-depolarizing muscle relaxants, etomidate, anticholinesterases, and inhalational agents.

—Barbiturates are contraindicated in three of the four hepatic porphyrias (acute intermittent porphyria, variegate porphyria, and hereditary coproporphyria). Porphyria cutanea tarda and the erythropoietic porphyrias are not exacerbated by barbiturates.

—It is theorized that barbiturates can provoke an attack of porphyria by inducing the enzyme aminolevulinic acid synthetase, which results in synthesis of more porphyrin compounds and their precursors.

Propofol and renal dysfunction

—Renal dysfunction has not been demonstrated to cause significant changes in pharmacokinetics or pharmacodynamics of benzodiazepines, narcotics (with the possible exception of butorphanol), barbiturates, or propofol.

—In patients with renal dysfunction, the above drugs may appear to have an increase in duration or intensity. This has been explained as a response to the systemic effects of renal dysfunction rather than specific effects on the metabolism of theses drugs.

—Some muscle relaxants are significantly affected by renal failure.

PROPRANOLOL (Betachron, Inderal)

Classification and indications

—Propranolol is a nonselective beta adrenergic blocking agent.

—It is indicated for the management of hypertension, angina, and tachyarrhythmias (ventricular and supraventricular).

Pharmacology

—Propranolol is a competitive inhibitor of beta receptors. Effects of beta 1 blockade include decreased heart rate and contractility, slowed conduction through the atrioventricular and sinus node, decreased automaticity, and decreased myocardial oxygen consumption.

—Beta 2 blockade results in some increase in peripheral vascular resistance (due to unopposed alpha stimulation). The overall effect of beta blockade and other less understood mechanisms causes a decrease in blood pressure.

—Bronchial constriction from beta 2 blockade may result in increased airway resistance, especially in patients with reactive airway disease (asthma, chronic obstructive pulmonary disease, bronchitis).

—Onset of action after administration of 0.5 mg intravenously is almost immediate and single doses have an approximate half-life of 2–3 hours.

—Elimination is almost completely dependent on liver metabolism.

Dose

—For tachyarrhythmias:

—Adults: 0.5–3 mg administered no faster than 1 mg/min.

—Children: 10–20 µg/kg infused over about 10 minutes, for life-threatening arrhythmias.

Propranolol Interactions with Anesthesia Drugs

Propranolol and calcium channel blockers (diltiazem, verapamil)

—Verapamil and diltiazem, particularly when used intravenously, can significantly potentiate the effects of beta blockers on cardiac conduction and contractility.

—Severe bradycardia and hypotension can occur when these medications are used concomitantly, especially in patients with abnormalities of cardiac conduction (sick sinus syndrome) or ventricular function (congestive heart failure).

Propranolol and chlorpromazine

—Large doses of propranolol given with chlorpromazine can increase the serum levels of both medications.

Propranolol and cocaine

—Beta blockers have been demonstrated to potentiate coronary vasoconstriction caused by cocaine.

—This interaction was documented in the cardiac catheterization lab using intranasal cocaine followed by administration of propranolol.

—Although the significance of this interaction to clinical practice is not clear, patients who develop hypertension, tachycardia, and angina from cocaine may be best treated by an agent such as labetalol, which has alpha blocking properties.

Propranolol and diazoxide

—The hypotensive response to diazoxide may be accentuated in patients taking beta blockers.

—This may be due to blunting of the normal sympathetic response that otherwise occurs.

Propranolol and dopamine, epinephrine, norepinephrine

—Use of esmolol or propranolol for treatment of supraventricular tachycardia may have undesirable effects in some patients; specifically, in patients requiring cardiovascular support with agents that are both inotropic and vasoconstrictive (dopamine, epinephrine, norepinephrine), blockade of beta receptors may result in decreased cardiac contractility in the face of systemic vasoconstriction, resulting in cardiac failure.

Propranolol and isoproterenol

—Patients who are receiving beta blockers may be more resistant to the bronchodilator effects of isoproterenol. The nonselective beta blockers, such as propranolol, are more likely to have an interaction of greater magnitude than selective blockers, such as metoprolol.

Propranolol and ketamine

—Ketamine may produce myocardial depression if there is interference with the normal sympathetic response, as seen in patients on beta blockers.

Propranolol and phenylephrine

—Phenylephrine produces mostly alpha stimulation and in patients who are receiving beta blockers has been associated with exaggerated hypertensive responses. This is due to the unopposed vasoconstriction from beta blockade. A similar response is seen with epinephrine.

—This interaction is more likely to occur with nonselective beta blockers such as propranolol, nadolol, timolol, or pindolol.

Propranolol Interactions with Diseases

Propranolol and asthma

—Use of beta blockers in patients with reactive airway disease (asthma, chronic obstructive pulmonary disease) can result in significant increases in airway resistance.

—Although noncardioselective beta blockers (labetalol, propranolol) are most likely to precipitate bronchospasm in these patients, even selective beta 1 blockers (esmolol) have enough beta 2 blocking properties to require caution.

Propranolol and congestive heart failure

—Beta blockers can precipitate congestive heart failure in patients with compromised cardiac function. In patients in congestive heart failure, there may be deterioration in cardiac status. The exception to these consequences might be the situation in which tachyarrhythmias may be precipitating acute cardiac decompensation by increasing the myocardial oxygen demand.

—Beta 1 adrenergic blockade reduces heart rate, myocardial contractility, and, therefore, cardiac ouput. Also, atrioventricular node conduction time is prolonged and sinus node automaticity is decreased.

Propranolol and heart block (second, third degree)

—Use of beta blockers in patients with second- or third-degree heart block can cause dangerous decreases in heart rate.

—Beta 1 adrenergic blockade results in a decrease in sinus node automaticity as well as a prolongation of atrioventricular conduction time.

—If beta blockers are used in patients with heart block, cardiac pacing may be necessary.

Propranolol and Raynaud's phenomenon

—Beta blockers must be used with extreme caution in patients with Raynaud's phenomenon because of the ability of these drugs to worsen or precipitate digital vasospasm.

—Arteriovenous shunts exist in the fingertips and dilate with beta adrenergic stimulation. Beta 1 blockade can result in vasoconstriction. Labetalol, because of its ability to block alpha receptors, would be less likely to cause this problem.

Propranolol and sick sinus syndrome

—Diltiazem, verapamil, and beta blockers should be avoided or used with extreme caution in patients with sick sinus syndrome (SSS).

—Use of these drugs, which depress sinus node automaticity, may cause severe bradycardia even in patients with SSS who are experiencing supraventricular tachycardia.

—Digitalis may be effective in controlling supraventricular tachycardias.

Propranolol and Wolf–Parkinson–White syndrome

—Verapamil, diltiazem, digitalis, beta blockers, and lidocaine should not be used to acutely treat wide complex tachyarrhythmias associated with the Wolf–Parkinson–White syndrome.

—In tachyarrhythmias with wide QRS complexes, antegrade conduction must be assumed to be taking place via accessory paths. Conduction through these paths can be accelerated by verapamil, diltiazem, digitalis, lidocaine, or propranolol. Intravenous procainamide is the treatment of choice.

—If the QRS complex is narrow, indicating antegrade conduction via normal conduction paths, treatment can be with agents that slow conduction through the AV node: verapamil, propranolol, digitalis, procainamide, or diltiazem.

Propranolol Interactions with Patient Drugs

Propranolol and amiodarone

—Metoprolol and propranolol have both been associated with life-threatening arrhythmias (severe bradycardia, cardiac arrest, or ventricular fibrillation) in patients taking amiodarone. In all cases, these arrhythmias developed within 1 hour to several hours after initiation of these beta blockers and after only one or two doses.

—Although these cases involved oral beta blockers, intravenous propranolol could have similar results.

—Other beta blockers have not been associated with this interaction.

Propranolol and dopamine

—Use of beta blockers for treatment of supraventricular tachycardia may have undesirable effects in some patients;

specifically, in patients requiring cardiovascular support with agents that are both inotropic and vasoconstrictive (dopamine, epinephrine, norepinephrine), blockade of beta receptors may result in decreased cardiac contractility in the face of systemic vasoconstriction, resulting in cardiac failure.

Propranolol and flecainide
—Flecainide can cause decreased myocardial contractility, particularly at the onset of intravenous therapy. Patients most significantly affected are those with compromised left ventricular function (ejection fraction <30%).
—Beta blockers and some calcium channel blockers may have added negative inotropic effects with flecainide.

Propranolol and mefloquine
—Mefloquine is a derivative of quinine and has rarely been associated with bradycardia and prolonged QT interval. Beta blockers and calcium channel blockers should be used with caution in patients on this medication.

Propranolol and methyldopa
—Patients taking methyldopa for hypertension may experience a hypertensive response when given beta blockers. This has been reported in a patient on methyldopa who was given a slow intravenous injection of propranolol.
—The mechanism for this response is thought to be related to the accumulation of methylnorepinephrine that is a result of methyldopa therapy. This substance has both vasoconstricting and vasodilating properties. The latter, when blocked by beta blockers, could leave unopposed vasoconstriction resulting in hypertension.

Propranolol and ritodrine, terbutaline
—Beta blockers may reverse the relaxation of bronchial and uterine smooth muscle produced by ritodrine and terbutaline.

PROTAMINE

Classification and indications
—Protamine is prepared from the testes or sperm of certain fish (salmon and some other species).
—It is indicated for the neutralization of heparin (either from heparin overdose or from reversal of anticoagulation for cardiopulmonary by-pass procedures).

Pharmacology

—Protamine inactivates heparin by binding to the heparin, forming a heparin–protamine complex.

—This occurs in part because protamine is a strong base, whereas heparin is strongly acidic.

—There are several severe reactions that can occur following administration of protamine. These include circulatory collapse and bradycardia and anaphylactic or anaphylactoid reactions. The precise mechanism of these responses is not clear.

—Certain patients appear to be at greater risk for hypersensitivity reactions to protamine. Patients with fish allergy, patients exposed previously to protamine from other surgery or through use of insulin preparations containing protamine, and vasectomized patients appear to be at higher risk.

—Onset of effect after intravenous administration is rapid and neutralization of heparin occurs within 5 minutes.

—Reheparinization can occur and may be either a result of mobilization of heparin from body tissues or breakdown of heparin–protamine complexes.

Dose

—Approximately 1 mg protamine for 100 units (1 mg) heparin).

Protamine Interactions with Diseases

Protamine and diabetes mellitus

—The presence of protamine in some insulin preparations has been implicated in allergic reactions to protamine used after cardiopulmonary bypass to reverse heparin. It has been suggested that the protamine in these insulin preparations used chronically in insulin-dependent diabetics may stimulate antibody formation. However, there is some controversy as to whether protamine exposure from insulin increases a patient's risk of such a reaction.

—The two most frequently used preparations are NPH (neutral protamine Hagedorn) and Lente insulin. NPH insulin is a suspension of insulin containing zinc, protamine, and a phosphate buffer. Lente insulin contains no protamine. The other form of insulin that contains protamine is the slow onset, PZI (protamine zinc insulin).

PYRIDOSTIGMINE (Mestinon)

Classification and indications

—Pyridostigmine is a synthetic parasympathomimetic agent.

—It is indicated for use as a reversal agent for non-depolarizing neuromuscular blocking agents (competitive inhibitors of acetylcholine). It is also used for testing for myasthenia gravis and has been used in the treatment of supraventricular tachycardias.

Pharmacology

—Pyridostigmine inhibits the destruction of acetylcholine by binding reversibly to acetylcholinesterase. As a result, acetylcholine accumulates at cholinergic synapses (such as the neuromuscular junction and the sinus node).

—Speed of reversal of the anticholinesterases depends on several factors, including depth of muscle blockade, neuromuscular blocker used, and dose and type of anticholinesterase.

—In general, onset of action is fastest with edrophonium, followed by neostigmine and pyridostigmine.

—At moderate levels of neuromuscular blockade (<90% twitch depression), neostigmine, edrophonium, and pyridostigmine are about equivalent in ability to induce reversal. When muscle blockade is profound (>90% twitch depression), edrophonium is not as effective as neostigmine.

—Pyridostigmine has the longest duration of action. Although edrophonium was thought to have a very short duration of action, studies with edrophonium doses of 0.5–1.0 mg/kg demonstrate a similar duration between edrophonium and neostigmine.

—Cardiac effects of parasympathomimetic agents, such as the anticholinesterases, result in bradycardia. To antagonize these responses, reversal agents are usually administered with either atropine or glycopyrrolate.

—Because of the rapid onset of edrophonium, atropine is usually recommended for coadministration, whereas glycopyrrolate (which is also slower in onset) is used for the slower onset of neostigmine and pyridostigmine.

Dose

—For reversal of neuromuscular blockade: Pyridostigmine, 0.1–0.25 mg/kg with glycopyrrolate, 7–15 µg/kg.

Pyridostigmine Interactions with Anesthesia Drugs

Pyridostigmine and succinylcholine

—Neostigmine, edrophonium, pyridostigmine, and any other anticholinesterase can significantly prolong the duration of neuromuscular blockade from succinylcholine.

—Since these medications are nonspecific anticholinesterases, they also inhibit plasma pseudocholinesterase and therefore delay metabolism of succinylcholine.

—The exact amount of time necessary to prevent this interaction after administering an anticholinesterase is not known. Because the duration of action of neostigmine is 50–90 minutes, this may be a minimum interval to avoid this interaction.

Pyridostigmine Interactions with Diseases

Pyridostigmine and acidosis (respiratory or metabolic)

—Alterations of the normal acid–base status may result in difficulty reversing non-depolarizing neuromuscular blockade.

—Respiratory acidosis ($pCO_2 > 50$) and metabolic alkalosis have been shown to prevent adequate reversal of pancuronium neuromuscular block. This interaction appears to be complex and is incompletely understood, but is probably related to changes in electrolytes and intracellular pH rather than simple changes in acid–base measurements.

Pyridostigmine and Eaton–Lambert syndrome

—Anticholinesterases are unreliable in reversing the muscle relaxation of non-depolarizing agents in patients with Eaton–Lambert syndrome.

—Patients with this syndrome may experience prolonged neuromuscular blockade with both non-depolarizing and depolarizing agents.

Pyridostigmine and hypocalcemia

—Reversal of neuromuscular blockade can be impaired in the presence of hypocalcemia.

—Stimulation of a motor nerve causes a nerve action potential that allows entry of calcium into the nerve ending. The calcium appears to cause release of acetylcholine from vesicles in the nerve ending into the neuromuscular junction, resulting in endplate depolarization.

—In the presence of inadequate ionized calcium, less acetylcholine is released, impairing the ability of acetylcholinesterase inhibitors to overcome the competitive blockade of acetylcholine receptors by neuromuscular blocking agents.

Pyridostigmine and hypokalemia

—Reversal of neuromuscular blockade in patients with hypokalemia may be more difficult. Although this has been demonstrated in animal studies, there is some controversy about the clinical importance of hypokalemia in reversal of muscle blockade in humans.

—Hypokalemia, particularly acute hypokalemia, can potentiate non-depolarizing neuromuscular blockers.

Pyridostigmine and hypothermia

—Non-depolarizing muscle blockade is prolonged by hypothermia. This interaction is a result of an effect on the neuromuscular blocking agents themselves rather than on the anticholinesterases used to reverse the neuromuscular blocking agents.

—Hypothermia appears to prolong the effect of the non-depolarizing agents by several mechanisms, including delayed metabolism into inactive metabolites as well as delayed excretion via the urinary and biliary routes.

Pyridostigmine and malignant hyperthermia

—Anesthetic agents considered safe for use in patients with known or suspected susceptibility for developing malignant hyperthermia (MH) include propofol, barbiturates, etomidate, ketamine, non-depolarizing neuromuscular blocking agents, narcotics, benzodiazepines, droperidol, epinephrine, norepinephrine, and anticholinesterases.

—Nitrous oxide is probably safe in the susceptible patient based on repeated use in MH-susceptible humans and swine.

—Local or regional anesthesia with either amide (such as lidocaine) or ester (such as procaine) anesthetics is now considered safe for MH-susceptible patients.

Pyridostigmine and myasthenia gravis

—Reversal of a non-depolarizing blockade in patients with myasthenia gravis is controversial.

—Because patients are treated chronically with anticholinesterases, anticholinesterase inhibition is already nearly maximized.

—Conservative recommendations are to not use anticholinesterases for reversal of muscle blockade but rather to allow spontaneous recovery.

ROCURONIUM (Zemuron)

Classification and indications

—Rocuronium is a non-depolarizing neuromuscular blocker.

—It is used for skeletal muscle relaxation during intubation and for maintenance of muscle relaxation during general anesthesia and surgery.

Pharmacology

—Rocuronium competes with acetylcholine at the neuromuscular junction of skeletal muscle by binding to acetylcholine receptors.

—There is no significant release of histamine, but at higher doses (0.6–1.0 mg/kg) there is a mild vagolytic effect. This may result in some increase in heart rate.

—Onset of skeletal muscle relaxation is more rapid than vecuronium, but less than succinylcholine. After a dose of 0.6 mg/kg, intubating conditions may be achieved in 60–90 seconds, with a clinical duration of about 31 minutes (25% recovery of twitch height).

—Though rocuronium undergoes no significant metabolism, elimination depends on renal and hepatic pathways. Patients with severe renal or hepatic dysfunction will likely have prolonged elimination times.

—Drug accumulation during prolonged infusion can occur, resulting in slower recovery from muscle relaxation.

—Elderly patients may experience longer clinical duration of muscle blockade than younger patients.

Dose

—Intubation: 0.6–1.0 mg/kg will have a clinical duration of about 45–75 minutes.

—Maintenance:

   —Bolus: 0.1–0.15 mg/kg will have a duration of about 15–25 minutes.

   —Infusion: 8–12 µg/kg/min.

Rocuronium Interactions with Anesthesia Drugs

Rocuronium and calcium channel blockers (diltiazem, nicardipine, nifedipine, verapamil)

—Calcium channel blockers have been associated with prolongation of neuromuscular blockade from non-depolarizing agents.

—This interaction is probably related to the depletion of intracellular calcium associated with chronic therapy. This can result in a decrease in acetylcholine release at the neuromuscular junction.

Rocuronium and inhalational anesthetics (desflurane, enflurane, halothane, isoflurane, sevoflurane)

—Desflurane, enflurane, halothane, isoflurane, and sevoflurane can significantly potentiate neuromuscular blockade, depending on the neuromuscular blocker used. Nitrous oxide has minimal effects.

—Tubocurarine and pancuronium are potentiated the most by inhalational agents, whereas atracurium and vecuronium are intensified significantly less.

—Potentiation by inhalational agents occurs through depression of spinal cord reflexes as well as effects at or distal to the neuromuscular junction.

Rocuronium and diphenylhydantoin, phenytoin

—Patients on chronic phenytoin therapy may be resistant to non-depolarizing muscle blockade. The studies involved metocurine and vecuronium, but may involve other non-depolarizing agents.

—The mechanism of this interaction is not known.

—Acute infusions of phenytoin may prolong non-depolarizing blockade. This was studied prospectively in a small number of patients who received a 10 mg/kg loading dose of phenytoin during steady-state muscle blockade with vecuronium. They had significant potentiation of their neuromuscular block compared to control patients.

Rocuronium and furosemide

—Furosemide may potentiate neuromuscular blockade from tubocurarine and succinylcholine.

—This is based on a case report of several patients given furosemide and tubocurarine during surgery and on animal studies.

—The implication for this interaction for other neuromuscular blocking drugs is uncertain and the mechanism is not known.

Rocuronium and lidocaine

—Most local anesthetics can block neuromuscular transmission from non-depolarizing agents as well as depolarizing muscle relaxants. Of clinical significance to the anesthesiologist, lidocaine, given as a 50- to 100-mg bolus or even by infusion, can significantly increase a non-depolarizer block or a phase II block from succinylcholine.

Rocuronium and procainamide

—Procainamide can potentiate muscle relaxation from non-depolarizing agents. This is probably a result of decreased acetylcholine release at the neuromuscular junction caused by procainamide.

Rocuronium and quinidine

—Quinidine, procainamide, propranolol, and most local anesthetics have been shown to enhance the neuromuscular blockade from depolarizing and non-depolarizing agents.

—A number of well-documented cases have illustrated the ability of these agents, when given in the immediate postoperative period, to convert subclinical muscle weakness from neuromuscular blocking drugs into significant muscle weakness requiring reintubation.

Rocuronium and succinylcholine

—Prior administration of succinylcholine has been shown to potentiate neuromuscular blockade of some non-depolarizing agents.

—Although this interaction has been documented with pancuronium, it was not seen with doxacurium and may not be a consistent finding with non-depolarizing agents.

Rocuronium Interactions with Diseases

Rocuronium and advanced age

—Prolonged duration of neuromuscular blockade can be seen in older patients with several different non-depolarizing agents including doxacurium, mivacurium, and rocuronium.

—In some cases, delayed onset of muscle relaxation also occurs. This has been attributed to decreased perfusion of the neuromuscular junction as a result of advanced age.

Rocuronium and burns

—Patients with burn injuries are susceptible to a life-threatening hyperkalemic response to succinylcholine and can have marked resistance to non-depolarizing muscle relaxants.

—Both of these altered responses to neuromuscular blocking agents have been attributed to proliferation of extrajunctional acetylcholine receptors, similar to that in the patient with a denervation injury.

—Resistance to non-depolarizing agents appears to increase with larger area burns and, in fact, may not be significant in patients with <30% body surface area burns. In addition to proliferation of extrajunctional acetylcholine receptors, this abnormal response is probably also related to the increased metabolic rate and hepatic and renal clearance seen in burn patients. Doses of non-depolarizing agents may need to be increased by as much as 300%.

—Duration of this resistance usually is 2 months following the injury but has been reported in a patient 463 days after the burn.

Rocuronium and cirrhosis, liver disease

—Prolonged neuromuscular blockade in patients with liver disease can be seen with doxacurium, mivacurium, vecuronium, pancuronium, rocuronium, and tubocurarine.

—This interaction is complex and may be due to decreased clearance, decreased hepatic uptake of the agent, or decreased synthesis of enzymes important for degradation of the neuromuscular blocker. An example of the latter is prolongation of mivacurium's duration of action as a result of decreased plasma cholinesterase from severe liver disease.

—Because of the increased volume of distribution of many drugs seen in patients with liver disease, initial doses of muscle relaxants may need to be larger than in healthy patients. Once neuromuscular blockade is achieved, recovery may be prolonged.

Rocuronium and Eaton–Lambert syndrome

—Patients with Eaton–Lambert syndrome are very sensitive to both depolarizing and non-depolarizing neuromuscular blockade.

—This disorder is similar to myasthenia gravis and patients complain of skeletal muscle weakness, but it is usually associated with carcinoma (especially small cell tumors of the lung).

—If the diagnosis is known or suspected prior to surgery, reduced doses of muscle relaxants should be used, but sometimes the diagnosis is first made when a patient has surgery for a lung tumor and has an unexpected, prolonged neuromuscular block.

—Anticholinesterases are unreliable in reversing muscle weakness.

Rocuronium and hyperthyroidism, thyrotoxicosis

—Muscle weakness is commonly seen with hyperthyroidism and affects proximal muscles, usually sparing respiratory function. In some cases, myopathy is the dominant feature of thyroid hormone excess and can resemble myasthenia. Lower doses of muscle relaxants may be indicated.

Rocuronium and hypokalemia

—Hypokalemia appears to potentiate the effects of neuromuscular blockade from non-depolarizing agents.

—The interaction is probably due to hyperpolarization of the muscle endplate and, therefore, resistance to depolarization. Hyperpolarization would more likely occur with more acute changes in potassium concentration because the potassium losses would be from the extracellular compartment rather than from intracellular sites.

—Chronic hypokalemia is more likely to be associated with potassium depletion from both extra- and intracellular compartments with no significant change in transmembrane potential. As a result, significant effects on neuromuscular blockade would be less likely.

Rocuronium and hypothermia

—Non-depolarizing muscle blockade is prolonged by hypothermia. This interaction is a result of an effect on the neuromuscular blocking agents themselves rather than on the anticholinesterases used to reverse the neuromuscular blocking agents.

—Hypothermia appears to prolong the effect of the non-depolarizing agents by several mechanisms, including delayed metabolism into inactive metabolites as well as delayed excretion via the urinary and biliary routes.

Rocuronium and malignant hyperthermia

—Anesthetic agents considered safe for use in patients with known or suspected susceptibility for developing malignant hyperthermia include propofol, barbiturates, etomidate, ketamine, non-depolarizing neuromuscular blocking agents, narcotics, benzodiazepines, droperidol, epinephrine, norepinephrine, and anticholinesterases.

—Nitrous oxide is probably safe in the susceptible patient, based on repeated use in MH-susceptible humans and swine.

—Local or regional anesthesia with either amide (such as lidocaine) or ester (such as procaine) anesthetics is now considered safe for MH-susceptible patients.

Rocuronium and myasthenia gravis

—Patients with myasthenia gravis are very sensitive to neuromuscular blockade from non-depolarizing agents.

—This is probably a result of decreased acetylcholine receptors from autoimmune destruction associated with myasthenia gravis.

—Although these patients are treated with the same or similar anticholinesterases used to antagonize muscle blockade, sensitivity (not resistance) to neuromuscular blockade is seen clinically.

Rocuronium and neuromuscular disease (amyotrophic lateral sclerosis, multiple sclerosis, syringomyelia)

—Patients with a wide variety of neuromuscular disorders may be more resistant than normal patients to the effects of non-depolarizing neuromuscular blockers.

—This includes patients with disuse atrophy of the muscles (such as bedridden patients with chronic disease) as well as patients with upper or lower motor neuron disease such as amyotrophic lateral sclerosis, multiple sclerosis, or syringomyelia.

—Disuse or denervation of muscle results in production of extrajunctional acetylcholine receptors on the muscle membrane. These receptors are less easily blocked by non-depolarizing agents but are activated by lower concentrations of depolarizing drugs (succinylcholine).

—When these receptors, which can be scattered over a large surface of the muscle, are depolarized by succinylcholine, ion flow takes place through the receptor channel. Large amounts of potassium may exit the muscle cell, causing hyperkalemia.

—Despite initial resistance to blockade, such patients may demonstrate prolonged neuromuscular weakness as a result of decreased muscle strength and mass.

Rocuronium and PIH (pregnancy-induced hypertension), preeclampsia/eclampsia, toxemia

—Patients with hypertensive disorders of pregnancy may require treatment with antihypertensives such as trimethaphan or magnesium sulfate (for preeclampsia/eclampsia). These medications can have significant interactions with anesthetic agents such as succinylcholine, non-depolarizing neuromuscular blocking agents, or calcium channel blockers.

—Neuromuscular blockade produced by both depolarizing and non-depolarizing agents can be potentiated in patients receiving magnesium sulfate. The mechanisms involved include a decreased amount of acetylcholine released by the nerve impulse at the motor nerve terminal and a decrease in the depolarizing action of acetylcholine on the muscle.

Rocuronium Interactions with Patient Drugs
Rocuronium and antibiotics

—A number of antibiotics have significant interactions with neuromuscular blocking agents.

—These include the aminoglycosides (amikacin, gentamicin, kanamycin, neomycin, paromomycin, netilmicin, neomycin, streptomycin, tobramycin), as well as polymyxin B, colistin, amphotericin B, clindamycin, bacitracin, and lincomycin.

—All of the above antibiotics may potentiate non-depolarizing agents, but some (aminoglycosides, amphotericin B, clindamycin, colistin) can also potentiate succinylcholine blockade.

—These antibiotics potentiate neuromuscular blockade by different mechanisms, making management of these problems difficult. Although treatment with anticholinesterases or calcium has been recommended, results are inconsistent.

Rocuronium and amphotericin B

—Prolonged neuromuscular blockade can occur with depolarizing and non-depolarizing agents in patients receiving amphotericin B.

—The mechanism for this interaction is thought to be associated with the hypokalemia that can be caused by amphotericin B therapy.

Rocuronium and beta blockers, propranolol

—Beta blockers may potentiate non-depolarizing neuromuscular blocking agents. This interaction has been reported between propranolol and tubocurarine.

—Other beta blockers are also capable of causing weakness in patients with myasthenia gravis, but the mechanism or significance of these interactions is unclear.

Rocuronium and calcium channel blockers (amlodipine, bepridil, diltiazem, felodipine, isradipine, lidoflazine, nicardipine, nimodipine, nisoldipine, nitrendipine, verapamil)

—Calcium channel blockers have been associated with prolongation of neuromuscular blockade from non-depolarizing agents.

—This interaction is probably related to the depletion of intracellular calcium associated with chronic therapy. This can result in a decrease in acetylcholine release at the neuromuscular junction.

Rocuronium and diphenylhydantoin, phenytoin

—Patients on chronic phenytoin therapy may be resistant to non-depolarizing muscle blockade. The studies involved metocurine and vecuronium, but may involve other non-depolarizing agents.

—The mechanism of this interaction is not known.

—Acute infusions of phenytoin may prolong non-depolarizing blockade. This was studied prospectively in a small number of patients who received a 10 mg/kg loading dose of phenytoin during steady-state muscle blockade with vecuronium. They had significant potentiation of their neuromuscular block compared to control patients.

Rocuronium and lidocaine

—Most local anesthetics can block neuromuscular transmission from non-depolarizing agents as well as depolarizing muscle relaxants. Of clinical significance to the anesthesiologist, lidocaine, given as a 50- to 100-mg bolus or even by infusion, can significantly increase a non-depolarizer block or a phase II block from succinylcholine.

Rocuronium and lithium

—Lithium has been reported to increase the duration of both non-depolarizing and depolarizing neuromuscular blocking drugs.

—The mechanism of this interaction is unknown and the clinical significance of this interaction is uncertain.

Rocuronium and magnesium sulfate

—Neuromuscular blockade produced by both depolarizing and non-depolarizing agents can be potentiated in patients receiving magnesium sulfate. The mechanisms involved include a decreased amount of acetylcholine released by the nerve impulse at the motor nerve terminal and a decrease in the depolarizing action of acetylcholine on the muscle.

Rocuronium and mexilitene

—Mexilitene, like lidocaine and most local anesthetics, can potentiate neuromuscular blockade from depolarizing and non-depolarizing agents.

Rocuronium and procainamide

—Procainamide can potentiate muscle relaxation from non-depolarizing agents. This is probably a result of decreased acetylcholine release at the neuromuscular junction caused by procainamide.

Rocuronium and quinidine

—Quinidine and quinine can potentiate muscle relaxation from both depolarizing and nondepolarizing agents.

—The mechanism of this interaction is a curare-like action at the myoneural junction. Also, plasma pseudocholinesterase is inhibited by quinidine (and quinine), resulting in possible prolongation of muscle relaxation from succinylcholine.

Rocuronium and tocainide

—Tocainide, an orally active form of lidocaine, can potentiate both depolarizing and non-depolarizing neuromuscular blockade. This is a property of most local anesthetics as well as a number of other medications.

SCOPOLAMINE (Transderm Scop)

Classification and indications

—Scopolamine is a belladonna alkaloid that is an inhibitor of acetylcholine. It is considered an antimuscarinic agent.

—It is indicated for sedation, both intraoperatively and preoperatively, for drying of respiratory tract secretions, and for preventing nausea and vomiting in the perioperative period.

Pharmacology

—Scopolamine is a competitive inhibitor of acetylcholine, primarily affecting the parasympathetic nervous system.

—Cardiac effects are dose-dependent, with mild bradycardia from central vagal stimulation at lower doses (0.1–0.2 mg) and tachycardia at higher doses.

—Gastrointestinal effects include drying of secretions, reduced gastric volume, and decreased intestinal motility.

—Respiratory tract secretions are also reduced and bronchial smooth muscles are relaxed.

—Scopolamine, but not other antimuscarinic agents, causes sedation and amnesia at usual doses. It blocks transmission of cholinergic transmission to the vomiting center from the vestibular nuclei and is therefore effective for treatment of motion sickness.

—Mydriasis is produced by scopolamine and may result in significant increases in intraocular pressure in patients with angle closure glaucoma. Patients with open angle glaucoma do not demonstrate this response.

—Onset of effects after intramuscular administration occurs in 30–60 minutes and peaks at 1–2 hours. The duration of effects is about 4–6 hours.

—Transdermal systems deliver an initial priming dose over about 6 hours, followed by a sustained release rate of 5 µg/hr for 66 hours.

Dose

—Adult:

—Parenteral (IV, IM, or SC): 0.3–0.65 mg.

—Transdermal: 0.5 mg patch will deliver medication for 72 hours. To optimally prevent motion sickness, patch should be placed 4 hours in advance.

—Pediatric: 6 µg/kg IV, IM, or SC.

Scopolamine Interactions with Diseases
Scopolamine and glaucoma
—Scopolamine, even in the form of transdermal patches, may cause significant increases in intraocular pressure in patients with narrow angle glaucoma. Patients with open angle glaucoma rarely experience a significant increase in intraocular pressure with scopolamine.

SEVOFLURANE (Ultane)

Classification and indications
—Sevoflurane is a nonflammable, halogenated ether (similar to isoflurane, ethrane, halothane).
—It is indicated for use as a general anesthetic.

Pharmacology
—The MAC of sevoflurane varies with age according to the following chart:

Age	Sevo/O_2	Sevo/N_2O[a]
0–1 mo	3.3%	
1–<6 mo	3.0%	
6 mo–3 yr	2.8%	2.0%
3–12 yr	2.5%	
25 yr	2.6%	1.4%
40 yr	2.1%	1.1%
60 yr	1.7%	0.9%
80 yr	1.4%	0.7%

[a]65% O_2/35% N_2O.

—The blood/gas solubility of sevoflurane is 0.63–0.69 (halothane, 2.4; enflurane, 1.9; isoflurane, 1.4; nitrous oxide, 0.47; desflurane, 0.42). Because of the low solubility, induction of anesthesia with sevoflurane is very rapid compared to more soluble agents such as isoflurane, halothane, or enflurane.
—Sevoflurane is metabolized by cytochrome P450 2E1 to hexafluoroisopropanol (HFIP), releasing fluoride ion and CO_2.
—HFIP is rapidly conjugated with glucuronic acid and is rapidly eliminated by renal excretion.
—Neither HFIP nor fluoride ion concentrations (even in excess of 50 μmol) have been demonstrated to have significant clinical effects associated with sevoflurane use.
—This is in contrast to methoxyflurane, where fluoride ion concentrations >50 μmol have been associated with polyuric renal failure.

—Direct contact of sevoflurane with soda lime or Baralyme results in production of compound A (pentafluoroisopropenylfluoromethyl ether), which has potential nephrotoxicity. Because accumulation of compound A increases with low gas flows, low–low anesthesia (<2 L/min) is not recommended. There is no evidence of nephrotoxicity in humans from compound A.

—Cardiovascular effects include a dose-related decrease in mean arterial pressure that is mainly the result of decreased systemic vascular resistance.

—Like other inhalational agents, sevoflurane causes dose-related cardiac depression, which may be offset by the decrease in systemic vascular resistance.

—Sevoflurane causes an increase in heart rate, but only above 2 MAC.

—All the inhalational agents cause a dose-related increase in cerebral blood flow. Halothane has the greatest effect followed by enflurane and then isoflurane. Desflurane and sevoflurane have effects similar to isoflurane.

Dose

—Inhalation induction:

—Sevoflurane, like halothane, is suitable for inhalation induction for adults and children because it is not irritating to the airway.

—The risk of laryngospasm, breath holding, and agitation is approximately equal to that with halothane.

—Maintenance: Use of other anesthetic agents (narcotics, benzodiazepines, nitrous oxide) can reduce the MAC of sevoflurane. As a result, depending on the anesthetic technique, the type of surgery, and the individual patient response, maintenance doses can vary significantly.

Sevoflurane Interactions with Anesthetics

Sevoflurane and clonidine

—Clonidine has been shown to reduce the MAC of inhaled and opioid anesthetics.

—This effect may be related to clonidine's inhibition of the sympathetic outflow from the vasomotor center in the medulla (clonidine is a central alpha 2 receptor agonist, which results in inhibition of CNS sympathetic centers).

Sevoflurane and epinephrine, norepinephrine

—Halothane and, to a lesser extent, isoflurane, ethrane, and sevoflurane reduce the threshold for arrhythmias from epinephrine and norepinephrine. The mechanism of this "sensitization" of the myocardium to these sympathomimetic amines includes an increase in automaticity and changes in depolarization.

—Although exact numbers are not agreed on, a general guideline for safe administration of epinephrine based on some clinical studies is to use no more than 10 mL of 1:100,000 (1 μg/mL) epinephrine solution every 10 minutes with a limit of 30 mL/hr. with isoflurane, sevoflurane, or ethrane, a slightly larger amount can probably be used.

Sevoflurane and muscle relaxants (atracurium, doxacurium, gallamine, metocurine, mivacurium, pancuronium, pipercuronium, rocuronium, tubocurarine, vecuronium)

—Sevoflurane, like other volatile anesthetics, has been shown to increase the intensity and duration of non-depolarizing muscle blockade.

—Although initial doses of non-depolarizing agents should be unchanged, repeat doses for maintenance may need to be reduced.

Sevoflurane and succinylcholine

—Although isoflurane and desflurane may cause prolongation of neuromuscular blockade from succinylcholine, this has not been documented with sevoflurane.

Sevoflurane Interactions with Diseases

Sevoflurane and cerebral edema, intracranial hypertension

—All commonly used inhalational volatile anesthetics (halothane > enflurane > isoflurane) cause an increased cerebral blood flow (CBF). Sevoflurane has effects similar to isoflurane. Nitrous oxide has minimal effects on CBF.

—The volatile anesthetics, although they depress cerebral metabolic rate, cause cerebrovascular dilation, which results in increased CBF. Hyperventilation to a $PaCO_2$ between 25 and 35 mm Hg will effectively prevent increased CBF from isoflurane and sevoflurane.

Sevoflurane and hepatitis

—All forms of anesthesia, including general, regional, and nitrous-narcotic, are associated with postoperative liver function test abnormalities. The exact mechanism of this reaction is not known but is likely related to reduced liver blood flow from anesthesia and surgery.

—The presence of hepatitis or any liver disease has been shown to increase the morbidity and mortality in patients receiving anesthesia. The mechanism of this increase in morbidity and mortality is not clear but is most likely related to changes in hepatic blood flow as a result of anesthesia and surgery.

—Because there is no known method of avoiding exacerbation of pre-existing liver disease by anesthesia, most recommendations are to postpone surgery in patients suspected of having acute hepatitis.

—There is no evidence that enflurane, isoflurane, desflurane, or sevoflurane is hepatotoxic. Halothane, however, can occasionally cause fulminant hepatic necrosis in both adults and children. A milder form of hepatotoxicity is also seen with halothane anesthesia.

Sevoflurane and malignant hyperthermia

—Halothane, isoflurane, enflurane, desflurane, sevoflurane, as well as other, older inhalational agents all are potent triggering agents of malignant hyperthermia in the susceptible patient.

—Succinylcholine, decamethonium, and possibly tubocurarine are also triggering agents.

—Anesthetic agents considered safe for use in patients with known or suspected susceptibility for developing malignant hyperthermia (MH) include propofol, barbiturates, etomidate, ketamine, non-depolarizing neuromuscular blocking agents, narcotics, benzodiazepines, droperidol, epinephrine, norepinephrine, and anticholinesterases.

—Nitrous oxide is probably safe in the susceptible patient based on repeated use in MH-susceptible humans and swine.

—Local or regional anesthesia with either amide (such as lidocaine) or ester (such as procaine) anesthetics is now considered safe for MH-susceptible patients.

Sevoflurane and myotonia

—Inhalational anesthetics may cause exaggerated cardiac depression in patients with myotonia dystrophica.

—Patients with myotonia dystrophica, but not the other myotonic syndromes, are likely to have some degree of cardiomyopathy even in the absence of clinical symptoms. As a result, these patients may be very sensitive to any myocardial depressant.

Sevoflurane and porphyria
—Inhalational agents are considered to be safe for use in patients with porphyria, as are narcotics, depolarizing and non-depolarizing muscle relaxants, etomidate, anticholinesterases, and propofol.

—Barbiturates are contraindicated in three of the four hepatic porphyrias (acute intermittent porphyria, variegate porphyria, and hereditary coproporphyria). Porphyria cutanea tarda and the erythropoietic porphyrias are not exacerbated by barbiturates.

—It is theorized that barbiturates can provoke an attack of porphyria by inducing the enzyme aminolevulinic acid synthetase, which results in synthesis of more porphyrin compounds and their precursors.

Sevoflurane and pregnancy
—Pregnancy is associated with significant reductions in minimal alveolar concentrations (MAC) for inhalational agents.

—In animal studies and some human studies, decreases in MAC of up to 40% have been documented.

—The suggested mechanism for this decreased MAC includes increases in progesterone and endorphin levels associated with pregnancy.

Sevoflurane and renal dysfunction
—Sevoflurane is probably safe for administration to patients with renal dysfunction.

—Although metabolism of sevoflurane results in production of fluoride ion at potentially nephrotoxic levels (50 μmol), there is no clinical evidence of renal toxicity from use of sevoflurane.

Sevoflurane Interactions with Drugs
Sevoflurane and amiodarone
—Amiodarone, an antiarrhythmic that increases refractoriness and slows conduction in most cardiac tissue, has been associated with severe cardiac complications including arrhythmias, low cardiac output, and decreased systemic vascular resistance in patients having general anesthesia with inhalational agents, although there is no specific documentation of this interaction with sevoflurane.

—The mechanism of these interactions is not known.

Sevoflurane and clonidine
—Clonidine has been shown to reduce the MAC of inhaled and opioid anesthetics.

—This effect may be related to clonidine's inhibition of the sympathetic outflow from the vasomotor center in the medulla (clonidine is a central alpha 2 receptor agonist, which results in inhibition of CNS sympathetic centers).

Sevoflurane and disulfiram

—Profound hypotension may occur when patients taking disulfiram are exposed to halogenated anesthetics (enflurane, isoflurane, halothane, desflurane, and sevoflurane).

SODIUM PENTOTHAL (Pentothal)

Classification and indications

—Thiopental, a short-acting barbiturate, is a nonanalgesic, intravenous anesthetic agent.

—It is indicated for intravenous induction of anesthesia. It is also an anticonvulsant and has been used as an infusion for maintenance of anesthesia.

Pharmacology

—The barbiturates are believed to exert their effects through the GABA receptor. Gamma aminobutyric acid (GABA) is the main inhibitory neurotransmitter in the CNS. Barbiturates augment the activity of GABA.

—CNS effects of thiopental include depression of the EEG, a decrease in the cerebral blood flow and metabolic rate, and a decrease in intracranial pressure (ICP). Cerebral perfusion pressure is maintained in spite of a decrease in mean arterial pressure because of a greater decrease in ICP.

—Cardiac effects following administration of thiopental include an initial decrease in blood pressure and a drop in cardiac output and contractility, but an increased heart rate. Although peripheral vascular resistance does not decrease, venodilation occurs.

—In patients who are very dependent on cardiac preload for hemodynamic stability (hypovolemia, congestive heart failure, tamponade, etc.), venodilation may result in profound decreases in cardiac output and blood pressure.

—Unlike etomidate, thiopental does not inhibit adrenocortical responses to surgical stress.

—Although thiopental causes a dose-related histamine release, the clinical significance is low and is still safe for use in asthmatic patients.

—Onset of effect after induction doses is within 1 minute with a duration of 5–15 minutes, depending on the dose and the individual. Termination of the effect is a result of redistribution.

—Contraindications to the use of thiopental are patients with acute intermittent, variegate, or hereditary coproporphyria.

Dose
—Induction:
—Adults: 2.5–5 mg/kg.
—Children: 5–6 mg/kg.

Sodium Pentothal Interactions with Diseases

Sodium pentothal and advanced age

—A reduced induction dose is recommended for thiopental, etomidate, and propofol in most elderly patients.

—Reduction in the dose requirements for these drugs may be a result of a decreased volume of distribution, decreased elimination, or a combination of effects brought about by aging.

Sodium pentothal and alcohol—acute intoxication

—Patients who are acutely intoxicated with alcohol (including chronic alcoholics) usually demonstrate increased sensitivity to general anesthesia.

—Although the precise mechanism of interactions are not agreed on, it appears that alcohol intoxication has additive CNS depression with barbiturates, benzodiazepines, and narcotics, as well as inhalational agents.

Sodium pentothal and alcohol—chronic abuse

—Chronic abuse of alcohol has complex and incompletely understood effects on a patient's response to anesthetic agents. In general, these patients tend to be more tolerant (in a nonintoxicated state) to barbiturates, benzodiazepines, narcotics, and inhalational agents.

—Exceptions to this generalization include the alcoholic patient with a cardiomyopathy who may demonstrate increased sensitivity to myocardial depression from inhalational agents.

—Also, the patient with severe liver disease may have impaired ability to metabolize succinylcholine due to decreased levels of plasma pseudocholinesterase.

Sodium pentothal and cerebral edema, intracranial hypertension

—Most intravenous anesthetics cause a reduction in cerebral blood flow and intracranial pressure (ICP) or have no effect on ICP. Although this effect is primarily from depression of cerebral metabolic rate, in some cases a direct vasoconstriction occurs.

—The exception to the above is ketamine, which causes an increased cerebral metabolic rate (CMR) and cerebral blood flow (CBF) with an increase in ICP.

—All of the narcotics, as well as barbiturates, etomidate, benzodiazepines, and propofol, have been associated with a reduction or maintenance of ICP during anesthesia.

Sodium pentothal and malignant hyperthermia

—Anesthetic agents considered safe for use in patients with known or suspected susceptibility for developing malignant hyperthermia (MH) include propofol, barbiturates, etomidate, ketamine, non-depolarizing neuromuscular blocking agents, narcotics, benzodiazepines, droperidol, epinephrine, norepinephrine, and anticholinesterases.

—Nitrous oxide is probably safe in the susceptible patient based on repeated use in MH-susceptible humans and swine.

—Local or regional anesthesia with either amide (such as lidocaine) or ester (such as procaine) anesthetics is now considered safe for MH-susceptible patients.

Sodium pentothal and porphyria

—Barbiturates are contraindicated in three of the four hepatic porphyrias (acute intermittent porphyria, variegate porphyria, and hereditary coproporphyria). Porphyria cutanea tarda and the ery-thropoietic porphyrias are not exacerbated by barbiturates.

—It is theorized that barbiturates can provoke an attack of porphyria by inducing the enzyme aminolevulinic acid synthetase, which results in synthesis of more porphyrin compounds and their precursors.

—Anesthesia can be safely administered to these patients using narcotics, depolarizing and non-depolarizing muscle relaxants, anticholinesterases, propofol, and inhalational agents.

—Questionable agents are benzodiazepines and ketamine.

Sodium pentothal and renal dysfunction

—Renal dysfunction has not been demonstrated to cause significant changes in pharmacokinetics or pharmacodynamics of benzodiazepines, narcotics (with the possible exception of butorphanol), barbiturates, or propofol.

—In patients with renal dysfunction, the above drugs may appear to have an increase in duration or intensity. This has been explained as a response to the systemic effects of renal dysfunction rather than specific effects on the metabolism of theses drugs.

—Some muscle relaxants are significantly affected by renal failure.

Sodium Pentothal Interactions with Patient Drugs
Sodium pentothal and monoamine oxidase inhibitors (isocarboxazid, phenelzine, selegilene, tranylcypromine)

—Barbiturates given to a patient receiving monoamine oxidase inhibitors may have a prolonged effect resulting in delayed awakening.

Sodium pentothal and probenecid

—Patients receiving probenecid may experience prolonged sedation after thiopental anesthesia.

—This interaction was studied prospectively in more than 80 patients.

SUCCINYLCHOLINE (Anectine, Quelicin, Sucostrin)

Classification and indications

—Succinylcholine is a depolarizing skeletal muscle relaxant.

—It is indicated primarily for intubation but can be used as an infusion for sustained muscle relaxation for surgery.

Pharmacology

—Succinylcholine has a high affinity for the acetylcholine receptor at the neuromuscular junction, where it produces depolarization of the motor endplate. Depolarization of the endplate results in fasciculation of muscles, most prominently the small, fast-twitch muscles of the face, eyes, and neck.

—After the fasciculations, skeletal muscle relaxation occurs. This occurs because the activity of succinylcholine at the neuromuscular junction is not rapidly terminated by acetylcholinesterase (succinylcholine is metabolized by plasma cholinesterase, not acetylcholinesterase).

—Succinylcholine molecules continue to interact with receptors, causing continued endplate depolarization. This activity interferes with the normal sequence of muscle depolarization, which depends on sequential receptor activation followed by rapid deactivation of the acetylcholine receptors at the motor endplate.

—Depolarization of acetylcholine receptors occurs at virtually all cholinergic autonomic receptors. Since acetylcholine is the mediator of parasympathetic nerves and at the prejunctional synapses of sympathetic nerves, these systems are also affected. The result is in some cases bradycardia (increased vagal tone) or ventricular arrhythmias (sympathetic stimulation).

—By administering a non-depolarizing agent (which can reduce some depolarization), fasciculations as well as autonomic effects (bradycardia) may be blunted. Administration of atropine can also block the bradycardia from succinylcholine.

—Patients with neuromuscular disease (upper and lower motor neuron abnormalities) can respond to succinylcholine with a dangerous, sometimes fatal hyperkalemia. This probably occurs because of proliferation of extrajunctional acetylcholine receptors on the muscle membrane. Depolarization of these receptors causes potassium leak through the muscle membrane.

—Succinylcholine is one of the drugs considered to be a triggering agent for malignant hyperthermia.

—After a dose of 1 mg/kg, intubating conditions are achieved in 60–90 seconds and full recovery occurs in 12–15 minutes.

—Elimination of succinylcholine depends on enzymatic degradation by plasma cholinesterase (pseudocholinesterase). Patients with genetic variants of this enzyme will have prolonged muscle relaxation from succinylcholine.

—The most important of these genetic variants of pseudocholinesterase is inhibited by dibucaine by about 20%, whereas the normal enzyme is inhibited by about 80%. The dibucaine number of a patient with two normal pseudocholinesterase genes will be 20–30 (representing the percentage inhibited by dibucaine). A patient who is homozygous for the abnormal gene will have a dibucaine number of 70–80 (representing the percentage inhibition by dibucaine). Heterozygous individuals will have intermediate dibucaine numbers (50–60).

—In addition to the presence of abnormal pseudocholinesterase, an important factor in metabolism of succinylcholine is the amount and activity of the enzyme. This is measured by the plasma cholinesterase activity. A number of factors influence the enzyme activity, including anticholinesterase medications, liver disease, pregnancy, and nutritional status.

Dose
—Intravenous:
   —Adults: 0.3–1.1 mg/kg (average dose 0.6 mg/kg) for intubation.
   —Children*: 1 mg/kg.
   —Infants (up to 2 years old)* and small children: 2 mg/kg.
—Intramuscular:
   —Children*: 2–3 mg/kg (up to 150 mg).
   —Infants (up to 2 years old)*: 4 mg/kg.

Succinylcholine Interactions with Anesthesia Drugs
Succinylcholine and digitalis
—Succinylcholine may precipitate cardiac arrhythmias in digitalized patients.
—Possible explanations of this interaction include the potential of succinylcholine to cause a shift of potassium from the intracellular- to-extracellular compartments in muscle tissue.

Succinylcholine and edrophonium, neostigmine, pyridostigmine
—Neostigmine, edrophonium, pyridostigmine, and any other anticholinesterase can significantly prolong the duration of neuromuscular blockade from succinylcholine.
—Since these medications are nonspecific anticholinesterases, they also inhibit plasma pseudocholinesterase and therefore delay metabolism of succinylcholine.
—The exact amount of time necessary to prevent this interaction after administering an anticholinesterase is not known. Since the duration of action of neostigmine is 50–90 minutes, this may be a minimum interval to avoid this interaction.

---

* Three important considerations exist for pediatric administration of succinylcholine:
—Bradycardia can occur and is more severe with second doses (atropine pretreatment may be necessary, particularly in younger patients).
—Fulminant pulmonary edema has occurred in patients 3–8 weeks old following succinylcholine administration. The etiology is unclear, but the edema responds to positive pressure ventilation.
—Succinylcholine is one of the triggering agents of malignant hyperthermia in susceptible patients.

Succinylcholine and inhalational anesthetics (enflurane, desflurane, halothane, isoflurane, sevoflurane)

—Succinylcholine neuromuscular blockade may be potentiated by desflurane and isoflurane. Halothane and enflurane probably have clinically insignificant interactions with succinylcholine.

—There is no documentation of significant interaction between succinylcholine and sevoflurane.

Succinylcholine and esmolol

—Coadministration of esmolol and succinylcholine may result in a slight (5–8 minute) prolongation of the neuromuscular blockade in some patients.

—The onset of the neuromuscular blockade is not affected.

Succinylcholine and furosemide

—Furosemide may potentiate neuromuscular blockade from tubocurarine and succinylcholine.

—This is based on a case report of several patients and on animal studies.

—The implication for this interaction for other neuromuscular blocking drugs is uncertain and the mechanism is not known.

Succinylcholine and lidocaine

—Most local anesthetics can block neuromuscular transmission from non-depolarizing agents as well as depolarizing muscle relaxants.

—Bolus doses of lidocaine may prolong neuromuscular blockade from succinylcholine, but large doses of lidocaine (>3 mg/kg) are required for clinically significant interaction.

—Phase II block from succinylcholine can be prolonged from normal bolus doses of lidocaine.

Succinylcholine and muscle relaxants (atracurium, doxacurium, gallamine, metocurine, mivacurium, pancuronium, pipercuronium, rocuronium, tubocurarine, vecuronium)

—Prior administration of succinylcholine has been shown to potentiate neuromuscular blockade of some non-depolarizing agents.

—Although this interaction has been documented with pancuronium, it was not seen with doxacurium and may not be a consistent finding with non-depolarizing agents.

Succinylcholine and quinidine
—Quinidine, procainamide, and most local anesthetics have been shown to enhance the neuromuscular blockade from depolarizing and non-depolarizing agents.

—A number of well-documented cases have illustrated the ability of these agents, when given in the immediate post-operative period, to convert subclinical muscle weakness from neuromuscular blocking drugs into significant muscle weakness requiring reintubation.

Succinylcholine and trimethaphan
—Trimethaphan can significantly prolong the effects of succinylcholine in some cases.

—Even though trimethaphan is metabolized by plasma cholinesterase, it inhibits this enzyme by an unknown mechanism.

Succinylcholine Interactions with Diseases

Succinylcholine and amyotrophic lateral sclerosis, Guillain–Barré syndrome, multiple sclerosis, muscular dystrophy, polyneuropathy, syringomyelia
—Chronic or progressive motor neuron disease places patients at continuous risk for hyperkalemia from succinylcholine. Syringomyelia, amyotrophic lateral sclerosis, multiple sclerosis, acute idiopathic polyneuritis (Guillain–Barré syndrome), and all forms of muscular dystrophy have been associated with this response.

—Patients with neuromuscular disease (upper and lower motor neuron abnormalities) can respond to succinylcholine with a dangerous, sometimes fatal hyperkalemia. This probably occurs because of proliferation of extrajunctional acetylcholine receptors on the muscle membrane. Depolarization of these receptors causes potassium leak through the muscle membrane.

Succinylcholine and burns
—A marked hyperkalemic response to succinylcholine can occur in burn patients. This response does not usually occur until 24 to 48 hours following the injury, but may persist for up to 1 year or more.

—The mechanism involved appears to be related to proliferation of extrajunctional acetylcholine receptors, similar to what occurs after denervation injuries. The extent of the burn is unreliable in predicting the extent of the hyperkalemic response.

Succinylcholine and cirrhosis, liver disease

—Termination of the effect of succinylcholine is dependent on plasma pseudocholinesterase which is synthesized in the liver. However, even in severe liver disease, plasma pseudocholinesterase levels are not depressed enough to prolong the effects of succinylcholine.

—Mivacurium is also cleared by plasma cholinesterase, but there is evidence that there is significant prolongation of action of mivacurium in patients with severe liver disease.

Succinylcholine and Eaton–Lambert syndrome

—Patients with Eaton–Lambert syndrome are very sensitive to both depolarizing and non-depolarizing neuromuscular blockade.

—This disorder is similar to myasthenia gravis and patients complain of skeletal muscle weakness, but it is usually associated with carcinoma (especially small cell tumors of the lung).

—If the diagnosis is known or suspected prior to surgery, reduced doses of muscle relaxants should be used, but sometimes, the diagnosis is first made when a patient has surgery for a lung tumor and has an unexpected, prolonged neuromuscular block.

—Anticholinesterases are unreliable in reversing muscle weakness.

Succinylcholine and glaucoma

—Succinylcholine can be used safely in certain patients with glaucoma. Although succinylcholine causes an increase in intraocular pressure, this pressure increase is transient.

—More importantly, certain medications used for treatment of glaucoma are anticholinesterases and can prolong the effect of succinylcholine due to a decrease in plasma cholinesterase. These miotic agents are echothiophate, demecarium bromide, and isoflurophate.

Succinylcholine and malignant hyperthermia

—Halothane, isoflurane, enflurane, desflurane, sevoflurane, as well as other, older inhalational agents, are all potent triggering agents of malignant hyperthermia in the susceptible patient.

—Succinylcholine, decamethonium, and possibly tubocurarine are also triggering agents.

—Anesthetic agents considered safe for use in patients with known or suspected susceptibility for developing malignant hyperthermia (MH) include propofol, barbiturates, etomidate, ketamine, non-depolarizing neuromuscular blocking agents, narcotics, benzodiazepines, droperidol, epinephrine, norepinephrine, and anticholinesterases.

—Nitrous oxide is probably safe in the susceptible patient based on repeated use in MH-susceptible humans and swine.

—Local or regional anesthesia with either amide (such as lidocaine) or ester (such as procaine) anesthetics is now considered safe for MH-susceptible patients.

Succinylcholine and myasthenia gravis

—The response of myasthenics to succinylcholine is usually similar to non-depolarizing agents in that a reduced dose is normally appropriate. However, one study has shown a resistance of myasthenics compared to normal patients. The clinical significance of this finding is not clear and most sources suggest lower doses of succinylcholine for patients with myasthenia gravis.

—Factors affecting patients' response to succinylcholine include treatment with anticholinesterase medications, which also reduce plasma pseudocholinesterase. As a result, duration of neuromuscular blockade from succinylcholine is usually prolonged.

—Also, significant clinical muscle weakness would dictate lower doses than in normal patients or myasthenic patients with good muscle strength.

Succinylcholine and myotonia

—Myotonic dystrophy includes three forms of the disease: myotonia dystrophica (most common form), myotonia congenita, and paramyotonia.

—All three forms can respond to depolarization from succinylcholine with persistent muscle contraction lasting several minutes. Use of non-depolarizing agents alone does not produce muscle contraction nor does reversal of neuromuscular blockade with anticholinesterases.

Succinylcholine and neuromuscular disease

—Patients with neuromuscular disease (upper and lower motor neuron abnormalities) can respond to succinylcholine with a dangerous, sometimes fatal hyperkalemia. This probably occurs because of proliferation of extrajunctional acetylcholine receptors on the muscle membrane. Depolarization of these receptors causes potassium leak through the muscle membrane.

—Patients with traumatic spinal cord damage can manifest this hyperkalemic response as early as 24–48 hours. The period of time that such patients remain at risk for this response is not clear. As in burn patients, the potential for hyperkalemia following succinylcholine may persist for over 1 year following the injury.

—Chronic or progressive motor neuron disease places patients at continuous risk for hyperkalemia from succinylcholine. Syringomyelia, amyotrophic lateral sclerosis, multiple sclerosis, acute idiopathic polyneuritis (Guillain–Barré syndrome), all forms of muscular dystrophy, and familial periodic paralysis (hyperkalemic form) have all been associated with this response.

Succinylcholine and PIH (pregnancy-induced hypertension), preeclampsia/eclampsia, toxemia

—Patients with hypertensive disorders of pregnancy may require treatment with antihypertensives such as trimethaphan or magnesium sulfate (for preeclampsia/eclampsia). These medications can have significant interactions with anesthetic agents such as succinylcholine, non-depolarizing neuromuscular blocking agents, or calcium channel blockers.

—Neuromuscular blockade produced by both depolarizing and non-depolarizing agents can be potentiated in patients receiving magnesium sulfate. The mechanisms involved include a decreased amount of acetylcholine released by the nerve impulse at the motor nerve terminal and a decrease in the depolarizing action of acetylcholine on the muscle.

Succinylcholine and periodic paralysis

—Succinylcholine should be avoided in patients with the hyperkalemic form of familial periodic paralysis. These patients can respond to succinylcholine with sustained muscle contraction, similar to patients with myotonia.

—Patients with the hypokalemic form have been given succinylcholine without complications.

Succinylcholine and pregnancy

—Plasma pseudocholinesterase levels in pregnant women have been shown to be significantly lower than in nonpregnant women. However, in a study of 50 women, the response to succinylcholine and recovery of twitch height were not significantly different in pregnant versus nonpregnant patients.

Succinylcholine and renal dysfunction

—Succinylcholine does not appear to result in significantly prolonged neuromuscular blockade in patients with renal failure unless given by infusion.

—Because one of the metabolites of succinylcholine is highly dependent on renal clearance, use of succinylcholine by infusion can result in prolonged neuromuscular blockade.

—Although there is controversy about decreased levels of plasma cholinesterase in patients with renal failure, recent studies have indicated that mivacurium elimination is prolonged in such patients because of decreased plasma cholinesterase.

Succinylcholine Interactions with Patient Drugs

Succinylcholine and amphotericin B

—Prolonged neuromuscular blockade can occur with depolarizing and non-depolarizing agents in patients receiving amphotericin B.

—The mechanism for this interaction is thought to be associated with the hypokalemia that can be caused by amphotericin B therapy.

Succinylcholine and antibiotics

—A number of antibiotics have significant interactions with neuromuscular blocking agents.

—These include the aminoglycosides (amikacin, gentamicin, kanamycin, neomycin, paromomycin, netilmicin, neomycin, streptomycin, tobramycin), as well as polymyxin B, colistin, amphotericin B, clindamycin, bacitracin, and lincomycin.

—All of the above antibiotics may potentiate non-depolarizing agents, but some (aminoglycosides, amphotericin B, clindamycin, colistin) can also potentiate succinylcholine blockade.

—These antibiotics potentiate neuromuscular blockade by different mechanisms, making management of these problems difficult. Although treatment with anticholinesterases or calcium has been recommended, results are inconsistent.

Succinylcholine and chlorambucil

—Some patients receiving the chlorambucil may have depressed levels of plasma pseudocholinesterase. In some cases, the result may be delayed metabolism of succinylcholine and a prolonged neuromuscular blockade.

Succinylcholine and cyclophosphamide
—Antipseudocholinesterases (echothiophate, phenelzine, nitrogen mustard, cyclophosphamide) prevent the metabolic destruction of succinylcholine and thus prolong its neuromuscular blocking properties.

Succinylcholine and demecarium bromide, echothiophate, isoflurophate
—The nonspecific anticholinesterase miotics (echothiophate, demecarium bromide, isoflurophate) used in treatment of glaucoma can result in significant depression of plasma pseudocholinesterase levels.

—Prolonged neuromuscular blockade can occur with succinylcholine in these patients. A period of 2–4 weeks may be necessary to restore plasma cholinesterase levels after discontinuing the anticholinesterase miotics.

Succinylcholine and digitalis
—Succinylcholine may precipitate cardiac arrhythmias in digitalized patients.

—Possible explanations of this interaction include the potential of succinylcholine to cause a shift of potassium from the intracellular to extracellular compartments in muscle tissue.

Succinylcholine and hexafluorenium
—Antipseudocholinesterases (echothiophate, hexafluorenium, phenelzine, tetrahydroaminocrine, nitrogen mustard, cyclophosphamide) prevent the metabolic destruction of succinylcholine and thus prolong its neuromuscular blocking properties.

Succinylcholine and ifosfamide
—Some patients receiving ifosfamide may have depressed levels of plasma pseudocholinesterase. In some cases, the result may be delayed metabolism of succinylcholine and a prolonged neuromuscular blockade.

Succinylcholine and lithium
—Lithium has been reported to increase the duration of both non-depolarizing and depolarizing neuromuscular blocking drugs.

—The mechanism of this interaction is unknown and the clinical significance of this interaction is uncertain.

Succinylcholine and mechlorethamine
—Some patients receiving mechlorethamine may have depressed levels of plasma pseudocholinesterase. In some cases, the result may be delayed metabolism of succinylcholine and a prolonged neuromuscular blockade.

Succinylcholine and melphalan
—Some patients receiving melphalan may have depressed levels of plasma pseudocholinesterase. In some cases, the result may be delayed metabolism of succinylcholine and a prolonged neuromuscular blockade.

Succinylcholine and mexilitene
—Mexilitene, like lidocaine and most local anesthetics, can potentiate neuromuscular blockade from depolarizing and non-depolarizing agents.

Succinylcholine and nitrogen mustard
—Antipseudocholinesterases (echothiophate, phenelzine, nitrogen mustard, cyclophosphamide) prevent the metabolic destruction of succinylcholine and thus prolong its neuromuscular blocking properties.

Succinylcholine and phenelzine
—Phenelzine is the only monoamine oxidase inhibitor associated with reduced plasma cholinesterase activity. This has been reported to be associated with a prolonged neuromuscular blockade in one patient.

Succinylcholine and quinidine
—Quinidine and quinine can potentiate muscle relaxation from both depolarizing and nondepolarizing agents.
—The mechanism of this interaction is a curare-like action at the myoneural junction. Also, plasma pseudocholinesterase is inhibited by quinidine (and quinine), resulting in possible prolongation of muscle relaxation from succinylcholine.

Succinylcholine and tetrahydroaminocrine
—Antipseudocholinesterases (echothiophate, hexafluorenium, phenelzine, tetrahydroaminocrine, nitrogen mustard, cyclophosphamide) prevent the metabolic destruction of succinylcholine and thus prolong its neuromuscular blocking properties.

Succinylcholine and tocainide
—Tocainide, an orally active form of lidocaine, can potentiate both depolarizing and non-depolarizing neuromuscular blockade. This is a property of most local anesthetics as well as a number of other medications.

SUFENTANIL (Sufenta)

Classification and indications
—Sufentanil is an opioid analgesic.
—It is indicated for use in patients being anesthetized for surgery. It can be used as part of a technique for general anes-

thesia (such as nitrous/narcotic) or as part of a regimen for intravenous sedation (such as with propofol or midazolam).

Pharmacology

—Sufentanil, like other narcotics, exerts its analgesic effects through opioid receptors in the CNS (brain and spinal cord).

—Although narcotics used in anesthesia are potent analgesics, there is controversy about the level of amnesia induced with even large doses of narcotics. To avoid awareness during anesthesia, use of other anesthetic agents (benzodiazepines, inhalation agents, etc.) is recommended.

—Somatosensory evoked potentials (SEPs) are not significantly affected by narcotics.

—Although there is some controversy about increases in intracranial pressure from opioids, in general, opioids cause slight decreases in cerebral blood flow, metabolic rate, and intracranial pressure.

—Cardiovascular effects of alfentanil, sufentanil, and fentanyl include variable degrees of bradycardia and hypotension. This is thought to be mostly from decreased central sympathetic outflow, although some direct effects have been suggested.

—Like other narcotics, sufentanil causes respiratory depression and reduced hypoxic ventilatory drive.

—Muscle rigidity, particularly of the chest wall, has been associated with rapid administration of narcotics. The mechanism of this action is not clear, but older patients seem more prone to this response. It has also been associated most frequently with alfentanil.

—Muscle rigidity can occur not only during induction but also on emergence from anesthesia or, rarely, hours after the last opioid dose.

—Onset of analgesia and anesthesia is in 1–3 minutes with a duration less than fentanyl but greater than alfentanil.

—For comparison, the elimination half-lives of fentanyl, sufentanil, and alfentanil are 219, 164, and 90 minutes, respectively.

—Elimination of alfentanil, sufentanil, and fentanyl is a result of hepatic metabolism.

—Older patients and those with liver disease may demonstrate prolonged effects from sufentanil due to decreased clearance of the drug.

Dose

—As part of a general anesthetic: Total doses should not exceed 1 µg/kg/hr.

—Bolus dosing: For procedures of 1 to 2 hours, initial dose can be up to 1 to 2 µg/kg, depending on other agents used. For procedures lasting longer, higher initial doses can be used.

—Infusion: The rate of infusion should be adjusted according to the initial dose so that the total amount administered is no more than 1 µg/kg/hr.

—Anesthetic dose (such as for cardiac surgery):

—Bolus dosing: 8–30 µg/kg can produce deep anesthesia. At this dosage level, other anesthetic agents are usually not necessary.

—Infusion: Depending on the initial dose, infusions should be adjusted according to patient responses to stimulation. Total dose for the procedure should not exceed 30 µg/kg.

—Epidural dose: For labor and delivery, 10–15 µg of sufentanil can be administered with 10 mL of bupivicaine 0.125%. A total of no more than 3 doses at 1-hour intervals is recommended.

Sufentanil Interactions with Anesthesia Drugs

Sufentanil and clonidine

—Clonidine has been shown to potentiate narcotics and reduce the MAC of inhaled anesthetics.

—This effect may be related to clonidine's inhibition of the sympathetic outflow from the vasomotor center in the medulla (clonidine is a central alpha 2 receptor agonist, which results in inhibition of CNS sympathetic centers).

Sufentanil and naloxone

—Cases of pulmonary edema, hypertension, and ventricular arrhythmias have occurred in postoperative patients receiving naloxone for reversal of respiratory depression induced by narcotics. The precise etiology of these reactions is not known.

Sufentanil Interactions with Diseases

Sufentanil and advanced age

—Elderly patients may require lower doses of narcotics than younger adults.

—This may be a result of reduced metabolism of this class of drugs or represent an increased brain sensitivity to narcotics as a result of aging.

Sufentanil and alcohol—acute intoxication

—Patients who are acutely intoxicated with alcohol (including chronic alcoholics) usually demonstrate increased sensitivity to general anesthesia.

—Although the precise mechanism of interactions is not agreed on, it appears that alcohol intoxication has additive CNS depression with barbiturates, benzodiazepines, and narcotics, as well as inhalational agents.

Sufentanil and alcohol—chronic abuse

—Chronic abuse of alcohol has complex and incompletely understood effects on a patient's response to anesthetic agents. In general, these patients tend to be more tolerant (in a nonintoxicated state) to barbiturates, benzodiazepines, narcotics, and inhalational agents.

—Exceptions to this generalization include the alcoholic patient with a cardiomyopathy who may demonstrate increased sensitivity to myocardial depression from inhalational agents.

—Also, the patient with severe liver disease may have impaired ability to metabolize succinylcholine due to decreased levels of plasma pseudocholinesterase.

Sufentanil and cerebral edema, intracranial hypertension

—Most intravenous anesthetics cause a reduction in cerebral blood flow and intracranial pressure or have no effect on ICP. Although this effect is primarily from depression of cerebral metabolic rate, in some cases a direct vasoconstriction occurs.

—The exception to the above is ketamine, which causes an increased CMR and CBF with an increase in ICP.

—All of the narcotics, as well as barbiturates, etomidate, benzodiazepines, and propofol, have been associated with a reduction or maintenance of ICP during anesthesia.

Sufentanil and malignant hyperthermia

—Anesthetic agents considered safe for use in patients with known or suspected susceptibility for developing malignant hyperthermia include propofol, barbiturates, etomidate, ketamine, non-depolarizing neuromuscular blocking agents, narcotics, benzodiazepines, droperidol, epinephrine, norepinephrine, and anticholinesterases.

—Nitrous oxide is probably safe in the susceptible patient based on repeated use in MH-susceptible humans and swine.

—Local or regional anesthesia with either amide (such as lidocaine) or ester (such as procaine) anesthetics is now considered safe for MH-susceptible patients.

Sufentanil and obesity

—The elimination half-life of sufentanil can be significantly prolonged in obese patients.

—A study of obese neurosurgical patients determined that the volume of distribution of sufentanil was increased, thereby delaying its elimination. The amount of increase in the volume of distribution was determined by the extent of obesity.

Sufentanil and porphyria

—Narcotics are considered safe anesthetics for use in porphyrias.

—Not all of the porphyrias have significance for the anesthesiologist. Three of the four hepatic porphyrias (acute intermittent, variegate, hereditary coproporphyria) and none of the erythropoietic porphyrias are associated with neurologic symptoms that can be triggered by certain medications: barbiturates, etomidate, and corticosteroids.

—Benzodiazepines and etomidate are considered to be questionable triggering agents, whereas safe anesthetics are inhalational agents, narcotics, muscle relaxants, anticholinesterases, and propofol.

Sufentanil and renal dysfunction

—Renal dysfunction has not been demonstrated to cause significant changes in pharmacokinetics or pharmacodynamics of benzodiazepines, narcotics (with the possible exception of butorphanol), barbiturates, or propofol.

—In patients with renal dysfunction, the above drugs may appear to have an increase in duration or intensity. This has been explained as a response to the systemic effects of renal dysfunction rather than specific effects on the metabolism of theses drugs.

—Some muscle relaxants are significantly affected by renal failure.

Sufentanil Interactions with Patient Drugs

Sufentanil and cimetidine

—Cimetidine may potentiate narcotics, causing greater respiratory depression and sedation than expected. This may be related to the alteration of hepatic metabolism of narcotics produced by cimetidine.

—This effect is seen less with morphine than other narcotics and is probably related to the fact that morphine undergoes a different metabolic process than some other narcotics such as fentanyl or meperidine.

—Ranitidine is not associated with this interaction.

Sufentanil and clonidine

—Clonidine has been shown to potentiate narcotics and reduce the MAC of inhaled anesthetics.

—This effect may be related to clonidine's inhibition of the sympathetic outflow from the vasomotor center in the medulla (clonidine is a central alpha 2 receptor agonist, which results in inhibition of CNS sympathetic centers).

THEOPHYLLINE (Aerolate, Aquaphyllin, Asmalix, Lanophyllin, Quibron, Respbid, Theo-24, Theo-Dur, Theo-Sav, Theochron, Theolair, Uniphyl)

Classification and indications

—Aminophylline is a xanthine derivative.

—It is used as a bronchodilator and also to treat apnea in infants and patients with Cheyne–Stokes respiration.

Pharmacology

—Aminophylline is a compound of theophylline with ethylenediamine, which makes theophylline more water-soluble.

—Theophylline competitively inhibits phosphodiesterase and increases intracellular cyclic AMP, resulting in bronchodilation and pulmonary arteriolar dilation.

—Theophylline is a CNS and cardiovascular stimulant. Partially offsetting the stimulating effect on the cardiovascular system is systemic arteriolar and venous dilation (as well as coronary artery dilation).

—Optimal bronchodilation usually requires serum theophylline levels between 10–20 μg/mL. Above 20 μg/mL, adverse effects of theophylline are likely to manifest (tachycardia, nausea, delirium, seizures, etc.).

—Elimination of theophylline is impaired in patients with congestive heart failure, chronic obstructive pulmonary disease, liver disease, or in geriatric patients.

Dose

—Intravenous therapy for acute bronchospasm in patients not receiving theophylline (aminophylline) requires a loading dose of approximately 6 mg/kg of aminophylline (which is the equivalent of 4.7 mg of theophylline).

—Maintenance doses vary according to age or presence of other medical conditions:

—Children and healthy, young adult smokers: 1–1.2 mg/kg/hr.

—Healthy, nonsmoking adults: 0.7 mg/kg/hr.

—Older patients or those with liver disease, lung, or heart disease: 0.5–0.6 mg/kg/hr.

Theophylline Interactions with Anesthesia Drugs

Theophylline and adenosine

—Adenosine is a nucleoside that slows conduction through the atrioventricular node. Xanthines such as theophylline, aminophylline, and caffeine can reverse or block the physiologic effects of adenosine.

Theophylline and cimetidine

—Cimetidine can significantly reduce hepatic metabolism of theophylline or aminophylline. This effect on theophylline metabolism is seen as soon as therapeutic levels of cimetidine are achieved.

Theophylline Interactions with Diseases

Theophylline and cirrhosis, liver disease

—Patients with severe liver disease (cirrhosis) or congestive heart failure may require reduced maintenance doses of theophylline (or its more water-soluble derivative, aminophylline). Initial loading doses for untreated patients, however, do not usually require adjustment.

—Reduction in maintenance dosing in the above type of patients is necessary because metabolism of theophylline takes place primarily in the liver.

Theophylline and congestive heart failure

—Patients with severe liver disease (cirrhosis) or congestive heart failure may require reduced maintenance doses of theophylline (or its more water-soluble derivative, aminophylline). Initial loading doses for untreated patients, however, do not usually require adjustment.

—Reduction in maintenance dosing in the above type of patients is necessary because metabolism of theophylline takes place primarily in the liver.

TRIMETHAPHAN (Arfonad)

Classification and indications

—Trimethaphan is a ganglionic blocking agent.

—It is indicated for management of hypertensive emergencies (such as autonomic dysflexia) or controlled hypotension for surgery.

Pharmacology

—Trimethaphan is a competitive inhibitor of acetylcholine at both sympathetic and parasympathetic ganglia. (Acetylcholine is the neurotransmitter at all presynaptic ganglia and the postsynaptic ganglia of the parasympathetic system. Norepinephrine is the neurotransmitter at most postsynaptic sympathetic ganglia.)

—Sympathetic blockade from trimethaphan results in arteriolar dilation, venodilation, and lowered blood pressure. It also has a direct vasodilating effect and causes some release of histamine.

—Parasympathetic blockade may result in tachycardia.

—Cerebral vasodilation rarely occurs because ganglionic blockade does not affect the cerebral circulation (unlike nitroprusside and nitroglycerin). Pupillary dilation from parasympathetic blockade may be problematic during intracranial surgery.

—Onset of hypotension is almost immediate and has a half-life of 1–2 minutes due to rapid inactivation by plasma cholinesterase.

Dose

—Intravenous infusion: 3–4 mg/min (usual dose) of a solution of 1 mg/mL trimethaphan. The dosage range may be from 0.3 to 6 mg/min or greater.

Trimethaphan Interactions with Anesthesia Drugs

Trimethaphan and succinylcholine

—Trimethaphan can significantly prolong the effects of succinylcholine in some cases.

—Even though trimethaphan is metabolized by plasma cholinesterase, it inhibits this enzyme by an unknown mechanism.

Trimethaphan and tubocurarine

—Trimethaphan can prolong the effects of tubocurarine neuromuscular blockade in some cases.

—Although the mechanism is not well understood, this may result from decreased perfusion of the neuromuscular junction. It is not known if other non-depolarizing agents are affected.

Trimethaphan Interactions with Diseases

Trimethaphan and cerebral edema, intracranial hypertension

—Most systemic vasodilators (nitroglycerin, nitroprusside, hydralazine, calcium channel blockers, and adenosine) can produce cerebrovascular vasodilation as well. As a result, cerebral blood volume is either maintained or increased even though systemic blood pressure is decreased.

—Trimethaphan, a ganglionic blocker, usually will not increase cerebral blood volume because ganglionic blockade normally does not cause vasodilation of the cerebral circulation.

Trimethaphan and PIH (pregnancy-induced hypertension), preeclampsia/eclampsia, toxemia

—Patients with hypertensive disorders of pregnancy may require treatment with antihypertensives such as trimethaphan or magnesium sulfate (for preeclampsia/eclampsia). These medications can have significant interactions with anesthetic agents such as succinylcholine, non-depolarizing neuromuscular blocking agents, or calcium channel blockers.

—Trimethaphan can significantly prolong the effects of succinylcholine but not of non-depolarizing agents.

—This interaction results from inhibition of plasma pseudocholinesterase by trimethaphan. The result is delayed metabolism of succinylcholine.

TUBOCURARINE (Curare)

Classification and indications

—Tubocurarine is a non-depolarizing neuromuscular blocker.

—Although it has been used for skeletal muscle relaxation for intubation and during surgery, it has been replaced by newer agents. It can be used as a defasciculating agent in small doses prior to use of succinylcholine.

Pharmacology

—Tubocurarine competes with acetylcholine at the neuromuscular junction of skeletal muscle by binding to acetylcholine receptors.

—After doses of 0.5–0.6 mg/kg, maximal muscle relaxation occurs in 2–5 minutes and may have a clinical duration of 60 minutes or more.

—Significant histamine release is caused by tubocurarine and may result in hypotension, especially when administered rapidly IV.

—Elimination of tubocurarine is primarily by renal excretion, although some of the drug is excreted via the liver. As a result, patients with renal or hepatic disease are likely to experience prolonged effects.

Dose

—Intubation: 0.5–0.6 mg/kg.

—Maintenance: 0.1–0.15 mg/kg.

Tubocurarine Interactions with Anesthesia Drugs

Tubocurarine and calcium channel blockers (diltiazem, nicardipine, nifedipine, verapamil)

—Calcium channel blockers have been associated with prolongation of neuromuscular blockade from non-depolarizing agents.

—This interaction is probably related to the depletion of intracellular calcium associated with chronic therapy. This can result in a decrease in acetylcholine release at the neuromuscular junction.

Tubocurarine and inhalational anesthetics (desflurane, enflurane, halothane, isoflurane, sevoflurane)

—Desflurane, enflurane, halothane, isoflurane, and sevoflurane can significantly potentiate neuromuscular blockade, depending on the neuromuscular blocker used. Nitrous oxide has minimal effects.

—Tubocurarine and pancuronium are potentiated the most by inhalational agents, whereas atracurium and vecuronium are intensified significantly less.

—Potentiation by inhalational agents occurs through depression of spinal cord reflexes as well as effects at or distal to the neuromuscular junction.

Tubocurarine and diphenylhydantoin, phenytoin

—Patients on chronic phenytoin therapy may be resistant to non-depolarizing muscle blockade. The studies involved metocurine and vecuronium but may involve other non-depolarizing agents.

—The mechanism of this interaction is not known.

—Acute infusions of phenytoin may prolong non-depolarizing blockade. This was studied prospectively in a small number of patients who received a 10 mg/kg loading dose of phenytoin during steady-state muscle blockade with vecuronium. They had significant potentiation of their neuromuscular block compared to control patients.

Tubocurarine and furosemide

—Furosemide may potentiate neuromuscular blockade from tubocurarine and succinylcholine. This is based on a case report of several patients given furosemide and tubocurarine during surgery and on animal studies.

—The implication for this interaction for other neuromuscular blocking drugs is uncertain and the mechanism is not known.

Tubocurarine and lidocaine

—Most local anesthetics can block neuromuscular transmission from non-depolarizing agents as well as depolarizing muscle relaxants. Of clinical significance to the anesthesiologist, lidocaine, given as a 50- to 100-mg bolus or even by infusion, can significantly increase a non-depolarizer block or a phase II block from succinylcholine.

Tubocurarine and procainamide

—Procainamide can potentiate muscle relaxation from non-depolarizing agents. This is probably a result of decreased acetylcholine release at the neuromuscular junction caused by procainamide.

Tubocurarine and quinidine

—Quinidine, procainamide, propranolol, and most local anesthetics have been shown to enhance the neuromuscular blockade from depolarizing and non-depolarizing agents.

—A number of well-documented cases have illustrated the ability of these agents, when given in the immediate postoperative period, to convert subclinical muscle weakness from neuromuscular blocking drugs into significant muscle weakness requiring reintubation.

Tubocurarine and succinylcholine

—Prior administration of succinylcholine has been shown to potentiate neuromuscular blockade of some non-depolarizing agents.

—Although this interaction has been documented with pancuronium, it was not seen with doxacurium and may not be a consistent finding with non-depolarizing agents.

Tubocurarine Interactions with Diseases

Tubocurarine and advanced age

—Prolonged duration of neuromuscular blockade can be seen in older patients with several different non-depolarizing agents, including doxacurium, mivacurium, and rocuronium.

—In some cases, delayed onset of muscle relaxation also occurs. This has been attributed to decreased perfusion of the neuromuscular junction as a result of advanced age.

Tubocurarine and burns

—Patients with burn injuries are susceptible to a life-threatening hyperkalemic response to succinylcholine and can have marked resistance to non-depolarizing muscle relaxants.

—Both of these altered responses to neuromuscular blocking agents have been attributed to proliferation of extrajunctional acetylcholine receptors, similar to that in the patient with a denervation injury.

—Resistance to non-depolarizing agents appears to increase with larger area burns and, in fact, may not be significant in patients with <30% body surface area burns. In addition to proliferation of extrajunctional acetylcholine receptors, this abnormal response is probably also related to the increased metabolic rate and hepatic and renal clearance seen in burn patients. Doses of non-depolarizing agents may need to be increased by as much as 300%.

—Duration of this resistance usually is 2 months following the injury but has been reported in a patient 463 days after the burn.

Tubocurarine and cirrhosis, liver disease

—Prolonged neuromuscular blockade in patients with liver disease can be seen with doxacurium, mivacurium, vecuronium, pancuronium, rocuronium, and tubocurarine.

—This interaction is complex and may be due to decreased clearance, decreased hepatic uptake of the agent, or decreased synthesis of enzymes important for degradation of the neuromuscular blocker. An example of the latter is prolongation of mivacurium's duration of action as a result of decreased plasma cholinesterase from severe liver disease.

—Because of the increased volume of distribution of many drugs seen in patients with liver disease, initial doses of muscle relaxants may need to be larger than in healthy patients. Once neuromuscular blockade is achieved, recovery may be prolonged.

Tubocurarine and Eaton–Lambert syndrome

—Patients with Eaton–Lambert syndrome are very sensitive to both depolarizing and non-depolarizing neuromuscular blockade.

—This disorder is similar to myasthenia gravis and patients complain of skeletal muscle weakness, but it is usually associated with carcinoma (especially small cell tumors of the lung).

—If the diagnosis is known or suspected prior to surgery, reduced doses of muscle relaxants should be used, but sometimes the diagnosis is first made when a patient has surgery for a lung tumor and has an unexpected, prolonged neuromuscular block.

—Anticholinesterases are unreliable in reversing muscle weakness.

Tubocurarine and hyperthyroidism, thyrotoxicosis

—Muscle weakness is commonly seen with hyperthyroidism and affects proximal muscles, usually sparing respiratory function. In some cases, myopathy is the dominant feature of thyroid hormone excess and can resemble myasthenia. Lower doses of muscle relaxants may be indicated.

Tubocurarine and hypokalemia

—Hypokalemia appears to potentiate the effects of neuromuscular blockade from non-depolarizing agents.

—The interaction is probably due to hyperpolarization of the muscle endplate and, therefore, resistance to depolarization.

—Hyperpolarization would more likely occur with more acute changes in potassium concentration because the potassium losses would be from the extracellular compartment rather than from intracellular sites.

—Chronic hypokalemia is more likely to be associated with potassium depletion from both extra- and intracellular compartments with no significant change in transmembrane potential. As a result, significant effects on neuromuscular blockade would be less likely.

Tubocurarine and hypothermia

—Non-depolarizing muscle blockade is prolonged by hypothermia. This interaction is a result of an effect on the neuromuscular blocking agents themselves rather than on the anticholinesterases used to reverse the neuromuscular blocking agents.

—Hypothermia appears to prolong the effect of the non-depolarizing agents by several mechanisms, including delayed metabolism into inactive metabolites as well as delayed excretion via the urinary and biliary routes.

Tubocurarine and malignant hyperthermia

—Anesthetic agents considered safe for use in patients with known or suspected susceptibility for developing malignant hyperthermia (MH) include propofol, barbiturates, etomidate, ketamine, non-depolarizing neuromuscular blocking agents, narcotics, benzodiazepines, droperidol, epinephrine, norepinephrine, and anticholinesterases.

—Nitrous oxide is probably safe in the susceptible patient based on repeated use in MH-susceptible humans and swine.

—Local or regional anesthesia with either amide (such as lidocaine) or ester (such as procaine) anesthetics is now considered safe for MH-susceptible patients.

Tubocurarine and myasthenia gravis

—Patients with myasthenia gravis are very sensitive to neuromuscular blockade from non-depolarizing agents.

—This is probably a result of decreased acetylcholine receptors from autoimmune destruction associated with myasthenia gravis.

—Although these patients are treated with the same or similar anticholinesterases used to antagonize muscle blockade, sensitivity (not resistance) to neuromuscular blockade is seen clinically.

Tubocurarine and neuromuscular disease (amyotrophic lateral sclerosis, multiple sclerosis, syringomyelia)

—Patients with a wide variety of neuromuscular disorders may be more resistant than normal patients to the effects of non-depolarizing neuromuscular blockers.

—This includes patients with disuse atrophy of the muscles (such as bedridden patients with chronic disease) as well as patients with upper or lower motor neuron disease such as amyotrophic lateral sclerosis, multiple sclerosis, or syringomyelia.

—Disuse or denervation of muscle results in production of extrajunctional acetylcholine receptors on the muscle membrane. These receptors are less easily blocked by non-depolarizing agents but are activated by lower concentrations of depolarizing drugs (succinylcholine).

—When these receptors, which can be scattered over a large surface of the muscle, are depolarized by succinylcholine, ion flow takes place through the receptor channel. Large amounts of potassium may exit the muscle cell, causing hyperkalemia.

—Despite initial resistance to blockade, such patients may demonstrate prolonged neuromuscular weakness as a result of decreased muscle strength and mass.

Tubocurarine and PIH (pregnancy-induced hypertension), preeclampsia/eclampsia, toxemia

—Patients with hypertensive disorders of pregnancy may require treatment with antihypertensives such as trimethaphan or magnesium sulfate (for preeclampsia/eclampsia). These medications can have significant interactions with anesthetic agents such as succinylcholine, non-depolarizing neuromuscular blocking agents, or calcium channel blockers.

—Neuromuscular blockade produced by both depolarizing and non-depolarizing agents can be potentiated in patients receiving magnesium sulfate. The mechanisms involved include a decreased amount of acetylcholine released by the nerve impulse at the motor nerve terminal and a decrease in the depolarizing action of acetylcholine on the muscle.

Tubocurarine Interactions with Patient Drugs

Tubocurarine and antibiotics

—A number of antibiotics have significant interactions with neuromuscular blocking agents.

—These include the aminoglycosides (amikacin, gentamicin, kanamycin, neomycin, paromomycin, netilmicin, neomycin, streptomycin, tobramycin), as well as polymyxin B, colistin, amphotericin B, clindamycin, bacitracin, and lincomycin.

—All of the above antibiotics may potentiate non-depolarizing agents, but some (aminoglycosides, amphotericin B, clindamycin, colistin) can also potentiate succinylcholine blockade.

—These antibiotics potentiate neuromuscular blockade by different mechanisms, making management of these problems difficult. Although treatment with anticholinesterases or calcium has been recommended, results are inconsistent.

Tubocurarine and amphotericin B

—Prolonged neuromuscular blockade can occur with depolarizing and non-depolarizing agents in patients receiving amphotericin B.

—The mechanism for this interaction is thought to be associated with the hypokalemia that can be caused by amphotericin B therapy.

Tubocurarine and beta blockers, propranolol

—Beta blockers may potentiate non-depolarizing neuromuscular blocking agents. This interaction has been reported between propranolol and tubocurarine.

—Other beta blockers are also capable of causing weakness in patients with myasthenia gravis, but the mechanism or significance of these interactions is unclear.

Tubocurarine and calcium channel blockers (amlodipine, bepridil, diltiazem, felodipine, isradipine, lidoflazine, nicardipine, nimodipine, nisoldipine, nitrendipine, verapamil)

—Calcium channel blockers have been associated with prolongation of neuromuscular blockade from non-depolarizing agents.

—This interaction is probably related to the depletion of intracellular calcium associated with chronic therapy. This can result in a decrease in acetylcholine release at the neuromuscular junction.

Tubocurarine and diphenylhydantoin, phenytoin

—Patients on chronic phenytoin therapy may be resistant to non-depolarizing muscle blockade. The studies involved metocurine and vecuronium, but may involve other non-depolarizing agents.

—The mechanism of this interaction is not known.

—Acute infusions of phenytoin may prolong non-depolarizing blockade. This was studied prospectively in a small number of patients who received a 10 mg/kg loading dose of phenytoin during steady-state muscle blockade with vecuronium. They had significant potentiation of their neuromuscular block compared to control patients.

Tubocurarine and lidocaine

—Most local anesthetics can block neuromuscular transmission from non-depolarizing agents as well as depolarizing muscle relaxants. Of clinical significance to the anesthesiologist, lidocaine, given as a 50- to 100-mg bolus or even by infusion, can significantly increase a non-depolarizer block or a phase II block from succinylcholine.

Tubocurarine and lithium

—Lithium has been reported to increase the duration of both non-depolarizing and depolarizing neuromuscular blocking drugs.

—The mechanism of this interaction is unknown and the clinical significance of this interaction is uncertain.

Tubocurarine and magnesium sulfate

—Neuromuscular blockade produced by both depolarizing and non-depolarizing agents can be potentiated in patients receiving magnesium sulfate. The mechanisms involved include a decreased amount of acetylcholine released by the nerve impulse at the motor nerve terminal and a decrease in the depolarizing action of acetylcholine on the muscle.

Tubocurarine and mexilitene

—Mexilitene, like lidocaine and most local anesthetics, can potentiate neuromuscular blockade from depolarizing and non-depolarizing agents.

Tubocurarine and procainamide

—Procainamide can potentiate muscle relaxation from non-depolarizing agents. This is probably a result of decreased acetylcholine release at the neuromuscular junction caused by procainamide.

Tubocurarine and quinidine

—Quinidine and quinine can potentiate muscle relaxation from both depolarizing and nondepolarizing agents.

—The mechanism of this interaction is a curare-like action at the myoneu1ral junction. Also, plasma pseudo-cholinesterase is inhibited by quinidine (and quinine), resulting in possible prolongation of muscle relaxation from succinylcholine.

Tubocurarine and tocainide

—Tocainide, an orally active form of lidocaine, can potentiate both depolarizing and non-depolarizing neuromuscular blockade. This is a property of most local anesthetics as well as a number of other medications.

Tubocurarine and trimethaphan

—Trimethaphan can prolong the effects of tubocurarine neuromuscular blockade in some cases.

—Although the mechanism is not well understood, this may result from decreased perfusion of the neuromuscular junction. It is not known if other non-depolarizing agents are affected.

VECURONIUM (Norcuron)

Classification and indications
—Vecuronium is a non-depolarizing neuromuscular blocking agent.
—It is indicated for skeletal muscle relaxation for intubation or during surgery.

Pharmacology
—Vecuronium is a competitive inhibitor of acetylcholine at the neuromuscular junction of skeletal muscles.
—Intubating conditions are achieved in 2.5–3 minutes after a dose of 0.1 mg/kg. At this dose, the duration of blockade (25% recovery of twitch height) is 25–40 minutes.
—There is no significant release of histamine associated with administration of vecuronium and no clinically significant effect on the cardiovascular system.
—Elimination and clinical duration of vecuronium are not significantly affected by renal failure, although anephric patients may show a prolonged effect.
—Patients with hepatic dysfunction are likely to have prolonged recovery times because elimination depends on biliary excretion.
—Although significant cumulative effects do not seem to occur under most circumstances in anesthesia, prolonged infusion of vecuronium to intensive care unit patients has resulted in prolonged blockade.

Dose
—Intubation: 0.08–0.1 mg/kg provides good intubating conditions in 2.5–3 minutes.
—Maintenance:
—Bolus: 0.01–0.015 mg/kg every 25–40 min.
—Infusion: 0.8–1.2 µg/kg/min.

Vecuronium Interactions with Anesthesia Drugs
Vecuronium and calcium channel blockers (diltiazem, nicardipine, nifedipine, verapamil)
—Calcium channel blockers have been associated with prolongation of neuromuscular blockade from non-depolarizing agents.

—This interaction is probably related to the depletion of intracellular calcium associated with chronic therapy. This can result in a decrease in acetylcholine release at the neuromuscular junction.

Vecuronium and inhalational anesthetics (desflurane, enflurane, halothane, isoflurane, sevoflurane)

—Desflurane, enflurane, halothane, isoflurane, and sevoflurane can significantly potentiate neuromuscular blockade, depending on the neuromuscular blocker used. Nitrous oxide has minimal effects.

—Tubocurarine and pancuronium are potentiated the most by inhalational agents, whereas atracurium and vecuronium are intensified significantly less.

—Potentiation by inhalational agents occurs through depression of spinal cord reflexes as well as effects at or distal to the neuromuscular junction.

Vecuronium and diphenylhydantoin, phenytoin

—Patients on chronic phenytoin therapy may be resistant to non-depolarizing muscle blockade. The studies involved metocurine and vecuronium but may involve other non-depolarizing agents.

—The mechanism of this interaction is not known.

—Acute infusions of phenytoin may prolong non-depolarizing blockade. This was studied prospectively in a small number of patients who received a 10 mg/kg loading dose of phenytoin during steady-state muscle blockade with vecuronium. They had significant potentiation of their neuromuscular block compared to control patients.

Vecuronium and furosemide

—Furosemide may potentiate neuromuscular blockade from tubocurarine and succinylcholine.

—This is based on a case report of several patients given furosemide and tubocurarine during surgery and on animal studies.

—The implication for this interaction for other neuromuscular blocking drugs is uncertain and the mechanism is not known.

Vecuronium and lidocaine

—Most local anesthetics can block neuromuscular transmission from non-depolarizing agents as well as depolarizing muscle relaxants. Of clinical significance to the anesthesiologist, lidocaine, given as a 50- to 100-mg bolus or even by infusion, can significantly increase a non-depolarizer block or a phase II block from succinylcholine.

Vecuronium and procainamide

—Procainamide can potentiate muscle relaxation from non-depolarizing agents. This is probably a result of decreased acetylcholine release at the neuromuscular junction caused by procainamide.

Vecuronium and quinidine

—Quinidine, procainamide, propranolol, and most local anesthetics have been shown to enhance the neuromuscular blockade from depolarizing and non-depolarizing agents.

—A number of well-documented cases have illustrated the ability of these agents, when given in the immediate post-operative period, to convert subclinical muscle weakness from neuromuscular blocking drugs into significant muscle weakness requiring reintubation.

Vecuronium and succinylcholine

—Prior administration of succinylcholine has been shown to potentiate neuromuscular blockade of some non-depolarizing agents.

—Although this interaction has been documented with pancuronium, it was not seen with doxacurium and may not be a consistent finding with non-depolarizing agents.

Vecuronium Interactions with Diseases

Vecuronium and advanced age

—Prolonged duration of neuromuscular blockade can be seen in older patients with several different non-depolarizing agents including doxacurium, mivacurium, and rocuronium.

—In some cases, delayed onset of muscle relaxation also occurs. This has been attributed to decreased perfusion of the neuromuscular junction as a result of advanced age.

Vecuronium and burns

—Patients with burn injuries are susceptible to a life-threatening hyperkalemic response to succinylcholine and can have marked resistance to non-depolarizing muscle relaxants.

—Both of these altered responses to neuromuscular blocking agents have been attributed to proliferation of extrajunctional acetylcholine receptors, similar to that in the patient with a denervation injury.

—Resistance to non-depolarizing agents appears to increase with larger area burns and, in fact, may not be significant in patients with <30% body surface area burns. In addition to proliferation of extrajunctional acetylcholine receptors, this abnormal response is probably also related to the increased metabolic rate and hepatic and renal clearance seen in burn patients. Doses of non-depolarizing agents may need to be increased by as much as 300%.

—Duration of this resistance usually is 2 months following the injury but has been reported in a patient 463 days after the burn.

Vecuronium and cirrhosis, liver disease

—Prolonged neuromuscular blockade in patients with liver disease can be seen with doxacurium, mivacurium, vecuronium, pancuronium, rocuronium, and tubocurarine.

—This interaction is complex and may be due to decreased clearance, decreased hepatic uptake of the agent, or decreased synthesis of enzymes important for degradation of the neuromuscular blocker. An example of the latter is prolongation of mivacurium's duration of action as a result of decreased plasma cholinesterase from severe liver disease.

—Because of the increased volume of distribution of many drugs seen in patients with liver disease, initial doses of muscle relaxants may need to be larger than in healthy patients. Once neuromuscular blockade is achieved, recovery may be prolonged.

Vecuronium and Eaton–Lambert syndrome

—Patients with Eaton–Lambert syndrome are very sensitive to both depolarizing and non-depolarizing neuromuscular blockade.

—This disorder is similar to myasthenia gravis and patients complain of skeletal muscle weakness, but it is usually associated with carcinoma (especially small cell tumors of the lung).

—If the diagnosis is known or suspected prior to surgery, reduced doses of muscle relaxants should be used, but sometimes the diagnosis is first made when a patient has surgery for a lung tumor and has an unexpected, prolonged neuromuscular block.

—Anticholinesterases are unreliable in reversing muscle weakness.

Vecuronium and hyperthyroidism, thyrotoxicosis

—Muscle weakness is commonly seen with hyperthyroidism and affects proximal muscles, usually sparing respiratory function. In some cases, myopathy is the dominant feature of thyroid hormone excess and can resemble myasthenia. Lower doses of muscle relaxants may be indicated.

Vecuronium and hypokalemia

—Hypokalemia appears to potentiate the effects of neuromuscular blockade from non-depolarizing agents.

—The interaction is probably due to hyperpolarization of the muscle endplate and, therefore, resistance to depolarization. Hyperpolarization would more likely occur with more acute changes in potassium concentration because the potassium losses would be from the extracellular compartment rather than from intracellular sites.

—Chronic hypokalemia is more likely to be associated with potassium depletion from both extra- and intracellular compartments with no significant change in transmembrane potential. As a result, significant effects on neuromuscular blockade would be less likely.

Vecuronium and hypothermia

—Non-depolarizing muscle blockade is prolonged by hypothermia. This interaction is a result of an effect on the neuromuscular blocking agents themselves rather than on the anticholinesterases used to reverse the neuromuscular blocking agents.

—Hypothermia appears to prolong the effect of the non-depolarizing agents by several mechanisms, including delayed metabolism into inactive metabolites as well as delayed excretion via the urinary and biliary routes.

Vecuronium and malignant hyperthermia

—Anesthetic agents considered safe for use in patients with known or suspected susceptibility for developing malignant hyperthermia (MH) include propofol, barbiturates, etomidate, ketamine, non-depolarizing neuromuscular blocking agents, narcotics, benzodiazepines, droperidol, epinephrine, norepinephrine, and anticholinesterases.

—Nitrous oxide is probably safe in the susceptible patient based on repeated use in MH-susceptible humans and swine.

—Local or regional anesthesia with either amide (such as lidocaine) or ester (such as procaine) anesthetics is now considered safe for MH-susceptible patients.

Vecuronium and myasthenia gravis

—Patients with myasthenia gravis are very sensitive to neuro-muscular blockade from non-depolarizing agents.

—This is probably a result of decreased acetylcholine receptors from autoimmune destruction associated with myasthenia gravis.

—Although these patients are treated with the same or similar anticholinesterases used to antagonize muscle blockade, sensitivity (not resistance) to neuromuscular blockade is seen clinically.

Vecuronium and neuromuscular disease (amyotrophic lateral sclerosis, multiple sclerosis, syringomyelia)

—Patients with a wide variety of neuromuscular disorders may be more resistant than normal patients to the effects of non-depolarizing neuromuscular blockers.

—This includes patients with disuse atrophy of the muscles (such as bedridden patients with chronic disease), as well as patients with upper or lower motor neuron disease such as amyotrophic lateral sclerosis, multiple sclerosis, or syringo-myelia.

—Disuse or denervation of muscle results in production of extrajunctional acetylcholine receptors on the muscle mem-brane. These receptors are less easily blocked by non-depo-larizing agents but are activated by lower concentrations of depolarizing drugs (succinylcholine).

—When these receptors, which can be scattered over a large surface of the muscle, are depolarized by succinylcholine, ion flow takes place through the receptor channel. Large amounts of potassium may exit the muscle cell, causing hyperkalemia.

—Despite initial resistance to blockade, such patients may demonstrate prolonged neuromuscular weakness as a result of decreased muscle strength and mass.

Vecuronium and PIH (pregnancy-induced hypertension), preeclampsia/eclampsia, toxemia

—Patients with hypertensive disorders of pregnancy may require treatment with antihypertensives such as trimetha-phan or magnesium sulfate (for preeclampsia/eclampsia). These medications can have significant interactions with anesthetic agents such as succinylcholine, non-depolarizing neuromuscular blocking agents, or calcium channel block-ers.

—Neuromuscular blockade produced by both depolarizing and non-depolarizing agents can be potentiated in patients receiving magnesium sulfate. The mechanisms involved include a decreased amount of acetylcholine released by the nerve impulse at the motor nerve terminal and a decrease in the depolarizing action of acetylcholine on the muscle.

Vecuronium Interactions with Patient Drugs

Vecuronium and antibiotics

—A number of antibiotics have significant interactions with neuromuscular blocking agents.

—These include the aminoglycosides (amikacin, gentamicin, kanamycin, neomycin, paromomycin, netilmicin, neomycin, streptomycin, tobramycin), as well as polymyxin B, colistin, amphotericin B, clindamycin, bacitracin, and lincomycin.

—All of the above antibiotics may potentiate non-depolarizing agents, but some (aminoglycosides, amphotericin B, clindamycin, colistin) can also potentiate succinylcholine blockade.

—These antibiotics potentiate neuromuscular blockade by different mechanisms, making management of these problems difficult. Although treatment with anticholinesterases or calcium has been recommended, results are inconsistent.

Vecuronium and amphotericin B

—Prolonged neuromuscular blockade can occur with depolarizing and non-depolarizing agents in patients receiving amphotericin B.

—The mechanism for this interaction is thought to be associated with the hypokalemia that can be caused by amphotericin B therapy.

Vecuronium and beta blockers, propranolol

—Beta blockers may potentiate non-depolarizing neuromuscular blocking agents. This interaction has been reported between propranolol and tubocurarine.

—Other beta blockers are also capable of causing weakness in patients with myasthenia gravis, but the mechanism or significance of these interactions is unclear.

Vecuronium and calcium channel blockers (amlodipine, bepridil, diltiazem, felodipine, isradipine, lidoflazine, nicardipine, nimodipine, nisoldipine, nitrendipine, verapamil)

—Calcium channel blockers have been associated with prolongation of neuromuscular blockade from non-depolarizing agents.

—This interaction is probably related to the depletion of intracellular calcium associated with chronic therapy. This can result in a decrease in acetylcholine release at the neuromuscular junction.

Vecuronium and diphenylhydantoin, phenytoin

—Patients on chronic phenytoin therapy may be resistant to non-depolarizing muscle blockade. The studies involved metocurine and vecuronium, but may involve other non-depolarizing agents.

—The mechanism of this interaction is not known.

—Acute infusions of phenytoin may prolong non-depolarizing blockade. This was studied prospectively in a small number of patients who received a 10 mg/kg loading dose of phenytoin during steady-state muscle blockade with vecuronium. They had significant potentiation of their neuromuscular block compared to control patients.

Vecuronium and lidocaine

—Most local anesthetics can block neuromuscular transmission from non-depolarizing agents as well as depolarizing muscle relaxants. Of clinical significance to the anesthesiologist, lidocaine, given as a 50- to 100-mg bolus or even by infusion, can significantly increase a non-depolarizer block or a phase II block from succinylcholine.

Vecuronium and lithium

—Lithium has been reported to increase the duration of both non-depolarizing and depolarizing neuromuscular blocking drugs.

—The mechanism of this interaction is unknown and the clinical significance of this interaction is uncertain.

Vecuronium and magnesium sulfate

—Neuromuscular blockade produced by both depolarizing and non-depolarizing agents can be potentiated in patients receiving magnesium sulfate. The mechanisms involved include a decreased amount of acetylcholine released by the nerve impulse at the motor nerve terminal and a decrease in the depolarizing action of acetylcholine on the muscle.

Vecuronium and mexilitene

—Mexilitene, like lidocaine and most local anesthetics, can potentiate neuromuscular blockade from depolarizing and non-depolarizing agents.

Vecuronium and procainamide

—Procainamide can potentiate muscle relaxation from non-depolarizing agents. This is probably a result of decreased acetylcholine release at the neuromuscular junction caused by procainamide.

Vecuronium and quinidine

—Quinidine and quinine can potentiate muscle relaxation from both depolarizing and non-depolarizing agents.

—The mechanism of this interaction is a curare-like action at the myoneural junction. Also, plasma pseudocholinesterase is inhibited by quinidine (and quinine), resulting in possible prolongation of muscle relaxation from succinylcholine.

Vecuronium and tocainide

—Tocainide, an orally active form of lidocaine, can potentiate both depolarizing and non-depolarizing neuromuscular blockade. This is a property of most local anesthetics as well as a number of other medications.

VERAPAMIL (Calan, Isoptin, Verelan)

Classification and indications

—Verapamil is a calcium channel blocker.

—It is indicated for the management of supraventricular tachyarrhythmias and for the short-term management of rapid ventricular rates associated with atrial fibrillation or flutter.

Pharmacology

—Depolarization of cardiac and smooth muscle cells is associated with ion movement (sodium, calcium, potassium, chloride) through ion channels. These channels are voltage-gated, meaning that they are opened and closed according to changes in transmembrane potentials.

—With depolarization, there is rapid movement of sodium through "fast" channels, whereas calcium moves much more slowly through "slow" channels. It is by interfering with calcium movement through these slow calcium channels that calcium channel blockers mainly exert their effects.

—Some of the calcium channel blockers have more pronounced effects on cardiac conduction (verapamil, diltiazem), whereas others have greater effects on vascular smooth muscle, resulting in lower blood pressure and coronary vasodilation (nifedipine, nicardipine).

—Verapamil may cause hypotension in some patients. Also, it has a negative inotropic effect (decreased contractility).

—Elimination of verapamil is a result of hepatic metabolism and urinary excretion. Patients with decreased hepatic or renal function may have prolonged effects from repeated or continuous infusions of verapamil, but single doses are neither potentiated or prolonged in such patients.

Dose

—Intravenous dose:

—Adult: 0.075–0.15 mg/kg (5–10 mg for average adult). A repeat dose of 0.15 mg/kg (10 mg average dose) may be given after 30 minutes if necessary.

—Pediatric: 0.1–0.3 mg/kg (maximum of 5 mg). A repeat dose may be given in about 30 minutes in the same dosage range, but the maximum dose may be increased to 10 mg.

Verapamil Interactions with Anesthesia Drugs

Verapamil and beta blockers (esmolol, labetalol, propranolol)

—Verapamil and diltiazem, particularly when used intravenously, can significantly potentiate the effects of beta blockers on cardiac conduction and contractility.

—Severe bradycardia and hypotension can occur when these medications are used concomitantly, especially in patients with abnormalities of cardiac conduction (sick sinus syndrome) or ventricular function (congestive heart failure).

Verapamil and calcium chloride, calcium gluconate

—Calcium may antagonize some effects of calcium channel blockers.

—In some patients, intravenous calcium has reduced the hypotensive effects of nifedipine but not its ability to prevent angina. In other cases, calcium has caused a return of an arrhythmia that had been controlled with a calcium channel blocker.

—Since the response to calcium may not be completely predictable in patients treated with calcium channel blockers, caution should be used when using intravenous calcium in such patients.

Verapamil and dantrolene

—There has been a report of hyperkalemia and cardiac decompensation in a patient receiving verapamil who was given prophylactic intravenous dantrolene on the basis of a history of malignant hyperthermia.

—This has not been reported with any other calcium channel blockers and the same patient did not have this response when again given dantrolene for another anesthetic while taking nifedipine.

Verapamil and etomidate

—A case report of two patients who received verapamil, one on a chronic basis and one who had received a 10-mg intravenous dose prior to anesthesia, described prolonged anesthesia and respiratory depression following etomidate.

—The mechanism of this interaction or its significance is not known.

Verapamil and muscle relaxants (atracurium, doxacurium, gallamine, metocurine, mivacurium, pancuronium, pipercuronium, rocuronium, tubocurarine, vecuronium)

—Calcium channel blockers have been associated with prolongation of neuromuscular blockade from non-depolarizing agents.

—This interaction is probably related to the depletion of intracellular calcium associated with chronic therapy. This can result in a decrease in acetylcholine release at the neuromuscular junction.

Verapamil Interactions with Diseases

Verapamil and atrial fibrillation or flutter

—Patients who have atrial fibrillation or flutter associated with Wolf–Parkinson–White syndrome should not be treated with verapamil or diltiazem.

—These medications may cause a worsening tachycardia that is thought to be due to reflex increases in sympathetic activity.

Verapamil and autonomic dysfunction, Shy–Drager syndrome

—Patients whose autonomic nervous system responses are impaired by disease (Shy–Drager) or medications (beta blockers) may be unable to adequately compensate for vasodilation or negative inotropic and chronotropic effects of calcium channel blockers.

—In these patients, exaggerated hypotension or bradycardia may be seen with calcium channel blockers.

—Verapamil may be associated with hypotension, myocardial depression, and bradycardia. Other calcium channel blockers have more selective actions, such as nifedipine, which would be more likely to be associated with only hypotension.

Verapamil and cerebral edema, intracranial hypertension

—Most systemic vasodilators (nitroglycerin, nitroprusside, hydralazine, calcium channel blockers, and adenosine) can produce cerebrovascular vasodilation as well. As a result, cerebral blood volume is either maintained or increased even though systemic blood pressure is decreased.

—Trimethaphan, a ganglionic blocker, usually will not increase cerebral blood volume because ganglionic blockade normally does not cause vasodilation of the cerebral circulation.

Verapamil and congestive heart failure

—Some calcium channel blockers have negative inotropic activity (decreased myocardial contractility) and can worsen or precipitate congestive heart failure.

—Verapamil should be avoided in patients with impaired ventricular function. Although diltiazem and nicardipine have less potent negative inotropic effect than verapamil, they should be used cautiously in patients with decreased ventricular function.

—Nifedipine appears to have only slight negative inotropic actions.

Verapamil and heart block (second, third degree)

—Patients with second degree, Mobitz II AV block or sick sinus syndrome may experience worsening conduction blockade from verapamil or diltiazem.

—Verapamil and diltiazem have both cardiac conduction and vascular actions. The other calcium channel blockers have primarily vascular actions (smooth muscle relaxation causing decreased blood pressure).

—The cardiac effects of verapamil and diltiazem include decreased sinus node automaticity, prolongation of AV nodal conduction time, an increase in the refractory time of the AV node, and depressed myocardial contractility.

Verapamil and muscular dystrophy

—Use of verapamil in patients with Duchenne's muscular dystrophy has resulted in respiratory failure.

Verapamil and PIH (pregnancy-induced hypertension), preeclampsia/eclampsia, toxemia

—Calcium channel blockers should be used cautiously in patients who have pregnancy-induced hypertension (preeclampsia, eclampsia, toxemia).

—Such patients are likely to be treated with magnesium sulfate which, combined with calcium channel blockers, can cause profound hypotension.

Verapamil and sick sinus syndrome
—Diltiazem, verapamil, and beta blockers should be avoided or used with extreme caution in patients with sick sinus syndrome (SSS).
—Use of these drugs, which depress sinus node automaticity, may cause severe bradycardia even in patients with SSS who are experiencing supraventricular tachycardia.
—Digitalis may be effective in controlling supraventricular tachycardias.

Verapamil and Wolf–Parkinson–White syndrome
—Verapamil, diltiazem, digitalis, beta blockers, and lidocaine should not be used to acutely treat wide complex tachyarrhythmias associated with the Wolf–Parkinson–White syndrome.
—In tachyarrhythmias with wide QRS complexes, antegrade conduction must be assumed to be taking place via accessory paths. Conduction through these paths can be accelerated by verapamil, diltiazem, digitalis, lidocaine, or propranolol. Intravenous procainamide is the treatment of choice.
—If the QRS complex is narrow, indicating antegrade conduction via normal conduction paths, treatment can be with agents that slow conduction through the AV node: verapamil, propranolol, digitalis, procainamide, or diltiazem.

Verapamil Interactions with Patient Drugs
Verapamil and amiodarone
—Amiodarone increases refractoriness and slows conduction in most cardiac tissue. A number of medications, including class I antiarrhythmics like lidocaine, calcium channel blockers, and beta blockers, which have similar effects, can precipitate severe bradycardia when given to a patient taking amiodarone.
—A case was reported of a patient with sick sinus syndrome on amiodarone who developed profound sinus bradycardia after local anesthesia with lidocaine.

Verapamil and beta blockers (acebutolol, atenolol, betaxolol, carteolol, labetalol, levobunolol, metoprolol, nadolol, penbutolol, pindolol, propranolol, timolol)
—Verapamil and diltiazem, particularly when used intravenously, can significantly potentiate the effects of beta blockers on cardiac conduction and contractility.
—Severe bradycardia and hypotension can occur when these medications are used concomitantly, especially in patients

with abnormalities of cardiac conduction (sick sinus syndrome) or ventricular function (congestive heart failure).

Verapamil and digitalis

—When verapamil is given to patients taking digoxin, toxic digoxin levels may occur. This may be due to several different mechanisms including displacement of digoxin from tissue binding sites.

Verapamil and flecainide

—Flecainide can cause decreased myocardial contractility, particularly at the onset of intravenous therapy. Patients most significantly affected are those with compromised left ventricular function (ejection fraction <30%).

—Beta blockers and some calcium channel blockers may have added negative inotropic effects with flecainide.

—Verapamil has more negative inotropic effect than diltiazem, nicardipine, or nifedipine.

Verapamil and magnesium sulfate

—Magnesium potentiates the effect of calcium channel blockers and the combination may result in profound hypotension.

Verapamil and mefloquine

—Mefloquine is a derivative of quinine and has rarely been associated with bradycardia and prolonged QT interval. Beta blockers and calcium channel blockers should be used with caution in patients on this medication.

Verapamil and rifampin

—Patients taking rifampin require significantly higher doses of calcium channel blockers. This interaction has been documented with verapamil, diltiazem, and nifedipine.

—The studies done demonstrated the increased requirement for both oral and intravenous forms of the calcium channel blockers, but requirements were higher for patients taking oral medications.

—The mechanisms of this interaction include an increased metabolism and reduced protein binding of the calcium channel blockers by rifampin.

INDEX